Organisational Culture

Organisational Culture

SECOND EDITION

Andrew D Brown

Judge Institute of Management Studies
University of Cambridge

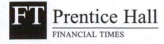
Prentice Hall
FINANCIAL TIMES

An imprint of **Pearson Education**

Harlow, England • London • New York • Boston • San Francisco • Toronto • Sydney • Singapore • Hong Kong
Tokyo • Seoul • Taipei • New Delhi • Cape Town • Madrid • Mexico City • Amsterdam • Munich • Paris • Milan

For Jess and Charles

PEARSON EDUCATION LIMITED
Edinburgh Gate
Harlow CM20 2JE
Tel: +44 (0)1279 623623
Fax: +44 (0)1279 431059
www.pearsoned.co.uk

First published in Great Britain in 1995
Second edition 1998

ISBN-13: 978-0-273-63147-7

British Library Cataloguing in Publication Data
A CIP catalogue record for this book can be obtained from the British Library

14 13 12 11
09 08 07

Typeset by PanTek Arts, Maidstone, Kent.
Printed and bound in Great Britain by Bell & Bain Ltd, Glasgow, Scotland.

The Publishers' policy is to use paper from sustainable forests.

CONTENTS

LIST OF FIGURES

LIST OF EXHIBITS

LIST OF MINI CASES

PREFACE

Three years after the publication of the first edition of *Organisational Culture*, culture is still a relatively new, controversial and little understood management concept. While business school academics continue to argue about what organisational culture really is, many business people claim to have successfully mastered and harnessed their organisation's culture for improved effectiveness. This book aims to provide a coherent overview of the principal ideas and frameworks for understanding culture, how and why cultures change, and the linkages between culture, strategy and performance. It is essentially a textbook for students who require an insight into this field of inquiry. In discussing the various concepts and models it also sheds some light on the reasons why there is so much scope for disagreement regarding the organisational culture perspective.

For a long time the management of organisations was considered to be a rational process that required managers to employ certain principles embodying good practice. Some well-known examples from Beach (1993) include:

- each subordinate should receive orders from only one superior;
- each superior should have no more than about six subordinates;
- authority and responsibility should flow from the top of the organisational hierarchy to the bottom;
- subordinates should make routine decisions, and unique, important decisions should be made by superiors;
- units within the organisation should specialise in particular activities;
- units should be organised as profit centres.

These classical principles have not been proved wrong so much as they have been superseded. There is now a greater recognition that different sorts of organisations require different structures and rules, that even ostensibly similar organisations can be successful using radically dissimilar methods, and that organisations in general are not always rational, machine-like entities. Rather, organisations are often irrational, hypocritical, uncoordinated, and highly political miniature societies. Much of the current interest in organisational culture stems from this realisation, because seeing organisations as cultures allows us to focus our attention on these hitherto neglected social and political processes. This interest has been bolstered by suggestions that once the non-rational, ambiguous and unpredictable nature of organisations is understood, we may then be able to offer design suggestions that improve their performance and effectiveness.

In dealing with these issues this book is divided into six main chapters, each of which is focused on a specific set of related concerns. All the chapters begin with a list of student objectives, and an introduction which provides a concise overview of its contents. Throughout the book the theoretical points made are illustrated with a wealth of case study material. Within each chapter are a series of *mini cases* drawn from a variety of different countries, while each chapter then concludes with a longer and more detailed case which provides ample opportunity for classroom discussion. In addition, the book contains a further five integrative cases which encourage reconsideration of material contained in several different chapters. Many of the mini cases and all the longer cases contain suggested questions for students. Each chapter also contains a final *summary/conclusions* section which summarises the main issues discussed, a list of *key concepts,* and a large number of questions for discussion. The book is, therefore, extremely 'student friendly', and it is hoped that it will appeal to students at undergraduate, graduate and post-experience level in business and management, and on related professional courses.

Chapter 1 'An introduction to organisational culture' provides a detailed and comprehensive yet immediately comprehensible introduction to what organisational culture is. Chapter 2 'Exploring organisational culture' builds on the ideas contained in the first chapter in its consideration of issues such as the sources from which an organisation derives its culture, how cultures develop and are perpetuated, typologies of cultures, and approaches for assessing the strength of a culture. Chapter 3, 'Discovering issues in organisation culture' considers issues of subculture and the functions that cultures are often said to play, and links culture to important aspects of organisation such as gender and learning. Chapter 4 'Understanding organisational culture change' describes and critiques five important models that have been devised to account for how cultures change. Chapter 5 'Managing organisational culture change' outlines some of the means available to executives intent on managing their organisation's culture. Chapter 6 'Organisational culture, strategy and performance' considers the interrelationships between culture, strategy and performance, and points out the difficulties involved with trying to manage culture to maximise economic effectiveness. Chapter 7 'Integrative case studies' consists of five more detailed cases to illustrate the material contained in the previous chapters. Chapter 8 'Conclusions' contains a summary statement and some brief conclusions.

Finally, it is worth noting that no single book can hope to fully cover such a vast and diverse field as that presented by organisational culture. Even as this book went to press new books and journal articles focused on almost all facets of organisational culture were continuing to appear, and indeed, only a fraction of that material produced up to the mid to late 1990s has been included. Any student whose interest in organisational culture is aroused by this book is therefore recommended not only to read some of the references referred to here, but to search out the wealth of fascinating material that continues to be produced by scholars worldwide.

ACKNOWLEDGEMENTS

A large number of people have helped me with the preparation of this book, not least Penelope Woolf at Financial Times Pitman Publishing whose assistance and advice guided my perceptions of what a good textbook should be. I am particularly indebted to Mick Rowlinson for his practical suggestions regarding how to make this book more intellectually coherent and accessible to students. My thanks also go to Roy Payne, Kevin Gaston and Ian Tanner who in various ways contributed to my understanding of organisational culture. I am similarly grateful to David Ellis and Tom Wilson for allowing me the leeway to pursue my interest in organisational culture while a doctoral student.

A variety of other individuals have provided me with ideas and material which appear in this book. Among these are Owen Atkin, Howard Bevan, Ioannis Giannopoulos, Jasmine Georgiou, Clarence Gan, Dawn Lyon and Muhammad Yaqoob and who are all here gratefully acknowledged.

Finally, I would like to thank my wife, BiYu, for her encouragement and interest in my work.

An introduction to organisational culture

To enable students to:

- explore the origins of the current interest in organisational culture;
- discover the intellectual progenitors of culture research and the relationship between culture and the broad spectrum of organisational theory;
- become familiar with examples of the many definitions of concepts of organisational culture and to present a rudimentary classification scheme for them;
- identify the contents of an organisational culture;
- learn about two simple models of organisational culture;
- make the distinction between espoused culture and culture-in-practice;
- understand the importance of interpretation and problems of meaning to the organisational culture perspective.

INTRODUCTION

This chapter provides an introduction to some fundamental issues in organisational culture. It begins by tracing the origins and intellectual traditions from which the culture perspective emerged. Attention is then focused on some of the many definitions of organisational culture that have been formulated by scholars in this field. The principal components of an organisational culture are considered in some detail, and a large number of examples which illustrate the theoretical points made are given. This chapter provides the basis on which Chapters 2 and 3 draw in their consideration of further issues in organisational culture.

ORGANISATIONAL CULTURE: ORIGINS OF THE CURRENT INTEREST

This section examines some of the reasons for the current interest in organisational culture, and traces the intellectual origins of the culture concept. Current interest in organisational culture stems from at least four different sources: climate research, national cultures, human resource management, and from a conviction that approaches which emphasise the rational and structural nature of organisation cannot offer a full explanation of organisational behaviour. We will briefly consider each of these in turn.

Organisational climate

The current fascination with organisational culture developed in part from work on organisational climate conducted during the 1970s. The phrase 'organisational climate' refers to the beliefs and attitudes held by individuals about their organisation. According to Tagiuri (1968) climate is a relatively enduring quality of an organisation that (1) is experienced by employees and (2) influences their behaviour. Climate studies using a variety of survey questionnaires such as the Business Organisational Climate Index (BOCI) are still being conducted, though their popularity has waned (see Chapter 2). The results of the climate research seemed to suggest that in many organisations there is little agreement between employees concerning what it is like to work for their organisation. But the real finding of the climate surveys was that a more sophisticated approach to understanding this aspect of organisation was required.

National culture

A further impetus to the development of a new trend in management thinking came with the realisation that organisations in different countries were often structured and behaved differently. These differences were most striking when they were detected in the subsidiary companies of the same multinational organisation, because they seemed to suggest that national cultural differences may help shape organisational design and behaviour at a local level. Hofstede's (1980) scholarly book, *Culture's Consequences*, was one of the first to draw attention to these issues. Given the dominance of American management thinking and Japanese corporations it was perhaps inevitable that popular interest should then focus on the differences between Japan and the USA with the publication of books such as Theory Z (Ouchi, 1981) and *The Art of Japanese Management* (Pascale and Athos, 1981). While Ouchi (and others) argued against trying to re-create Japanese culture in America, he suggested that it was possible to adopt some of their business practices and to change the culture of individual corporations. The scene was thus set for books such as Deal and Kennedy's (1982) *Corporate Cultures*, Kanter's (1983) *The Change Masters* and Peters and Waterman's (1982) *In Search of Excellence*, which shifted attention away from national cultures and focused specifically on organisational culture.

Human resource management

The vast literature on organisational culture has evolved hand in hand with the equally large and still burgeoning literature on human resource management (HRM). Together the development of the culture and HRM literatures are evidence of an intellectual refocusing on people in organisations as the means by which sustainable competitive advantage can be achieved – rather than information technology, products, or other intrinsic elements of an organisation such as its structures. The relationship between the culture and HRM literatures is, however, even closer than this may suggest, with many (maybe most) human resource specialists claiming that organisational culture is the territory of the human resource manager. Textbooks and popular journal articles now commonly exhort those working in the field of human resource management to be sensitive to the values and beliefs of their organisation's culture, and recommend that it should be managed through human resource policies, programmes and systems (see Chapter 5).

Explaining performance

Organisational culture is currently one of the major domains of organisational research, together with studies of formal structure, organisation–environment relations, and bureaucracy. In fact, it is arguable that organisational culture has become the single most active research arena. One reason for this is that organisations that differ widely in terms of a variety of performance measures have often been found to have very similar formal characteristics. For practical as well as theoretical purposes it is very important to be able to explain why organisations enjoy different rates of profitability, turnover and market share. It was the apparent failure of traditional approaches, which stressed the importance of formal organisational structure and environment relations, to offer convincing explanations that persuaded many commentators to consider organisational culture seriously. This said, it should also be borne in mind that its popularity owes much to the fact that it is easily understood (at least in its most superficial form), that many commentators have used it to construct 'formulae for success' which have great appeal to business people, and that the idea has been well marketed by the consulting group McKinseys (Guest, 1992).

Davis (1984) has argued that the reason why our old models of organisation are no longer appropriate is that the economy of the developed world (particularly America) has undergone a radical transformation: 'We are operating in a post-industrial, service-based economy, but our companies are managed by models developed in, by, and for industrial corporations. This makes as much sense as managing an industrial economy with agrarian models' (Davis, 1984: 2). In the view of Davis and a variety of other commentators, Western managers have over-relied on complex structures, elaborate systems and formalistic planning mechanisms, with disastrous results. The current interest in organisational culture thus stems from the fact that it offers a non-mechanistic, flexible and imaginative approach to understanding how organisations work. The fact that most Western countries have experienced a dramatic downturn in their economies which has placed the structure of Western capitalism under severe pressure has also probably been an impetus to scholars in emphasising cultural problems (Meek, 1988).

INTELLECTUAL ORIGINS

A new field of management inquiry cannot develop *ex vacuo*; it builds on what has gone before. In fact, many of the central themes and concepts employed by specialists in organisational culture are not entirely novel. What has happened over the past fifteen years or so is that a rich mixture of ideas, theories and frameworks have been drawn together under the single unifying heading of 'organisational culture'. These notions have principally been derived from two intellectual traditions: anthropology and organisational sociology.

Anthropology

In 1871 Edward B. Tylor, one of the first anthropologists, introduced the term 'culture' into the English language. He defined the word as referring to 'that complex whole which includes knowledge, beliefs, art, morals, law, custom and any other capabilities and habits acquired by man as a member of society'. Since the nineteenth century, anthropologists have enormously elaborated and refined Tylor's original conception of culture. The contemporary anthropologist who has probably had the most important influence over the evolution of our interest in organisational culture is Clifford Geertz (1973). Geertz suggested that studies of culture should focus on the 'native's point of view', that is, what the people living the culture consider to be significant about the way they live. This approach is often called 'semiotic' because it concentrates on language and symbols in order to understand a given social situation. Other features of organisational life such as rites, rituals and social structures are also integral elements of a culture for anthropologists. All these aspects of culture are considered in more detail in subsequent sections.

Organisational sociology

The influence of sociology on the study of organisational culture has been broad and direct. Indeed, according to some authors, the study of organisational culture is rooted more deeply in sociology than any other intellectual tradition (Ouchi and Wilkins, 1985). As long ago as the late nineteenth century an influential sociologist called Emile Durkheim proposed that symbols, myths and rituals were important means of understanding social reality. In the early twentieth century the German sociologist Max Weber proposed the idea of charismatic leadership as a concept for understanding how certain individuals managed to exercise authority without reliance on formal structures or tradition. Since then a host of sociologists have identified other features of organisational life – such as informal norms, folkways, ambiguity, apparent irrationality – which are central to our current interest in organisational culture. Again, all these elements are reviewed in greater detail in later sections.

Anthropology and organisational sociology, together with many other intellectual traditions, have had a considerable influence on the development of the broad field of organisational theory. Such is the diversity of ideas that have helped organisational theory develop as a field of inquiry that a large number of schools of thought or perspectives have developed. The next section attempts to situate organisational culture within the context of organisational theory and to illustrate some of the common bonds between them and the culture perspective.

ORGANISATIONAL CULTURE AND ORGANISATIONAL THEORY

Organisational culture is the newest perspective in organisational theory. It is at the same time both a radical departure from the mainstream of contemporary organisational behaviour studies, and a continuation and elaboration of long-established traditions. On the one hand it is a departure from the preoccupation with the formal and rational aspects of organisation, and on the other hand, it is a reworking of many of the concerns of established perspectives focused on group dynamics, power and politics. The growing body of scholarly work conducted under the banner of culture research is testament both to disillusionment with 'standard' approaches and excitement that a new and more fruitful means of understanding organisations has evolved. The view that organisations are like miniature societies with unique configurations of heroes, myths, beliefs and values has proved popular with practitioners as well as academics. In fact, it is in part this broad spectrum of interested parties (academics, business people and students) that has propelled culture into an increasingly dominant position over the past fifteen years.

There are an enormous number of different perspectives on organisations, many of which share common threads both with each other and with the cultural perspective. Here we will briefly consider four schools of thought, and what they have contributed to the study of organisational culture: human relations, modern structural theory, systems theory, and power and politics.

Human relations

This school developed in the late 1950s and 1960s, and is associated with scholars such as Chris Argyris and Warren Bennis. It developed on the basis of new theories of motivation and group dynamics, and adopted a frame of reference which emphasised that organisations exist to serve human needs. A great deal of work on beliefs, values and attitudes was done by the human relations school, the results of which have helped to shape the culture perspective.

Modern structural theory

Modern structural theory is a phenomenon of the 1960s, when it was popularised by authors such as Lawrence and Lorsch. It considered organisations to be rational, goal-oriented and mechanistic, and focused on issues of authority and hierarchy as manifested in organisational charts. While it emphasised the importance of such concepts as differentiation and integration that culture theorists are also interested in, this school has had a rather minimal influence on the development of the culture perspective.

Systems theory

While many of the ideas entertained by the systems school had first been developed by Wiener in the 1940s, it was not until the 1960s that this perspective was (and remains) widely adopted. With the publication of Katz and Kahn's *The Social Psychology of Organizations* (1966) the notion that organisations were best thought of as interdependent systems linked by inputs, outputs and feedback loops became dominant. Indeed, some culture theorists today write of 'cultural systems' rather than cultures. In fact, while most culture specialists eschew the view that organisations can be controlled through feedback loops, the culture perspective has certainly been influenced by systems theory's outlook on organisational life: both emphasise the importance of analysing the organisation in its environment, the stresses placed on organisations due to uncertainty, and the limited scope employees have for exercising their individuality.

Power and politics

This perspective is of comparatively recent origin, having been developed in the late 1970s by authors such as Pfeffer. This school suggests that organisations are complexes of individuals and coalitions with different and often competing values, interests and preferences. The power and politics perspective has a great deal in common with the culture perspective. Both argue that organisations often act irrationally, that their goals and objectives emerge through a process of negotiation and influence, and that organisations are composed of groups (coalitions or subcultures). As these two schools of thought share so many common assumptions concerning how organisations work, so eminent authors such as Kanter and Mintzberg have found it natural to research from within both perspectives.

What this brief review of some of the recent history of perspectives in organisational behaviour has illustrated is that culture is merely the latest in a long series of movements. Furthermore, it suggests that far from being an aberration, the culture perspective has drawn on a number of well-established ideas, and is very closely related to at least one other school ('power and politics'). Some authors have suggested that the current interest in organisational culture reflects the mood and concerns of our times. Ott (1989), for example, has argued that the 1980s were (and, we might add, the 1990s are) a time of intense questioning concerning how we interpret social institutions, the extent to which we and our organisations are rational entities, and the role beliefs, values and assumptions have in influencing our behaviour. Our current preoccupation with organisational culture may, therefore, be thought of as a reformulation of existing models and theories to satisfy changing views of how organisations work, and which is likely to enjoy its pre-eminence for a finite period of time.

ORGANISATIONAL CULTURE: DEFINITIONS OF A CONCEPT

Definitions of the concepts we employ in our attempts to understand organisations are important because they influence how we think about the phenomena they refer to. Definitions focus our attention on some parts of a phenomenon at the expense of others; that is, they are selective. In the case of some organisational concepts, such as 'formalisation' and 'specialisation' there is consensus on appropriate definitions.[1] With regard to organisational culture, however, no such consensus has yet emerged, with the available literature offering the interested reader an embarrassment of definitional riches. It is unsurprising that there should be a great diversity of opinion concerning what the phrase 'organisational culture' refers to. This is because even before the terms 'culture' and 'organisation' were used in combination, the term 'culture' had been defined in literally dozens of different ways. In fact, as long ago as 1952 the anthropologists Kroeber and Kluckhohn isolated 164 different definitions of culture. Today there are almost certainly even more definitions of organisational culture than there were of culture in 1952. A selection of some of the best-known and widely promulgated definitions is contained in Exhibit 1.1.

Exhibit 1.1
Definitions of organisational culture

The culture of the factory is its customary and traditional way of thinking and of doing things, which is shared to a greater or lesser degree by all its members, and which new members must learn, and at least partially accept, in order to be accepted into service in the firm. Culture in this sense covers a wide range of behaviour: the methods of production; job skills and technical knowledge; attitudes towards discipline and punishment; the customs and habits of managerial behaviour; the objectives of the concern; its way of doing business; the methods of payment; the values placed on different types of work; beliefs in democratic living and joint consultation; and the less conscious conventions and taboos. (*Jaques, 1952: 251*)

The culture of an organization refers to the unique configuration of norms, values, beliefs, ways of behaving and so on that characterize the manner in which groups and individuals combine to get things done. The distinctiveness of a particular organization is intimately bound up with its history and the character-building effects of past decisions and past leaders. It is manifested in the folkways, mores, and the ideology to which members defer, as well as in the strategic choices made by the organization as a whole.
(*Eldridge and Crombie, 1974: 89*)

A set of understandings or *meanings shared* by a group of people. The meanings are largely *tacit* among members, are clearly *relevant* to the particular group, and are *distinctive* to the group. Meanings are *passed* on to new group members. (*Louis, 1980*)

Culture . . . is a pattern of beliefs and expectations shared by the organization's members. These beliefs and expectations produce norms that powerfully shape the behaviour of individuals and groups in the organization. (*Schwartz and Davis, 1981: 33*)

A quality of perceived organizational specialness – that it possesses some unusual quality that distinguishes it from others in the field. (*Gold, 1982: 571–2*)

Organizational culture is not just another piece of the puzzle, it is the puzzle. From our point of view, a culture is not something an organization has; a culture is something an organization is.
(*Pacanowsky and O'Donnell-Trujillo, 1982: 126*)

Exhibit 1.1 continued

Corporate culture may be described as a general constellation of beliefs, mores, customs, value systems, behavioral norms, and ways of doing business that are unique to each corporation, that set a pattern for corporate activities and actions, and that describe the implicit and emergent patterns of behavior and emotions characterising life in the organization. (*Tunstall, 1983: 15*)

I will mean by 'culture': a pattern of basic assumptions – invented, discovered, or developed by a given group as it learns to cope with its problems of external adaptation and internal integration – that has worked well enough to be considered valid and, therefore, to be taught to new members as the correct way to perceive, think, and feel in relation to those problems. (*Schein, 1985b: 9*)

The culture metaphor points towards another means of creating organized activity: by influencing the language, norms, folklore, ceremonies, and other social practices that communicate the key ideologies, values, and beliefs guiding action. (*Morgan, 1986: 135*)

By culture I mean the shared beliefs top managers in a company have about how they should manage themselves and other employees, and how they should conduct their business(es). These beliefs are often invisible to the top managers but have a major impact on their thoughts and actions. (*Lorsch, 1986: 95*)

Corporate culture is the *implicit, invisible, intrinsic* and *informal* consciousness of the organization which guides the behaviour of the individuals and which shapes itself out of their behaviour. (*Scholz 1987: 80*)
'Culture' refers to the underlying values, beliefs, and principles that serve as a foundation for an organization's management system as well as the set of management practices and behaviours that both exemplify and reinforce those basic principles. (*Denison, 1990: 2*)

Culture represents an interdependent set of values and ways of behaving that are common in a community and that tend to perpetuate themselves, sometimes over long periods of time. (*Kotter and Heskett, 1992: 141*)

Culture is 'how things are done around here'. It is what is *typical* of the organization, the *habits*, the prevailing *attitudes*, the grown-up pattern of *accepted* and *expected* behaviour. (*Drennan, 1992: 3*)

Culture is the commonly held and relatively stable beliefs, attitudes and values that exist within the organization. (*Williams et al.,1993*

These definitions reflect very different understandings of what culture is. An attempt to clarify some of the issues at stake here by providing a rudimentary classification system is provided by Fig. 1.1. This illustrates that there is a fundamental distinction to be made between those who think of culture as a metaphor, and those who see culture as an objective entity. The idea that culture is just the latest in a whole series of metaphors to be developed for understanding how organisations work has been admirably expressed by Morgan (1986) in his book *Images of Organization*. In the field of organisation studies it has long been recognised that metaphors allow us to understand organisations in terms of other complex entities.[2] Historically, two of the most important of these metaphors have been the 'machine' and the 'organism'. Scholars using these metaphors have thus been able to point out in what ways organisations are similar to machines and organisms in their attempts to explain the essence of human organisation. Other metaphors which have been employed to elaborate aspects of organisational life include the 'theatre' (Mangham and Overington, 1983), the 'political arena' (Pfeffer, 1981a) and the 'psychic prison' (Marcuse, 1955). Indeed, in one sense at least, the term 'organisation' is itself a metaphor referring to the experience of collective co-ordination and orderliness (Smircich, 1983).

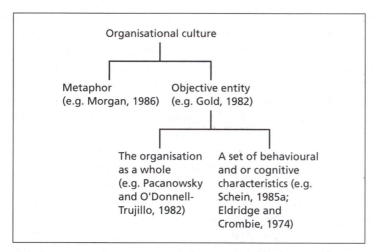

Fig. 1.1 Classifying definitions of organisational culture

Most commentators have, however, chosen to think of culture as an objective entity. Agreement on this point still leaves room for a broad spectrum of opinion on other details. According to Pacanowsky and O'Donnell-Trujillo (1982) an organisation is, quite literally, a culture, and all features of an organisation including its systems, policies, procedures and processes are elements of its cultural life. While this is an intellectually coherent position many theorists have resisted this view, because if everything is culture, then it is not possible to use the concept to frame causal explanations of other aspects of organisational activity. In effect, the idea that organisations are cultures is almost indistinguishable from the view that culture is best interpreted as a metaphor for understanding organisations. In contrast, other authors such as Schein (1985a) have suggested that culture is best thought of as a set of psychological predispositions (which he calls 'basic assumptions') that members of an organisation possess, and which leads them to think and act in certain ways. While the view that culture is essentially a cognitive phenomenon that resides in the psychology of organisational participants is widespread, many theorists, Eldridge and Crombie among them, acknowledge that patterns of behaviour are equally important. How we choose to define culture has considerable implications for how we attempt to examine and study it. Unless otherwise stated the definition of organisational culture adopted in this book is as follows:

Organisational culture refers to the pattern of beliefs, values and learned ways of coping with experience that have developed during the course of an organisation's history, and which tend to be manifested in its material arrangements and in the behaviours of its members.

CULTURE AS METAPHOR

The idea that culture is most appropriately regarded as a metaphor for understanding organisations has received increasing attention from academics in recent years. More generally, following the publication of Morgan's (1986) book *Images of Organization,* there has been considerable interest in the argument that organisation theory consists of a series of metaphors for understanding organisations. A metaphor allows us to comprehend one element of experience in terms of another, and is thus an important organising device in our thinking and talking about the world. The metaphors we use for understanding organisations are subject to change over time as new insights are sought. The view that organisations are best thought of as machines or organisms has, in recent years, been overtaken by the argument that organisations are best regarded as political arenas and, more recently still, cultures.

The view that organisations can profitably be understood in terms of the culture metaphor has been forcibly supported by authors such as Smircich (1983) and Morgan (1996). According to this position, culture is not an objective, tangible or measurable aspect of an organisation, but an intellectual device which helps us to comprehend organisations in terms of a specific vocabulary (such as norms, beliefs, values, symbols and so forth). From this perspective every aspect of an organisation is a part of its culture so that debates regarding how 'culture' influences 'strategy' or 'technology' impacts on 'culture' are not possible. Indeed, they are considered misleading because they fail to recognise that strategy and technology, together with everything else that makes up an organisation, are elements of culture. The fact that many cultural concepts such as rites, rituals, ceremonies, stories, myths and legends do not lend themselves to quantification or operationalisation as variables in cause–effect relationships suggests that there are good reasons for regarding culture as a metaphor.

Some authors have, however, expressed considerable reservations about the use of metaphors in organisation theory. It has been argued that metaphors cannot be translated into precise and objective language, cannot therefore be rigorously measured or tested, and so cannot help us to develop a science of organisations. Others have suggested that any given metaphor is incomplete, biased and potentially misleading. Alvesson (1993) has argued that there are grave dangers associated with choosing inappropriate metaphors that do not yield important insights into organisations. Reed (1990) suggests that a focus on metaphors is problematic because in themselves they give no insight into the historical development of organisation theory. These well-made points are not in themselves arguments against examining the role of metaphor in organisation theory or regarding culture as a useful metaphor for analysis. They do, however, remind us that in using metaphors to help further our understanding of organisations we should be both critical and self-aware.

CONTENTS OF AN ORGANISATIONAL CULTURE

While definitions can usefully focus our attention on the kernel of the subject matter here, they are necessarily concise. In this section we will expand the definitions to examine the contents of an organisation's culture. A large number of different aspects or elements of organisational culture generally have been identified by theorists, including:

- artefacts;
- language in the form of jokes, metaphors, stories, myths and legends;
- behaviour patterns in the form of rites, rituals, ceremonies and celebrations;

- norms of behaviour;
- heroes;
- symbols and symbolic action;
- beliefs, values and attitudes;
- ethical codes;
- basic assumptions; and
- history.

Although these categories of things and events are often described as if they were distinct classes, it is important to note that there is overlap between them. For instance, some researchers consider language and behaviour patterns to be forms of artefact, while basic assumptions may be thought of as particular configurations of beliefs and values. In order to minimise these potential sources of confusion and impose some order on the complexities of culture research, authors have sought to build these elements of culture into various models. Two of the best-known models of organisational culture are illustrated in Figs. 1.2 and 1.3. While these simple hierarchies of cultural variables are extremely appealing, we should always recall that actual organisational cultures are not as neat and tidy as the models seem to imply. The complexity of real-life cultures and the uncertainties and ambiguities actual cultures exhibit are indicated by the case studies at the end of each chapter in this book.

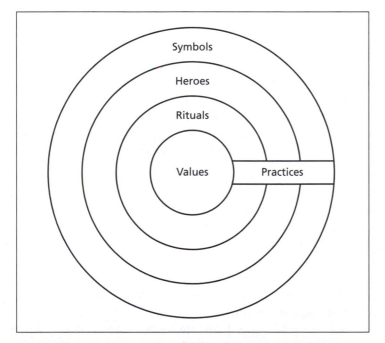

Fig. 1.2 Manifestations of culture: from shallow to deep

Source: reprinted from 'Measuring organizational cultures: A qualitative and quantitive study across twenty cases' by Hofstede *et al.* published in *Administrative Science Quarterly*, Vol. 35, Iss. 2 (1990) by permission of *Administrative Science Quarterly*

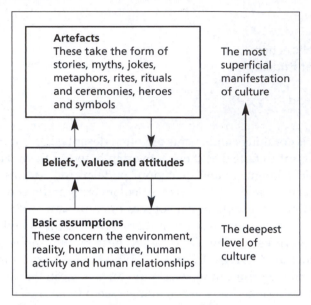

Fig. 1.3 Levels of culture and their interaction
Source: adapted from Schein (1985b)

Artefacts

These are often said to be the most visible and most superficial manifestations of an organisation's culture. The category 'artefacts' generally refers to the total physical and socially constructed environment of an organisation. Dictionary definitions of the word *artefact* generally assert that it is a product of human action, has an aim (such as solving a problem or satisfying a need), and has a physical presence. Students of organisational culture often describe as artefacts objects and physical arrangements, patterns of behaviour, and abstract linguistic expressions such as stories and jokes. Some fundamental subcategories of artefacts include:

- *Material objects* For example, annual reports, the products an organisation makes, and sales and advertising brochures.
- *Physical layouts* For example, how office space is used (open or closed plan, shared or individual working spaces), the quality and functionality of the furnishings, dress codes (whether formal or informal), the relative location of different departments, and the general appearance of the buildings and car parks.
- *Technology* In the form of information technologies such as computers, fax machines, photocopiers and telephones, and any equipment the organisation employs to manufacture its products.
- *Language* For instance, jokes, anecdotes, stories, metaphors and jargon terms.
- *Behaviour patterns* For example, rites, rituals, ceremonies and celebrations.
- *Symbols* A very general category that encompasses material objects, physical layouts and other things and events such as posters and one-off actions by executives made to demonstrate a particular point.

- *Rules, systems, procedures and programmes* For example, human resource systems dealing with compensation, appraisal and promotion, rules governing the structure, composition and periodicity of committee meetings, and quality assurance programmes, to name but a few.

There are obviously a vast array of different types and forms of artefact observable within organisations. Indeed, the classification system here is by no means fully exhaustive. Their importance stems from the link they are assumed to have with the 'deeper' levels of an organisation's culture, of which they are generally thought to be indicators. The argument is that the 'cultural essence' of an organisation will, all things being equal, be evident in the choices it makes concerning such things as its use of language, behaviour patterns and technologies. For example, in most universities academics tend to be accommodated in individual offices, reflecting not only the nature of the work they conduct but an ethic of individual autonomy and independence. In contrast, in an organisation like Digital Equipment Corporation most office space is open-plan, reflecting a cultural inclination for co-operation and teamwork, and for control through peer pressure. For those able to decipher them, then, artefacts may be used as a powerful guide for understanding the nature of an organisational culture. Indeed, according to Wuthnow *et al.* (1984: 4): 'A simple artifact often holds the essence of a whole social system.' It is therefore a little puzzling that scholars of organisational culture have tended to pay lip service to artefacts while neglecting them in substance (Gagliardi, 1990).

Material objects: corporate logos and mission statements

Two products that often provide good insights into the deep structure of an organisation's culture are logos and mission statements. Consider, for example, Hampden-Turner's (1990) useful analysis of the logos of Apple, Honda, Volvo and Tandem Computers. Apple uses the multicoloured image of the forbidden fruit of Eden, from which a bite has been taken. This presumably symbolises the birth of new knowledge. Honda's logo is an H expressed in the form of the *tori* gates that stand at the entrance to Japanese shrines, and which are supposed to unite earth and sky. Volvo employs the symbol of hands holding wrists, an overt expression of the value of co-operative relationships. Finally, Tandem Computers uses its name to convey a sense of two-in-one and thus mutual support and synchrony. While we should be careful not to read too much into artifices which may have been developed by astute advertising agencies rather than the organisations themselves, they should not be dismissed as meaningless and inconsequential.

The same is true of mission statements. A mission statement defines the long-term vision of the organisation in terms of where it wants to be and whom it wants to serve. Mission statements often make reference to the purposes of the organisation, its principal business aims, the key beliefs and values of the company, definitions of its major stakeholders, and ethical principles which govern codes of conduct. Organisational mission statements can thus be an excellent source of initial information regarding culture, as the examples provided in Exhibit 1.2 make clear. If a word of warning is required here, it is that there is often a substantial gap between the good intentions expressed in the mission statement and the reality of an organisation's management practices.

Exhibit 1.2
Mission statements

We are an international retailing group specialising in high technology consumer electronics, photography, office and home equipment and domestic appliances. We trade in the United Kingdom . . . and in the United States . . . We aim to offer unrivalled value to our customers through the range and quality of the products we sell, the competitiveness of our prices and the high standards of in-store and after sales service we provide . . . (*Dixons Group*)

The NatWest way is to bring:
　　QUALITY TO OUR CUSTOMERS . . .
　　QUALITY TO OUR INVESTORS . . .
　　QUALITY TO OUR PEOPLE . . .
　　QUALITY TO OUR COMMUNITY . . . (*National Westminster Bank*)

Ford Motor Company is a worldwide leader in automotive and automotive-related products and services as well as in new industries such as aerospace, communications, and financial services. Our mission is to improve continually our products and services to meet our customers' needs, allowing us to prosper as a business and to provide a reasonable return for our stockholders, the owners of our business. (*Ford Motor Company*)

We all want a company that our people are proud of and committed to, where all employees have an opportunity to contribute, learn, grow, and advance based on merit, not politics or background. We want our people to feel respected, treated fairly, listened to and involved. Above all, we want satisfaction from accomplishments and friendships, balanced personal and professional lives, and to have fun in our endeavours . . . (*Levi Strauss*)

Corporate architecture and corporate identity

Modern organisations are paying increasing attention to their physical appearance. Examples of organisations that have invested vast amounts of money in stylish buildings, office layouts, landscape gardening and corporate uniforms can be found in most industrial sectors. For instance, in the oil industry Mobil has launched a corporate identity programme, in the airline industry British Airways has a visual identity programme, and in the telecommunications industry BT and KTAS Copenhagen have developed image enhancement programmes. It has been argued that this emphasis on corporate surfaces is a purposeful adaptation to a post-modern society in which organisations are judged in terms of their appearance (which is often equated with credibility) as well as performance. A preoccupation with corporate image and identity, however, is not a new phenomenon, as Olins (1978) has illustrated with reference to the old UK railway industry (see Exhibit 1.3).

Some recent research by Berg and Kreiner (1990) has led them to make the following six suggestions concerning the functions and efficacy of corporate architecture.

1 The architecture of corporate buildings has a significant influence on human behaviour in terms of how we interact, communicate and perform our work tasks. That attempts have been made to mould employee behaviour through architecture is illustrated by the comments of the architect who designed the corporate headquarters of ABV, a leading Swedish contractor: 'The ABV building is . . . a friendly, pink building with an inviting main entrance which leads directly into the glass-covered courtyard,

Exhibit 1.3
Corporate architecture in British Railway companies

Before British Rail was formed a number of large railway companies ran the UK rail network. Each of these attempted to differentiate itself from its rivals. Olins (1978) has described the results.

The individuality of the great [British Railway] companies was expressed in styles of architecture, typography and liveries of engines and carriages, even down to the knives and forks and crockery used in refreshment rooms and dining cars. The Midland favoured Gothic, and so, in a less expensive way, did the Great Eastern. The Great Western remained its strong Gooch-and-Brunel self. Greek learning dominated the London and North Western. The Great Northern went in for a reliable homeliness rather than beauty. The Midland Railway was the line for comfort rather than speed. It introduced dining cars in the very early days and its rolling stock was always particularly agreeable to travel on, although rarely quite as fast as its competitors. St Pancras Station, its scarlet brick terminal in London, was much grander than next door's King's Cross, London terminal of the rival Great Northern Railway. The Great Northern was, as Betjeman says, 'noted more for its trains than its buildings'. The Midland put Sir Gilbert Scott's fantastical Gothic palace in front of Barlow's magnificent engine shed, but the Great Northern's workman-like King's Cross was designed by Lewis Cubitt with the minimum delay, cost and fuss.

Source: Olins (1978)

an oasis for visitors, coffee-drinking restaurant guests, and passing personnel. A lot of offices and almost all the conference rooms face the yard and give life to it. From the yard one can see the glass lift cages going up and down which contributes to the vitality of the yard. A ride in the lift gives the people working in the building as well as the visitors a stimulating impression of the company as a whole and its activities.' Berg and Kreiner speculate that the impression of vitality given by the building has a complementary effect on visitors and employees of ABV.

2   Buildings may serve as totems or uniting symbols of corporate identity for employees. This is evidenced by the tendency for many organisations to use pictures of their buildings in advertising and in their annual reports and accounts.

3   Buildings can act as symbols of an organisation's strategic profile. For example, Round Office, a leading Swedish office furniture manufacturer, has incorporated many 'round office' ideas into its furniture, graphics and design of its headquarters in Orebo. Thus semi-circular furniture in the offices is complemented by the structure of the building, which has a domed roof, rounded doors and some rounded corners. In these ways a strong corporate identity is presented both to the outside world and to employees.

4   Buildings can in effect become part of an organisation's product. Organisations as varied as consumer oil companies to purveyors of fast food have reconstituted their buildings to make a visit to them distinctive for customers. The packaging that surrounds a Macdonald's hamburger, for instance, includes not just the plastic wrapper that keeps it warm, but the ambience created by the standard tables, chairs, pot plants, lighting and so forth.

5   Buildings can be symbols of organisational and individual opulence, status, potency and good taste among other things. For example, large organisations often commission well-known architects to produce buildings which become 'landmarks' in

big international cities, while the executives who populate them will often vie for the most prestigious offices and furniture.

6   Buildings are often intimately bound up with the history and development of an organisation, and changes in location often mark radical alterations in the strategic direction or general character of a company. For example, following enforced decentralisation and the deregulation of the telephone industry in the USA, AT&T constructed a new headquarters in New York. In other instances buildings can be used to symbolise history and tradition. IKEA, for example, uses pictures of the old barn where the company originated in its publicity and information material. Indeed, within IKEA buildings from the company's early days 'are almost regarded as sacred places and symbolize the historical roots of the company' (Berg and Kreiner, 1990).

While a close study of an organisation's architecture and other symbols of corporate identity can provide fascinating insights into its cultural life, we should always recall that buildings are seldom left to speak for themselves. Rather, they are described, reviewed and interpreted by employees, customers and the general public who reach their own conclusions based on their experience, knowledge and feelings. Designing a building to make a highly specific statement or to convey a particular message may, therefore, be extremely difficult, if not impossible.

Language

The language we employ is not merely a means of communication, it is also a fundamental determinant of how we comprehend the world we live in. The idea that words generate understanding has important implications for the study of organisational culture. It should make us aware that the cultural approach adopted here defines a particular way of understanding how organisations work that is constrained by its central concepts. In other words, the culture perspective makes use of notions such as 'artefacts', 'symbols' and 'basic assumptions' which are useful descriptive categories, but there are other equally valid ways of analysing organisations that employ a different vocabulary and emphasise different aspects of organisational reality. After all, while organisational culture has only been a popular subject of debate since the early 1980s, scholars have been theorising about organisational behaviour and design for centuries. What is more, as students of organisational culture it is incumbent on us not to forget that our own thoughts on the subject are themselves largely culturally bound, and that we are arguably the intellectual prisoners of our socio-historical context.

Much the same argument can be applied at the level of the individual organisation. It has been suggested that in order to work together in an organisational setting people must develop mutual understanding through the common use of language and conceptual categories. They are encouraged to arrive at joint understanding for commercial reasons (efficiency, effectiveness, and ultimately survival of the venture), and by human psychology, by which people naturally tend to want to reduce their levels of anxiety caused by misunderstanding and ambiguity. As Schein (1985a) has pointed out, abstractions such as a 'good service', 'high quality' and 'excellence', which are commonly used to frame strategic and operational objectives in organisations, can (and do) mean different things in different organisational cultures. Quite evidently serious organisational communication problems can arise if different people (or departments) in the same organisation choose to interpret these and other ideas in incompatible ways. Disputes between production and quality control departments over what constitutes 'acceptable quality', and between production and sales departments over an 'optimum product price' are just two of the many well researched forms in which different culturally based understandings disrupt organisational life.

Metaphors

A metaphor is a word or phrase applied to an object or action which it does not literally denote. Metaphors can be powerful means of communicating ideas, and are in common use in many organisations. Some of the most dominant metaphors employed in organisational life are those associated with the game of chess, the military and the church. If, in an organisation where the use of the chess metaphor dominates, personnel are sent from head office to sort out an underperforming subsidiary company, they may be referred to as 'white knights', junior members of staff as 'pawns in the game', strategy documents as 'game plans', redundant staff as 'sacrifices' and powerless senior executives in the subsidiary as having been 'checkmated'. In organisations which make use of the military metaphor conversations may include talk of 'attacks', 'forays', 'retreats', 'orders', 'defences', 'victories' and 'defeats'. In contrast, in organisations where the church metaphor predominates one is likely to hear that 'we are a broad church', new leaders may be hailed as 'prophets' and discredited leaders dismissed as 'false prophets', and managers do not deliver briefings but instead give 'sermons'. Exhibit 1.4 provides a further illustration of the use of metaphors as they are used by those involved in corporate takeovers.

Exhibit 1.4
The language of corporate takeovers

The world of corporate takeovers is a tough and emotional one. Not only are large sums of money often involved, but people's jobs, pride and reputations are also generally on the line. Maybe this in part explains the richness and diversity of the language employed by those who make corporate takeovers their business.

The *game* (takeover activity) usually begins with the identification of a *target* (potential acquisition). Particularly vulnerable companies are referred to as *pigeons* and especially desirable firms are termed *sleeping beauties*. If an intermediary such as a broker is involved, then they might be said to be *playing cupid* or acting as a *matchmaker*. If after an extended period of negotiations between two organisations there is no positive result, then this is a case of *sex before marriage*.

In those situations where the intended takeover is hostile there is a *pursuit, warfare* then breaks out, a *siege* situation ensues and the *raiders/pirates* (i.e. the offensive company) together with their *hired guns* (lawyers and other specialist staff) force the situation toward a *shootout* (the climax of a takeover), with the result that the acquired company is *raped* and the two organisations are *married*.

An astute organisation that seeks to avoid being taken over might attempt to find a *safe harbour* or set up *barricades* (impediments to takeover). Alternatively, if faced with a particularly aggressive and unwelcome threat of takeover a firm might seek a *white knight* (friendly acquirer).

Once an acquisition has been made a period of euphoria may set in that is referred to as *afterglow*. These feelings of elation are frequently soon eroded especially for those in the acquired company, where *mushroom treatment* (keeping them in the dark and feeding them on manure) may be evident. In fact, it is not unknown for executives in the acquired company to develop health and career problems and thus find themselves on the *wounded list*.

These are just a few of the many linguistic expressions employed in this field. What makes them so interesting is the variety of metaphors that they embrace: courtship, warfare, westerns, chivalry and nautical.

Source: adapted from Hirsch and Andrews (1983)

While there are organisations in which just one metaphor is prevalent, in most organisations different metaphors are used to describe different sorts of activities. In some organisations metaphors have been extended into specialist organisational vocabularies. For example, at Digital Equipment Corporation (UK) an extensive dictionary of terms called 'DecSpeak' is circulated to teach new recruits that instead of using the term 'feedback' one refers to 'pushback', Digital employees are called 'Deckies', and verbal assaults result in one being 'beaten up'. Other forms of extended metaphor and linguistic expressions include jokes, technical vocabularies, stories and myths. Of these stories and myths deserve special attention.

Stories

Organisational stories have been defined by Martin *et al.* (1983) as narratives which focus on a single, unified sequence of events, and which are apparently drawn from the institution's history. Stories have long been recognised to be an integral feature of organisational life. People tend to tell stories not just because the performance is itself enjoyable, but in order to influence other people's understanding of situations and events, to illustrate their knowledge and insight into how their organisation works, and to show that they are loyal members of the team. In analysing organisational stories we should be careful to note that accounts of the same story given by different individuals are likely to differ. Stories, therefore, have a plastic quality which often makes their relation with historical 'fact' difficult to verify. They are nevertheless important as indicators of:

- cultural values and beliefs;
- formal and informal rules and procedures;
- the consequences of deviance from, and compliance with, the rules; and
- social categories and status, and thus the power structure of an organisation.

Stories also perform a vital 'third order' control function in organisations, by which is meant that they exercise control over the fundamental premises which govern decision making (Perrow, 1979). In other words, they are not just indicators of cultural values and beliefs, but guardians of them as well. Stories are a particularly effective control mechanism because (1) they facilitate recall of information (i.e. are memorable); (2) they tend to generate belief; and (3) they encourage attitudinal commitment by appealing to legitimate values (Wilkins, 1983). This is an important point, which the stories in Exhibit 1.5 help to clarify. First, consider the Revlon story. The latent message here seems to be that while rules should be strictly obeyed by most people, they do not apply to those of high status and need not be enforced where they are concerned. In contrast, the lesson from the Illinois Bell story is that even the most senior executives know their job and will give good service. Finally, the story from AT&T is strongly suggestive that managers should support and protect their staff against 'the system', and that this action will result in success for all concerned. As these stories are told and retold within an organisation they create and reinforce cultural preferences for certain types of action and decision. While most organisational stories circulate uncontrolled, the ease with which stories such as these are remembered, their emotional appeal and their vividness make them potentially powerful tools of management (see Chapter 5).

Exhibit 1.5
Organisational stories

Revlon

At the Revlon Corporation the story is told about Charles Revlon, the head of the group, who insisted that employees arrived for work on time, but seldom arrived himself much before noon. One day Charles wandered in and began to look over the sign-in sheet, only to be interrupted by a receptionist who had strict orders that the list should not be removed. Both insisted that they were in the right until finally Charles said 'Do you know who I am?' And she said 'No sir, I don't'. 'Well, when you pick up your final paycheck this afternoon, ask 'em to tell ya'. (*Tobias, 1976*)

Illinois Bell

At Illinois Bell a story is told about their CEO of the late 1960s, Charles Brown. During a crippling strike 'Charlie', as he was known, would himself repair telephones. On one occasion the country club to which he belonged complained about a broken telephone. Without even changing his clothes Charlie went out and fixed the apparatus, despite suffering from fairly serious teasing from other club members. (*Kleinfield, 1981*)

AT&T

At AT&T the story is told of a senior manager known for supporting his subordinates. A female employee is remembered telling how 'they (headquarters) offered me a position as a general manager in a small town, and this was a promotion. But at the time I was single and working towards my MBA at night. It was a terrible ordeal, because I'd always heard that if you turned down a promotion you'd never be considered again; that you could kiss your career at AT&T goodbye. But I knew my social life and future education would be nil in this small town . . . I explained this situation to Ralph and, while he didn't agree, he understood. He represented my position to headquarters and the offer was withdrawn. Six months later I got a promotion right there in the big city. I know it was because he put his career on the line for me. I've always tried to back subordinates up like he did, and it has paid off.' (*Sutton and Nelson, 1990*)

A final point worth noting is that organisational cultures often carry a claim to uniqueness that stories help to corroborate for members of a culture. Many culture researchers have discovered that organisations like to think of themselves as in some way unique. In this way organisations are like individuals, for whom one aspect of emotional maturing is individuation, that is, coming to distinguish oneself from other members of society. Stories are one means by which organisations make their uniqueness claim, often by incorporating distinctive personalities and specific organisationally relevant events and activities. Martin *et al.* (1983), however, have suggested that while the details of organisational stories do differ, it is nevertheless possible to identify certain common themes between them. Their analysis of a variety of organisational stories led them to discover seven types of story that frequently occur in public and private organisations (see Exhibit 1.6). Just how common these sorts of stories are and whether there are other basic story types is still a matter for further research.

Myths

Myths are generally circulated in organisations in the form of narratives and are often indistinguishable from stories, except that the events they describe are wholly fanciful. While they are often incorporated into stories, organisational myths may also exist as individual beliefs about how the world works. Myths, then, are unjustified beliefs, often enshrined in stories, and which influence how organisational actors understand and react to their social situation. Boje *et al.* (1982) have suggested that there are four basic types of organisational myth, each of which deserves brief consideration.

Exhibit 1.6
Common organisational stories

Martin *et al.* (1983) identified seven basic types of stories prevalent in organisations. These stories provided the answers to fundamental questions about how employees should conduct themselves and what they could expect of their bosses. The seven questions were:

1 Can employees break the rules?
2 Is the big boss human?
3 Can the little person rise to the top?
4 Will I get fired?
5 Will the organisation help me when I have to move?
6 How will the boss react to mistakes?
7 How will the organisation deal with obstacles?

Question

1 Can you identify which questions the organisational stories in Exhibit 1.5 provide answers for?

Source: adapted from Martin *et al.* (1983) by permission of the publisher, from *Organisational Dynamics*, Autumn 1983 © 1983. American Management Association, New York. All rights reserved.

1 *Myths that create, maintain and legitimise past, present or future actions and consequences.* A good example of this is the use consultants make of the myths of 'newness' and 'rational scientific principles' to lend their activities legitimacy, and help gain access to client organisations. Another example has been pointed out by Mintzberg (1973), who has suggested that many executives accept the mythological view that they are rational planners, forecasters, budgeters and controllers, while in fact they tend to make snap decisions, work at a fast pace, tolerate frequent interruptions and do little that can be identified under the traditional categories of management.

2 *Myths that maintain and conceal political interests and value systems.* Myths are intimately related to the power structure of an organisation, and are often used to justify actions that may appear unfair, selfish or unethical. Vast differences in pay rates are sometimes justified on mythological grounds such as the 'special' skills possessed, 'experience' or 'unusual' demands of the job, when no unique skills, experience or job demands are actually involved. Myths can also affect the decision-making capabilities of whole industries. For example, for a long time the US auto industry refused to believe that domestic car buyers would ever purchase small, compact vehicles in large numbers. This myth was underpinned by the failure of a few models such as the Vega and the Pinto, which left internal planners and external critics arguing in vain for a change in strategy. It was only when the myth became untenable in the face of deteriorating profitability that car manufacturers came to reconsider the 'big car' myth, and by then foreign competitors had stolen much of the market.

3 *Myths that help explain and create cause and effect relationships under conditions of incomplete knowledge.* Individuals often suffer from incomplete information about how and why certain organisational phenomena occur, and in these circumstances myths can fill the knowledge gap. For instance, one widespread myth is that women are unreliable workers because they treat their career as secondary to getting married and having children. This myth provides the rationale for precluding women from promotion to better and higher-paying jobs. A self-fulfilling prophecy has thus developed in some organisations with women choosing to leave those places where they cannot progress. To employees in these organisations the data seem to support the dominant myth.

4 *Myths that rationalise the complexity and turbulence of activities and events to allow for predictable action taking.* Faced with apparently random actions and events people tend to impute rationality to them in an attempt to reduce their uncertainty and anxiety. For instance, organisational members like to think of their place of work as easily identifiable, measurable, analysable and changeable, despite all the difficulties associated with these tasks. The resort to ethical codes of conduct or standards of acceptability by members of some organisations to deal with complex situations is another manifestation of this sort of myth.

Ceremonies, rites and rituals

Recurrent patterns of behaviour are a feature of organisational life. Of these, *ceremonies* are often the most vivid and memorable for employees. *Ceremonies* may be thought of as celebrations of organisational culture, or collective acts of cultural worship that remind and reinforce cultural values. Among the more extravagant ceremonies are the annual presentations held at the Mary Kay Cosmetics organisation. These are described by the founder as 'a combination of the Academy Awards, the Miss America Pageant, and a Broadway opening' (Ash, 1981). They involve several nights of well-orchestrated presentations, prizes (including mink coats and diamonds), and speeches by high achievers telling how they succeeded. The proceedings are capped by the crowning of the Director, Consultant Queens and Supersaleswomen in various categories. The message is unmistakable: selling is the goal of the organisation, and everyone within the company has the ability to succeed.

Rites and *rituals* may be defined as 'relatively elaborate, dramatic, planned sets of activities that consolidate various forms of cultural expression into organised events, which are carried out through social interaction, usually for the benefit of an audience' (Beyer and Trice; 1988: 142). Some examples of these behaviours are provided in Exhibit 1.7. *Rites of passage* ease transitions in social roles and status. *Rites of questioning* can be employed by managers to facilitate change by challenging the existing order of things. *Rites of renewal* assist the smooth functioning of an organisation by bringing people together. Rather like stories and myths, ritualised behaviour is important not just for the messages it communicates to individuals who participate in the culture, but also for the power it exercises over them. Among other things, rites structure our understanding of how our organisations work, what is acceptable behaviour, and how to manage change (see Chapter 5).

Exhibit 1.7
Three examples of organisational rite

Type of rite	Examples	Possible functions
Rites of passage	Training programmes Induction programmes Retirement dinners	These facilitate changes in social role and status
Rites of questioning	Use of external consultants Commissioning of critical reports Circulation of critical stories	These challenge the established order of an organisation
Rites of renewal	Office parties Job redesign programmes Employee opinion surveys	These rejuvenate and refurbish the status quo

Source: adapted from Trice and Beyer (1984)

Norms of behaviour

Norms are rules for behaviour which dictate what are considered to be appropriate and inappropriate responses from employees in certain circumstances. They develop over time as individuals negotiate with each other in their attempts to reach a consensus on how to deal with specific problems of organisation. For example, in all organisations there are certain norms concerning the basis on which individuals command respect that have fundamental implications for the dominant patterns of power and deference that emerge. In technically oriented organisations respect may tend to be based on the possession of expertise, while in many traditional UK manufacturing companies respect is often based on length of service (sometimes described as 'experience'). In contrast, in bureaucracies the norm is frequently that individuals command respect by virtue of the position they hold in the hierarchy of management, whereas in other organisations it may be charisma and the possession of good interpersonal skills that people use to determine who should be respected. Something of the broad scope and variety of organisational norms is illustrated in Exhibit 1.8, which provides a summary of norms in the Los Angeles Olympic Organizing Committee. Norms are vital to organisations as they regulate much of the day-to-day behaviour of employees. They function as the providers of coherence and structure to the cultural life of an organisation and thus facilitate predictable and stable patterns of behaviour.

Symbols

Symbols are words, objects, conditions, acts or characteristics of persons that signify something different or wider from themselves, and which have meaning for an individual or group. Typical examples include the speeches of senior executives designed to symbolise their commitment to particular products or policies, corporate logos which symbolise a company, and employees working overtime in order to symbolise their loyalty to an organisation. While some authors have chosen to describe symbols as a clear and distinct subset of cultural elements, it is more useful to think of symbols as a very broad category that includes stories, myths and rites. The point is that almost every

Exhibit 1.8
Organisational norms developed by the Los Angeles Olympic Organizing Committee

The Los Angeles Olympic Organizing Committee (LAOOC) was formed in order to organise and operate the Games of the XXIIIrd Olympiad, which were held between 28 July and 12 August 1984. The organisation had a total history of just over a thousand days, and then virtually ceased to exist. During this time it grew from a handful of individuals to 20 000 employees complemented by 50 000 volunteers. In order to ensure that the enormous task of running an Olympic Games was conducted smoothly and efficiently the organisation had to develop an appropriate set of behavioural norms as quickly as possible. Some of the most important of these included:

- The athlete comes first.
- The Games must be private sector financed.
- New building must be strictly limited.
- The organisation should be decentralised.
- Where possible, services should be contracted to private organisations.
- Staff badges are indicators of seniority and status.
- Men should wear ties and must not wear beards.
- Women should wear dresses and stockings.
- Employees must appear busy at all times.
- High-tension situations and conflicts can legitimately be resolved by jokes including near-the- mark practical jokes.

These rules for good behaviour, some encrypted in an organisational rules book and others informal, helped the LAOOC to run their Olympic Games more efficiently and effectively than would otherwise have been possible.

Source: adapted from McDonald (1991)

aspect, event and process that occurs within an organisation is open to interpretation as a symbol. The more difficult task for any given organisation is to identify its most significant symbols, work out what they mean for organisational participants, and decide how they relate to each other and to the total cultural fabric of the organisation.

In order to facilitate such analyses, classification schemes such as that provided in Exhibit 1.9 have been devised. This suggests that there are three basic types of symbol (verbal, actions and material), and three functions that symbols perform within organisations (description, the control of energy, and system maintenance). Descriptive symbols are shorthand means of conveying what it is like to work in an organisation, or a part of it. Some symbols also have a motivating/demotivating role to play in organisations, and thus help control the flow of energy in them. Finally, there are the system maintenance symbols that help stabilise and justify aspects of organisational activity by offering reasons and guidelines for action. Symbols, then, are an integral feature of cultural life which play vital roles in the smooth functioning of organisations.

Heroes

In the early 1980s authors such as Peters and Waterman (1982) and Deal and Kennedy (1982) began identifying *corporate heroes,* who they claimed were key to the success of their organisations. According to Deal and Kennedy: 'The hero is a great motivator. The magician, the person everyone will count on when things get tough . . . America's boardrooms need heroes more than Hollywood's box offices need them. Heroism is a leadership component that is all but forgotten by modern management.'

Exhibit 1.9
A classification of functions and types of organisational symbolism

	Verbal	*Actions*	*Material*
Descriptive			
Providing an experienced expression of the organisation	Some stories and myths	Celebrations and ceremonies	Corporate logos
Energy controlling			
Increasing tension	Some speeches of senior executives	Rites of conflict and questioning	Some posters and reports
Decreasing tension	Some jokes	Rites of integration and renewal	Some posters and reports
System maintenance			
Giving reasons Providing coherence, order and stability	Some speeches of senior executives	Training and induction programmes	Organisational histories
Giving guidelines Providing acceptable patterns for change	Some stories and myths	Rites of passage	Company handbooks and codes of ethics

Source: adapted from Dandridge *et al.* (1980)

A cursory examination of some of the more populist books and articles on the subject of organisational culture reveals a wealth of claims to have identified organisational heroes. Those named are frequently also the organisation's founders. For example, Bill Hewlett and Dave Packard at Hewlett-Packard are said to be legends in their own lifetime to the employees of that company. Their status as corporate heroes is more or less assured by the formal socialisation processes (see Chapter 2), which include new employees being shown a slide presentation of 'Bill and Dave' making some of the first products using the Hewlett oven. Some organisations go to extraordinary lengths to create their own heroes. At Digital Equipment Corporation (UK), for instance, the author was surprised to find a booklet with brief biographies of half a dozen so-called 'corporate heroes' in circulation. Such attempts to manufacture heroes are largely a response to claims made by authors such as Deal and Kennedy that heroes fulfil certain vital functions in organisations, namely:

- they make success seem attainable and human for ordinary employees;
- they provide role models who set high standards of performance for others to follow;
- they symbolise the organisation to external constituencies;
- they preserve and enhance cultural values, and enshrine what is unique about an organisation;
- they encourage greater commitment to the organisation, and urge people to identify their personal achievements with the organisation's success; and
- they motivate employees.

Mini Case 1.1

Jan Carlzon: A hero in decline at SAS?

Scandinavian Airlines System (SAS) is the national airline of Denmark, Norway and Sweden, and the Governments of these three countries own some 50 per cent of the share equity of the corporation. SAS employs around 25 000 people, many of whom are based in the Stockholm headquarters (Sweden) and its main airport in Copenhagen (Denmark). In 1981 Jan Carlzon was appointed managing director of SAS. This followed an extremely difficult period in which the company had posted losses of about 75m Danish Kroner (approximately £7.5m) in each of the last two financial years. Carlzon's brief was to turn around the financial performance of SAS.

Using his excellent communication skills and flair for handling the media Carlzon established a reputation as a shrewd operator. Typical of his use of symbolic acts and events was his stage-managed attempt to assist loading an SAS flight at Copenhagen Airport. This event generated huge publicity for SAS, demonstrated to employees the importance of routine tasks, and effectively illustrated the principle that SAS employees should work together to help the organisation to succeed.

Carlzon was not merely sensitive to the importance of symbols, he also had a particular vision of how SAS could win back market share. He centred his attention on the frontline personnel who dealt direct with customers, and who he thought were the keys to the success or failure of the corporation. Carlzon recognised that there was a strong need for authority to be delegated to these people, so that when customer problems arose they would have the decision-making power required to satisfy them without recourse to senior managers. The importance of these employees to the success of the company was reinforced through both internal SAS magazines and the mass media.

Employees at SAS reacted to Carlzon with enthusiasm, and the organisation came to be noted for its hard-working, highly motivated and committed staff. The financial implications of this sea-change in attitudes became clear in 1982/3 when SAS declared an operating surplus of 620m Danish Kroner. SAS, it seemed, had changed from being a technical-oriented organisation to a service-oriented airline ('the businessman's' airline), which in 1982 was recognised as being the most punctual airline by the European Flight Association. Carlzon himself was not just regarded as a very successful leader, but 'was seen as a hero by employees who would, if need be, go to hell and back for him'.

In the early 1990s, however, SAS was again in financial difficulties, partly due to a worldwide depression of the airline business following the Gulf War, partly as a result of the company's preparation for the European Community Internal Market, which increased competitive pressures for airlines, and partly as a result of some poor strategic decisions. The most costly of these failed strategies involved purchasing a 40 per cent stake in International Hotels, and a share in the American company Continental Airlines. In 1991 SAS cut 3500 jobs in a bid to reduce operating expenses, a move that many employees hold Carlzon personally responsible for. The level of disillusionment with Carlzon was aptly expressed by John Vangen, spokesmen for a Danish trade union for cabin crew (Flightpersonnel): 'None of Carlzon's strategies have succeeded since 1984. He has to take responsibility for that. If he cannot make the company run he should leave it. We need a management we can trust.'

Questions

1 If Carlzon could fall from grace so quickly, is it fair to describe him as once having been a hero, or was he just a temporarily esteemed leader?

2 What steps, if any, could Carlzon have taken to ensure that he preserved his 'hero' status?

Source: adapted from P. Darmer (1994), 'SAS – Mergers in the Air', in Derek Adam-Smith and A. Peacock (eds) (1994)

More recently, however, theorists such as Wilkins *et al.* (1990) have argued that there may be dangers associated with deliberately attempting to create heroes. There are, for example, many collaborative cultures where teamwork and co-operation are prized more than individual excellence. In these organisations efforts to manufacture heroes may be dysfunctional. In addition, few groups like to be told who their heroes should be. The process of hero formation thus requires very careful handling. There are also obvious dangers of choosing the 'wrong' people to transform into heroes. Making someone a hero inevitably gives him or her a lot of power, which may in turn make them overconfident and intimidating. Such people may also create disunity if they come to represent just one section of an organisation such as engineering or marketing, or the 'old' way of doing things. Organisational heroes, then, are a mixed blessing, for they may be demotivating for average performers, symbols of identification and loyalty for those resistant to change, and politically dangerous. Some of the problems with heroes are exemplified by the American businessman Roy Ash. Having developed a high-profile reputation in business and politics he became chairman and CEO of Addressograph-Multigraph with plans to turn it into the next IBM. He changed the name of the organisation to AM International and publicised a strategic vision which captivated corporate America. By 1982 the dream had effectively died. Roy Ash's confidence and enthusiasm had proved beguiling not just to investors but to himself, with impatience and inattention to detail undermining what had looked like a sound business proposition (Wilkins *et al.*, 1990). A more detailed account of the decline of a corporate hero is provided by Mini Case 1.1.

Values, beliefs and attitudes

Values and beliefs are part of the cognitive sub-structure of an organisational culture. *Values* are intimately connected with moral and ethical codes, and determine what people think *ought* to be done. Individuals and organisations which value honesty, integrity and openness consider that they (and others) should act honestly, openly, and with integrity because that is the right thing to do. *Beliefs*, on the other hand, concern what people think is and is not true. The beliefs that increasing expenditure on advertising will lead to increased sales, and that paying people according to their performance will improve output, are two widely held examples. In practice, beliefs and values are often hard to distinguish between, because beliefs about how the world works frequently involve values, that is, views about what should or ought to be done. For instance, individuals may both value honesty, openness and integrity and believe that it is only by acting honestly, openly and with integrity that organisations can function effectively. In such cases it is difficult to know whether honesty, openness and integrity are valued for their own sake, or because of the belief that they promote organisational wellbeing. Moreover some authors have defined values as particular sorts of belief. For example, Rokeach (1973: 5) has suggested that 'a value is an enduring belief that a specific mode of conduct or end-state of existence is personally or socially preferable to an opposite or converse mode of conduct or end-state of existence'. Difficulties such as these make it tempting to speak of 'belief/value clusters', thus obviating the need for specificity in the face of considerable organisational complexity. A selection of some of the most commonly subscribed to belief/value clusters in commercial organisations is contained in Exhibit 1.10.

According to Schein (1985a) an organisational leader's beliefs can be transformed into collective beliefs over time through the medium of values. He suggests that when faced with a problem the leader of an organisation will propose a solution, such as

Exhibit 1.10
A selection of beliefs/values commonly found in commercial organisations

Belief/value	Definition
Adaptability	To be able to change in response to new stimuli
Autonomy	To be able to work independently
Co-operation	To be able to work well with others
Creativity	To be able to generate new ideas and develop innovative approaches
Equality	Everyone has equal rights and opportunities
Honesty	To be open, candid and ethical in work activities
Rationality	To be analytical and logical

'increase productivity', because of a belief such as 'increased productivity means increased profitability'. Other members of the organisation, however, will hear this view not as a statement of belief (to which they may not subscribe) but as an assertion of the leader's values, namely, that one should or ought to increase productivity when one is experiencing problems. If this solution works (or, more correctly, is perceived to work), then the group may gradually accept the value as an accurate description of how the world works. As the value comes to be taken for granted and is seen to work reliably, then social validation may transform it into a rarely questioned belief. The fact that many UK manufacturing organisations respond to market uncertainties by increasing their productive efforts rather than by investing in new product development or marketing is testament to how firmly ingrained such beliefs can become. When beliefs have achieved this status they may be considered basic assumptions (see below).

Attitudes connect beliefs and values with feelings. An attitude may be thought of as a learned predisposition to respond in a consistently favourable or unfavourable manner to a particular thing or idea. Attitudes, therefore, involve evaluations based on feelings. For example, senior managers may believe that quality circles tend to lead to increased commitment from employees and thus enhance productivity and quality. If these people evaluate commitment, productivity and quality positively, then they can be said to hold a positive attitude towards quality circles. In contrast, middle management may believe that quality circles will lead to time-wasting discussion, increased friction in the workplace, and an undermining of their authority. In this instance the middle managers are likely to have a negative attitude towards quality circles. Attitudes are developed over time, and, like opinions, are often held as a result of prejudices and stereotypes rather than actual information. Unlike opinions, however, they are held relatively consistently, and have a more enduring impact on employee motivation.

Basic assumptions

A basic assumption is a taken-for-granted solution to an identifiable problem. Schein (1981) has proposed the idea that a culture may be defined in terms of its basic assumptions. A near synonym for 'basic assumptions' is 'theories-in-use' (Argyris, 1976). Both refer to the implicit, deeply rooted assumptions people share, and which guide their perceptions, feelings and emotions about things. Basic assumptions differ from ordinary beliefs in three ways. First, beliefs are held consciously and are relatively easy to detect, whereas basic assumptions are held unconsciously and are very difficult to surface. Second, beliefs are confrontable, debatable and therefore easier to modify than basic assumptions, which are by definition neither confrontable nor debatable. Third, beliefs are simple cognitions compared with basic assumptions, which involve not just beliefs but interpretations of those beliefs plus values and emotions. Basic assumptions, then, are pre-conscious, non-confrontable and highly complex aspects of human group psychology.

Schein (1985a) has suggested a typology of basic assumptions with five dimensions: humanity's relationship to nature, the nature of reality and truth, the nature of human nature, the nature of human activity, and the nature of human relationships. Each of these will be briefly considered here.

Humanity's relationship to its environment

Organisations differ greatly in terms of the extent to which they perceive themselves to be in control of their own destiny. Some organisations assume that they are able to dominate their environment; some that they must harmonise with it, often by finding an appropriate niche. Others, however, assume that they are dominated by their environment; and must accept whatever niche is available.

The nature of reality and truth

There are a great many ways of establishing 'truth' and reaching decisions in organisations. In some organisations truth is decided by pure dogma based on tradition or the supposed wisdom of trusted leaders. In other organisations decisions are arrived at through a 'rational-legal' process involving sophisticated rules and procedures. In still other organisations truth is said to be that which survives conflict and debate. Finally, there are organisations in which the pragmatic criterion of 'if it works, then it's the truth' is assumed.

The nature of human nature

Different assumptions about human nature dominate in different organisations. In some organisations people are regarded as being fundamentally lazy (McGregor's Theory X), while in others people are considered to be highly self-motivated (McGregor's Theory Y). In some organisations humans are thought to be motivated by monetary considerations, while in others employees are thought to be motivated by the need for social approval or the potential for self-actualisation.[3]

The nature of human activity

In the West the dominant assumption is that people should be proactive achievers who, through hard work and diligence, are able to achieve given objectives. Contrasting with this 'doing' orientation is the 'being' assumption, which espouses a more fatalistic approach to work life. Lastly, there is what Schein refers to as a 'being-in-becoming' orientation which emphasises self-actualisation and self-development through detachment, meditation and control. Of related interest here is the divide between those organisations in which work is primary, those organisations in which the private lives of employees are more valued, and those which assume that a balanced and integrated combination of both work and private life is feasible and desirable.

Mini Case 1.2

Philips Electronics

Introduction

Philips Electronics has its origins in a company started on 5 May 1891 by Gerard and his father Frederik Philips. Gerard's brother Anton joined the business in 1895, and it was agreed that he would take charge of commercial strategy while Gerard would be responsible for technical research. A century later Philips had a stock market value of £2.4bn, a workforce of 273 000,[1] and a turnover of £17bn. Although the company had been highly profitable for many years, in recent times profits had slumped in the face of severe competition, and attempts to rectify matters had had little impact. Some commentators (within as well as outside the firm) suggested that Philips' culture was a prime cause of the organisation's poor performance.

Philips' relationship to its environment

The overwhelming view within Philips is that the organisation is the world's foremost designer and manufacturer of high-quality, innovative consumer electronics, components, information technology and lighting products. In support of this self-perception the company can point to music cassettes, video cassette recorders and compact discs, all of which it has invented. These and other cultural artefacts have become the foci of identification and loyalty for Philips employees. Almost inevitably the markets relevant to such a vast organisation are not just social, economic and technological, but political too. It was, for example, apparent that Philips had managed to manipulate the political environment in Europe to win protection from imports, though this political influence seems to be waning. Curiously, there are many in Philips who think of the company as primarily a Dutch/European organisation rather than a true multinational, and some commentators have suggested that this is a limiting factor in the firm's culture. The fact that Philips is dominated by its competitive environment rather than the dominating force within it was, by the mid-1990s, apparent to all.

The nature of truth and reality

Philips prides itself on taking decisions by consensus, and sticking to them over the long term. This is, however, only part of the picture. Philips is also still constrained by the technological/commercial divide initiated by Gerard and Anton 100 years ago, and what is more, the technological arm still has greater kudos and attracts better recruits. In short, Philips is an organisation obsessed by technology rather than markets or profitability. Statements such as 'research is Philips' technological conscience' abound in the company's own literature. The result is that the consensual decisions taken have tended to ignore product design and marketing, and have overlooked the overwhelming evidence that consumer electronics is driven by fashion not technology. Philips' cultural inclination to define truth and reality according to its technological bias has led critics to charge that it is complacent, lethargic, inward-looking and risk-averse. There is, though, evidence that these basic assumptions are changing under the leadership of Jan Timmer and undeniable evidence of economic failure. For example, line managers have recently been made more accountable and are now immersed in their business on a day-to-day basis, while the profile of product design and marketing has also been raised.

The nature of human nature

Philips' culture views employees as essentially good, perfectible and deserving of reward. These assumptions are reflected in the company's history of benevolence and paternalism. Perhaps the clearest indication of this element of the organisation's culture is in its treatment of employees at its headquarters in Eindhoven. Despite declining profitability and the need to shed staff, very little has changed in Philips' HQ. Here the same cliquish rules and conventions still govern life among the company's elite as they have done for years. Neither has the axe fallen on large numbers of more junior employees, the suggestion being that this would have meant 'that top managers would have to drive through the town every day, passing people on the street they had made redundant', something that Philips' culture could not tolerate. These relaxed and cosy assumptions about the essential worth of people may well be connected with the fact that many senior executives had worked in developing countries in their formative years, and brought back a form of 'colonial outlook' to the Netherlands on their return. It should, however, be noted that the company's paternalism was most notable with respect to Dutch employees, especially those in Eindhoven, and that evidence for ruthlessness could be found elsewhere around the globe.

The nature of human activity

Traditionally Philips has paid lip service to the idea of being proactive shapers of the commercial environment, while limiting the scope of its proactivity to the technological sphere. The fact that most of the organisation's senior executives are Dutchmen who have spent their entire working lives with the company has not helped to breed a radical external orientation. A long history of economic success and insulation from the threat of takeover by formidable defences have also done little to encourage dynamism. Even faced with its current problems an executive was recently quoted as saying 'Philips doesn't panic. That's not part of its culture'. This said, there are indications that Philips' parochial perspective is altering under the influence first of Cor van der Klugt and latterly of Jan Timmer. The organisation has changed its name, instituted a massive downsizing programme, sold off many peripheral businesses, implemented a number of structural changes, and closed dozens of European factories in favour of plants in Mexico and south-east Asia. There is, however, still a sense that Philips is primarily reacting to events rather than helping to create the future, a feeling which is reinforced by its persistent complaints of unfair competition from Asian countries such as the Japanese (who they claim have rigged their domestic market against competition), and the South Koreans (whose cheap labour costs and currencies are claimed to be an unfair advantage).

The nature of human relationships

Philips' culture was built on the idea that teamwork and employee participation were commercially utilitarian. As Frederik Philips (1978: 257) stated in his autobiography: 'I believe participation is not so much a matter of structures as of attitudes. We can start where we are. Do we include people in our own decisions? Participation has to start from the top, but it also has to percolate right through from top to bottom. And we need to work hard to make this a reality.'[2] A few years ago this ethic of teamworking was apparent, but only within the organisation's patchwork of fiercely independent national suborganisations, each responsible for product development, manufacturing and marketing in its own country. The Japanese exposed the weaknesses in this fragmented and uncoordinated approach which could not make use of potential economies of scale. Jan Timmer has sought to regroup the company along product divisions, and in time the culture of teamworking fostered by the founders of the organisation can be expected to manifest itself once again. Some, however, have argued that there are too many weak points in Philips' culture to be confident concerning its future. As one former executive said: 'Timmer will succeed only if he can break through the Philips culture. And the only way to do that may be to destroy it.'

Questions

1 In your opinion, are all Philips' basic assumptions complementary, that is, do they fit together in a coherent way? Is there any potential for conflict between these assumptions?

2 What belief/value clusters would you expect to be associated with each of Philips' basic assumptions?

3 Which basic assumption do you feel is likely to have been most responsible for damaging Philips' economic performance in recent years?

Notes

1 In 1988 the company had employed 337 000 personnel.
2 Frederik Philips was the son of Anton Philips, and had been chairman of the board of governors of the holdings compan

Source: compiled from F. Philips (1978), J. Heskett (1989), *Financial Times*, 22 July 1988; 25 May 1990, 17; 2 July 1990; *Guardian*, 1 March 1991, 14

The nature of human relationships

Organisations differ greatly in the way they assume people should relate to each other. For example, some organisations tend to foster individualism whereas others favour collective action and co-operation. Further, there are organisations that are run as autocracies, some are paternalistic, others are democratic. Focusing specifically on role relationships we can detect organisations in which people interact as friends and those in which emotions are minimised (see Mini Case 2.1 for an illustration of this point).

Finally, it is important to note that basic assumptions are often mutually reinforcing and highly interdependent. Thus in order to be able to interpret an organisation's culture, it is necessary to unravel very complex sets of beliefs, values and emotions. This analytical task is made still more difficult by the fact that cultures are not static entities, but evolve over time. See Mini Case 1.2 for an exploration of basic assumptions at Philips Electronics.

History

While not strictly speaking a component of an organisation's culture it is generally agreed that a culture can only be fully understood as the product of a historical process. The idea that organisational cultures develop and change over time has been explicitly recognised by many theorists who have built a temporal element into their culture definitions. In fact, the scope that the cultural perspective offers for studying the history of organisations is one of the exciting possibilities opened up by this field of inquiry. The point is that most other perspectives on organisational behaviour are ahistorical, preferring to examine organisations as they are now rather than as the end result of complex evolutionary processes. Generally speaking, sociologists and psychologists have not, therefore, turned their critical attention on organisational history. Interestingly, some authors, such as Rowlinson and Hassard (1993), have argued that the full potential of the culture perspective for scrutinising the history of organisations has not yet been realised. They claim that the result is an undue emphasis on the founders of organisations as the shapers of culture, and stories and myths as the means by which culture is perpetuated. Their argument is that leaders, stories and myths have been mistakenly identified as core determinants of a culture, when a more thorough historical analysis may often reveal far more complexity than is at first apparent. This view is illustrated with reference to the Cadbury organisation in Mini Case 1.3.

ESPOUSED CULTURE AND CULTURE-IN-PRACTICE

A distinction can be drawn between the beliefs and values an organisation espouses and those which its employees actually use on a day-to-day basis to guide their work activities. Argyris and Schon (1978) have described this distinction as the difference between 'espoused theory' and 'theory-in-practice'. The idea is that through their formal documentation (such as publicity material and annual reports and accounts) and the speeches of senior executives, organisations present a particular view of their culture. This espoused culture refers to a normative or *desired state* vision of the organisation, that is, what the organisation should be. In contrast, an organisation's culture-in-practice is its actual culture as experienced by employees. The difference between an organisation's espoused culture and culture-in-practice can be dramatic. For example, some universities espouse concern for teaching quality ('we are a teaching-oriented institution') while in practice they recruit and promote employees on the basis of their research endeavours. Other instances of organisations espousing commitment to specific values, such as equal opportunities or concern for the environment, but acting according to very different value sets, are widespread.

Cadbury

Rowlinson and Hassard's (1993) study of Cadbury provides a powerful argument why we should seek to understand an organisation's culture through an examination of its history. They have illustrated how organisations impose the timing and significance of historical events such as centenaries upon history, rather than history imposing these events upon organisations. They have also shown how organisations are able to impose their prejudiced interpretations of why certain things were done. Culture, then, cannot be taken at face value, but must rather be thoroughly researched if useful and accurate accounts of it are to be drawn.

Cadbury, now part of Cadbury Schweppes, is a UK-based chocolate manufacturer which until 1962 had been largely owned and continuously managed by members of the Cadbury family. It was established by John Cadbury in 1824 in the centre of Birmingham, and taken over by his sons Richard and George who revived the firm's fortunes, partly by expanding from the tea and coffee trade into cocoa and chocolate production. Somewhat curiously, the company decided to celebrate its centenary in 1931, a date commemorated by the commissioning of two publications, *The Firm of Cadbury 1831–1931* and A Century of Progress 1831–1931. An incredible 180 000 copies of *A Century of Progress* were produced by Cadbury's Advertising Department at a cost of more than £7500, and distributed to the company's customers. A more modest number of *The Firm of Cadbury* were printed and distributed to Cadbury's long-serving employees. Both works unashamedly attempted to construct a history of the organisation which stressed unity and continuity, and the virtues of its Quaker leaders and working practices.

So successful were Cadbury's attempts to invent its history that subsequent historians sought to explain events at the organisation in terms of the leaders' Quaker beliefs. The organisation was helped in this by various publications produced by the Society of Friends and its members which emphasised the enlightened nature of Quaker business enterprises. There is, however, an alternative view at least as plausible as that promulgated by Cadbury. This holds that significant developments in the organisation's labour–management relations occurred in response to contemporary social movements, that is, external pressures rather than enlightened moral conviction. For example, Cadbury built and sold houses to its workers in Bournville and provided them with mortgages. A Charitable Trust was then formed to look after the interests of the owner-occupiers which was nominally independent of Cadbury and democratic in its vision. While Cadbury liked to suggest that religious and moral principle guided their actions, it is arguable that the character of the Bournville village owed more to the influence of the early town-planning movement than to the inspiration of Quakerism. The same is true of other Cadbury work practices, which probably derived more from developments in American corporations, the influence of a 'new' social science approach to managing organisations called 'scientific management',[1] and accepted business practice in the UK, than they did from the Quaker faith.

The point is that Cadbury used its privileged position to make known a version of its history that provided it with legitimacy in a period of change. It is tempting to suggest that in an increasingly secular society the apparent conformity of Cadbury to a religious ideal gave the company an identity which made it special, and leant it a morality that seemed to be lacking elsewhere. The history of organisations may themselves, under certain conditions, be thought of as cultural artefacts.

Questions

1 Do you think it is appropriate for organisations to place their own interpretations on historical facts and events in order to show them off in a positive light? Explain your answer.

2 Do you think that there are any potential dangers associated with an organisation wilfully misinterpreting its own history?

Note

1 Founded by F.W. Taylor *scientific management* was a movement that favoured the 'scientific' selection and training of workers. Further, it suggested that work tasks should be highly specialised, and that management was the preserve of managers, who should control the work of employees according to rigid procedures, which were to be discovered by observation and measurement.

Source: adapted from Rowlinson and Hassard (1993) ' The invention of corporate culture: A history of the histories of Cadbury', *Human Relations*, Vol. 46, No. 3, pp. 299–326

The recognition of the existence of separately identifiable espoused cultures and cultures-in-practice in organisations helps us to understand why so many organisational cultures appear confused and contradictory. Interestingly, large numbers of individuals seem able to tolerate high degrees of inconsistency between the espoused and actual cultures of the organisations in which they work. In some instances this will be because individuals have mentally conflated the espoused and the actual, thus failing to distinguish between fact and fiction. Such people do not perceive any internal conflicts in their organisation. Others may well recognise such discrepancies, but interpret them as being part of the psychological contract they have entered into on joining the organisation. That is, they accept that organisations often tend to portray themselves as they would like to be (or be seen to be) rather than as they actually are, as legitimate or even good business practice.

CULTURE, INTERPRETATION AND MEANING

It is through the medium of culture that we are able to make sense of our world and by means of organisational culture that we appreciate and attribute meaning to our organisational experiences. This may seem like an obscure academic point, but it is in fact very important to our understanding of organisational culture. The main idea is that organisational culture provides the basic theoretical processes upon which we rely to organise our experiences of working life. Our basic assumptions give us guidelines for understanding why individuals and groups behave the way they do, and our beliefs and values allow us to give explanations for actions and events which would otherwise perplex us. Similarly, stories and myths provide coherent accounts of people and phenomena that would otherwise remain mysterious.

Furthermore, because culture is shared, people within the same organisation will often possess quite similar views concerning, for instance, how an organisation is performing, who is in control, and how we should best behave. No culture, however, is shared absolutely, that is, without variation, and this can result in different interpretations being placed on the same behaviours, actions and events. These different interpretations are most notable between different subcultures, as we have seen in this chapter. The vital lesson for us here is that organisational culture is important because it influences how we interpret organisational life and the meaning that we place on organisational activities.

SUMMARY AND CONCLUSIONS

In this chapter four main themes were elaborated.

1 Something of the origins and history of the culture perspective were summarised. The origins of the current interest in organisational culture were found to have their roots in research into organisational climate and national cultures, and to be related to increased interest in human resource management and new explanations of corporate performance. The culture perspective was discovered to have been principally derived from two intellectual traditions: anthropology and organisational sociology. The place of organisational culture within the broad field of organisational theory was then discussed. It was found to have some similarities with four other schools of thought, namely, human relations, modern structural theory, systems theory and, especially, power and politics.

2 Some definitions of organisational culture were reviewed and some culture models illustrated. It was found that there is no consensus on how culture should be defined, and that scholars have variously defined it as a metaphor, an objective property of organisations, and as a psychological phenomenon. For the purposes of this book organisational culture was defined as: *the pattern of beliefs, values and learned ways of coping with experience that have developed during the course of an organisation's history, and which tend to be manifested in its material arrangements and in the behaviours of its members.*

3 The contents of an organisational culture were examined in some detail. It was suggested that at the most superficial level culture consists of material artefacts like corporate logos, mission statements and corporate architecture, linguistic artefacts such as metaphors, stories and myths, behavioural artefacts such as rites, rituals and ceremonies, and miscellaneous artefacts such as heroes and various organisational symbols. At a deeper level a culture may be thought of as consisting of the beliefs, values, attitudes and norms of behaviour that predominate, and which may be incorporated into ethical codes. According to some authors the most fundamental and important level of a culture is its basic assumptions, which are deeply held preconscious orientations about how the world functions, and which develop over time.

4 Readers were advised that organisational cultures are highly complex phenomena. It was argued that organisational culture is important because it is through the medium of culture that employees make sense of their working lives and attribute meaning to organisational experiences.

There is one final theme to note here. In order to provide a comprehensible and coherent account of organisational culture this chapter has to some extent underplayed the dynamic nature of cultural processes. Before we go on to consider further issues in this field, it is worth briefly considering this point. Organisational cultures are rarely completely static over long periods of time. Rather, they are subject to continuous processes of development and change due to organisational learning, which occurs as employees seek answers to problems of external adaptation and internal integration. In fact, different elements of a culture are likely to be differentially resistant to change, with basic assumptions being the least likely to alter radically and artefacts being the most prone to evolutionary processes. These issues are considered in more detail in Chapters 4 and 5.

KEY CONCEPTS

Organisational climate	Human relations	Myths	Norms
National culture	Modern structural	Rites	Rules
Human resource	theory	Rituals	Ethical codes
management	Power and politics	Ceremonies	Morals
Performance	Metaphors	Heroes	Basic assumptions
Anthropology	Artefacts	Symbols	History
Organisational	Language	Beliefs	Meaning
sociology	Jokes	Values	Interpretation
Organisational theory	Stories	Attitudes	

QUESTIONS

1 Why is there such great interest in organisational culture?

2 Why are there so many different definitions of organisational culture? Does it matter that there is currently no consensus on how the phrase should be defined?

3 Do you think organisational culture should be thought of as primarily a behavioural phenomenon (to do with rites, rituals, ceremonies and other patterns of behaviour) or a psychological phenomenon (concerned with beliefs, values, attitudes and assumptions)?

4 Is culture something an organisation is or something an organisation possesses?

5 Describe the artefacts of an organisational culture you know well. What light do they shed on the organisation's basic assumptions?

6 What are the advantages and disadvantages associated with corporate heroes?

7 Is it possible to understand an organisation's culture if you are unaware of its history? Discuss with reference to the Cadbury Mini Case and/or other organisations you know well.

A CULTURE IN TRANSITION: BASSETT FOODS PLC

Introduction

Based in the UK, Bassett (now Trebor Bassett) consisted of a holdings board and five principal subsidiaries. In addition, Bassett owned a small distributing company in the US and part-owned two others in West Germany and Hong Kong. The holdings board was composed of four executive and two non-executive directors, and each of the principal subsidiaries was operated by a small team of between three and five executive directors (see Fig. 1.4). The group employed approximately 3000 people of whom the vast majority were women and more than half of whom were part-timers. It was, however, noticeable that men were more likely to be employed on a full-time basis than women, and that there were no female executive directors either on the holdings board or the subsidiary boards. The shareholder profile for the organisation revealed that no single individual owned more than 10 per cent of the issued share capital, with private individuals being the largest share-owning sector with 38.88 per cent.

Bassett was principally concerned with the manufacture, distribution and sale of sugar confectionery worldwide. Within the UK it had two products in the top twenty selling sugar confectionery brands in 1988. The organisation's place in the industry was as one of the leading manufacturers of sugar confectionery (after Trebor and Rowntree, who accounted for 27 per cent of sales between them) in a market dominated by manufacturers of chocolate. While some sectors of the market had contracted steadily for a decade, in 1988 the UK market for sugar confectionery was still worth approximately £1 billion. Nevertheless nothing could disguise the fact that this had been a declining market, and in 1988 there were 40 fewer manufacturers of sugar confectionery registered with the Confectionery Alliance than in 1980. Historically, Bassett's performance within the industry had been weak. On an annual turnover which approached £100 million, profitability was currently less than half the £10 million target that the chief executive had set the organisation.

The impact of history

Originally formed in 1842 by George Bassett and Samuel Johnson, by 1862 Bassett employed nearly 150 people. Following the end of the First World War the company (and its profits) expanded dramatically and in June 1926 it was floated as a public company. By the time of the outbreak of the Second World War the labour force had increased to approximately 900 persons. Following the war, and the abolition of rationing and other controls over raw materials in 1953, the business was built up through acquisitions and organic growth to its current proportions. It should be noted that due to a preference share arrangement the descendants of one of the original partners retained effective control of the business

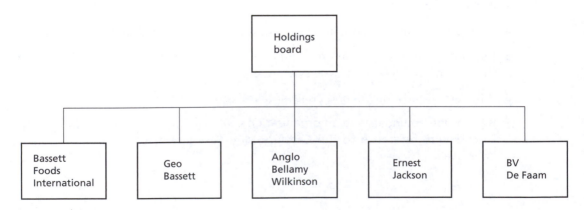

Fig. 1.4 Bassett Foods plc

until 1978 when they finally ceded control to a board of professional managers.

The period 1956–1980 had been a particularly traumatic one for Bassett. From 1956 until 1961 the company experienced an alarming decline in profitability due to increased competition, especially from manufacturers of chocolate. While profits took an upward turn in 1961 they remained shaky throughout the 1960s, compelling a radical reappraisal of the organisation's strategy. At first the company sought to strengthen itself by consolidating its position in the liquorice market and broadening its manufacturing base. However, from 1976 Bassett embarked on a disastrous policy of diversification into other markets including the import of toys, audio and TV games, and electronic calculators. The consequence was that in 1980 the company declared a loss of £1.22 million. There followed a period of considerable change: the main board was replaced with a younger team, many of the more recently acquired subsidiaries were sold off, and the core of the sugar confectionery business was restructured. Under the new management Bassetts' profitability began to improve dramatically, leading a local paper to assert that 'the board has done wonders in the last couple of years in reviving what looked like a shipwreck of a business in the 70s into the viable concern it is today'.[4]

The view from the top

The holdings board were housed in their own building three miles away from the group's largest subsidiary. While not especially palatial the building was luxuriously decorated with high-quality office furnishings that were less than a year old. The four executive directors had extensive office space and appeared to have generous secretarial support facilities. I was shown into Bev's (the chairman and chief executive) office by a glamorous receptionist, and coffee appeared a few minutes later served in an attractive china set. Exuding charm and confidence, Bev described how he had sought to fashion culture at Bassett. The starting point for his analysis was that:

> It takes a long time to change the corporate culture of a company. Status was all important in the 1970s. You know you just had to be important . . . . I think Bassett

had more managing directors than any other company in terms of how people described themselves: you know the marketing director would describe himself as MD, the production director would change his name to 'manufacturing director' so he could describe himself as 'MD'. I'm trying to get that out of the system.

On his own admission status seeking was still a problem in some areas, and this seemed to be linked to personal and political antagonisms that bedevilled relationships between some of the subsidiaries. Bev, however, thought that these internal squabbles were a less important element of Bassett's culture than the benevolent corporate attitude taken towards individual employees. This view was shared by all the other members of the holdings board, and one of the non-executive directors commented that:

> It's been promulgated on more than one occasion by the chairman that sure we have responsibilities to the shareholders, but we also have responsibilities to our people, and we should not consciously try to do things with the minimum of people. One of our roles, particularly in the Sheffield of the late twentieth century, is to provide jobs.

However, while Bev suggested that this was a wholly positive cultural trait other members of the holdings board talked about it being a mixed blessing that had led to a build-up of less than competent staff, slowed the ability of the company to respond to change, and adversely affected profitability. The idea that the rights and welfare of the workforce should figure prominently in the calculations of senior executives was, though, a tradition that dated back to the founding of the company, and seemed impervious to change, at least in the short term. Indeed, Bev and the other members of the holdings board all remarked on the one major positive that Bassett gained from its caring attitude: a tremendous loyalty to the organisation and its products from the great mass of its workforce. Perhaps this characteristic was related to the informality that Bev recognised as pervading his organisation, and the evidently relaxed pace of life at which most employees conducted their work activities. The company secretary, who was a relatively new member of the holdings board, spoke in general terms of people being 'laid-back' and 'slovenly', while the group finance director identified an older cadre of middle managers in the subsidiaries who needed to be 'replaced by the younger school'.

Despite some residual difficulties Bev and his fellow holdings board colleagues were absolutely convinced that the organisation had improved and was continuing to improve against a variety of performance indicators. They talked at length of the Bassett of three years ago where no one cared about constructing reasonable budgets or setting targets, and when they were set took little notice of them. No one had any illusions about the current state of the organisation, however, and all suggested that things had to get even better if Bassett was to survive. The development director admitted that he thought things were still a little 'cosy' and the company secretary noted an absence of people willing 'to say "that's my ball and I'm going to run with that one"'. Some senior executives thought that these attitudes could be related to the extremely democratic nature of the organisation, in which issues tended to be settled by consensus, and authority was massively delegated by the holdings board to the subsidiaries. As one of the non-executive directors said, 'within the limit of the framework of what has been agreed I think it's up to us to let them [the subsidiaries] go ahead and operate'.

Bev and his fellow holdings board directors were adamant that work activity within Bassett should (and did) emphasise co-operation rather than competition between individuals, departments and whole subsidiaries. In fact, some members of the holdings board, such as the development director, expressed something bordering on horror at the thought of competitive behaviour ('Competition between individuals is not a good thing'), which seemed to have its roots in the recent history of political in-fighting within the organisation. Many individuals at holdings board and subsidiary level could recall the days when ideas and information were used overtly politically to further the careers of some at the expense of others. This, I was informed, no longer occurred. There were, nevertheless, obvious signs of tension and conflict between some of the subsidiaries which may have been damaging Bassett's profitability. These were most evident between Geo Bassett (GB) and Anglo Bellamy Wilkinson (ABW), and between the Dutch subsidiary De Faam (DF) and Bassett Foods International (BFI). ABW had been created 18 months previously and was highly dependent on GB which was its principal market. Before the restructuring process had begun

ABW had been a directly managed site under the control of GB, and while the staff at ABW were obviously enjoying their new-found freedom many at GB wanted to turn back the clock. The conflict between DF and BFI seemed to centre on DF's managing director's perception that the international division was not selling enough of his company's products. He complained that at BFI 'There's no manager . . . there is no discipline, there are no orders and they don't work'. The general holdings board view was summed up by one of the non-executive directors, who considered that the problems were a complex mixture of 'personality, language, culture, competition, mistrust . . .'.

Most members of the holdings board recognised that Bassett was a highly introspective organisation, with terms such as 'blinkered', 'narrow' and 'introspective' being liberally employed. The non-executive directors were particularly concerned that too many internal promotions meant that talented individuals from outside the company could not be appointed, and that exporting goods internationally was given an insufficiently high priority. Bev was certain that these attitudes were changing, and spoke enthusiastically about his attempts to make Bassett a 'marketing-led' organisation, sensitive and aware of its external environment. The non-executive directors were rather more sceptical, and claimed that the mentality in the subsidiaries was still very much 'if in doubt keep the wheels churning and we'll find a way of selling it'. They were also acutely aware that Bassett was 'a comparatively small fish' in a highly competitive and increasingly difficult market, something the executive directors seemed less concerned about. The dictates of a past philosophy, it seemed, were not so easy to escape from as some members of the holdings board would have liked.

The view from the subsidiaries

The senior executives in each subsidiary company held remarkably similar views both to the senior executives in the other subsidiaries and to those on the holdings board. The perceptions and understandings expressed here are taken from employees in Geo Bassett, the largest Bassett subsidiary, which in 1988 achieved sales of £55 million and a trading profit of £2 million. Walking on to the factory site I was struck by the untidy, old-fashioned and ramshackle nature of many of the buildings, a perception that was reinforced by a later tour of the whole complex. Originally Geo Bassett had been the head office site for the chairman, and the board of Geo Bassett had controlled the whole Bassett operation. In 1986 a holdings board had been created and had taken itself off-site, while the international arm (BFI) and ABW had been taken out of Geo Bassett's control and set up as distinct companies. The managing director of Geo Bassett commented that:

> Because this site was the head office and the chairman, MD and everybody were here, I think we allowed overhead to build up when this was the Group . . . . You really can't knock the top off a building, you really can't clear people out for clearance sake – it needs half a generation or whatever to do that . . . . So I think it has its own specific problems being the body that's left when people keep tearing the arms and legs off it, and there's a limit to how fast you can react . . . . It is also a problem for the senior management who came to be managers of a multiple business: now they are managers of one site.

All the employees interviewed (from the MD to the most junior line worker) agreed that Geo Bassett was a caring employer. However, some middle and senior managers complained that what this really meant was that poor performers were tolerated, and high performers were left to get on with their jobs with little or no recognition. The spirit of egalitarianism that characterised the company was, it appeared, demotivating because it set such low expectations concerning the amount and quality of an individual's work output. While there was evidently intense loyalty to Geo Bassett, and there had been only one major strike in living memory, there was also great dissatisfaction. The comments of one junior manager give a flavour of the tensions and frustrations that younger staff felt as they suffered under the yoke of a large cadre of older managers 'on the glide path to retirement'. He suggested that the prevailing ethos of Geo Bassett was not so much relaxed as 'does it matter? – it doesn't matter to me', that 'there is no one throwing up trees out there', and that anyone seen trying to compete and 'get ahead' was 'usually regarded with suspicion'.

Even older and more established senior executives such as the production director recognised that the organisation suffered from a lack of well-qualified, highly motivated professionals. Nevertheless,

he was still inclined to describe the painstakingly slow and often tortuous route that important decisions had to take as 'subtly clever'. In contrast, the obviously more able of the middle managers were more likely to state that people were frightened to make decisions and even that they actively sought to evade responsibility: 'Some people are actually frightened to admit to themselves that they are responsible for something not having gone right. And historically they have never been found out in that sense, and nobody's really slapped them down really hard . . .' (General Manager, Trade & Development). Part of the problem here seemed to be Bassett's commitment to democratic, consensual and participative decision making which meant that ideas tended to be 'thrashed about' for long periods of time until either the issue went away or consensus was reached. Almost everyone expressed a similar opinion to the finance director, namely that the organisation was 'a little too democratic', but no impression was given that any action was going to be taken. Unfortunately, the heavy emphasis on procedural democracy was often employed by individuals to fight political battles. According to the managing director the element of fear that once permeated Geo Bassett had now gone, but full-scale wars were still fought between the production and engineering and between the sales and marketing departments.

One of the principal outcomes was an extremely slow pace of work activity in some parts of the business, and indeed this was true of the company as a whole. According to the production director, Geo Bassett 'always seems to move only when it is safe to do so, and always with balance': the great corporate phrase is 'balance'. This may have been one reason why despite senior executive claims that the organisation was becoming progressively more marketing-led the company was still dominated by its production department. It may also partially account for the introspective nature of the organisation and its people as described by even its most senior personnel. Nevertheless there was a great deal of confidence at all managerial levels that the organisation was improving, and would continue to perform well in the marketplace. Even the most complaining managers readily agreed that compared with just a few years ago the business was far healthier, leaner and fitter. Most important of all, it was argued, were the difficulties of finding a new strategic direction. As one of the operations managers admitted, 'We still seem to be flying around and we don't seem to have sorted out quite where we want to go'.

The future

In 1988 the future presented not only opportunities but considerable threats. Four years before, Bassett had fought off a hostile takeover bid from Avana, and the threat of takeover was possibly the single greatest worry of those on the holdings board.[5] Younger members of the organisation in the subsidiaries, however, talked of the possibility of being taken over with enthusiasm, imagining injections of cash into the business, and increased opportunities for transfer and promotion. Everyone, though, was concerned about a long-term trend in consumer tastes (bolstered by dental health issues) that threatened the whole sugar confectionery industry. Yet while the nature of the strategic concerns may have differed it was apparent that the culture of Bassett was little changed from 146 years ago:

> The same basic principles that animated George Bassett animate his successors today. Central to those principles is a recognition of the Company's simultaneous

obligations to its consumers, customers, employees, shareholders and the communities in which it works. Implicit in such recognition is the concept of management not as the employer – that is the role of the consumer – but an agent whose function it is to serve the interests of all these parties and to weld them into a harmony that provides pleasure for all. For in a competitive economy, those who live to please must please to live![6]

Questions

1 What are the key elements of Bassett's cultural profile as revealed by the case? Use Schein's model of culture to structure your answer.

2 Is Bassett's emphasis on the rights of individual employees the principal organisational dynamic shaping its culture? Is this a positive or negative aspect of the organisation's culture.

3 Despite the fact that Bassett had a lengthy history, only a relatively weak organisational culture had developed: there were, for example, no obvious corporate heroes and no highly elaborated ceremonies. Is this a problem that Bev should address?

4 Is Bassett's culture adversely affecting the organisation's scope for strategic manoeuvre? Explain your answer.

5 You have been retained as a highly paid consultant to Bassett. What advice would you give to Bassett's' chief executive?

NOTES

1 *Formalisation* is concerned with the amount of written documentation in an organisation. The more job descriptions, procedures, policy manuals and so forth there are, the greater is the extent of the organisation's formalisation. *Specialisation* refers to the extent to which organisational tasks are subdivided into separate jobs. The wider the range of tasks performed by employees, the lower the extent of organisational specialisation.

2 It has been suggested that the metaphoric process, involving seeing one thing in terms of another, is a fundamental aspect of human cognition, i.e. is the process by which we come to know and understand our world

(Lakoff and Johnson, 1980). According to this view, perception and knowing are linked in a metaphorically structured interpretative process which allows us to understand one domain of experience in terms of another (Koch and Deetz, 1981; Smircich, 1983).

3 According to Maslow's (1943) theory of motivation, individuals have a need to realise their potential and to continue to develop their skills and abilities. This phenomenon he describes as a need for self-actualisation.

4 *Morning Telegraph*, 21 June 1984.

5 Bassett Foods is now part of Cadbury Schweppes plc.

6 D.G. Johnson, *History of George Bassett & Co.*, September 1974.

CHAPTER 2

Exploring organisational culture

OBJECTIVES

To enable students to:

- identify the sources from which an organisation derives its culture;
- become familiar with the processes by which organisational cultures are perpetuated;
- explore some means for examining and researching organisational cultures;
- consider accounts of some important typologies of organisational cultures;
- understand some approaches for assessing the strength of organisational cultures.

INTRODUCTION

This chapter builds on the introduction to organisational culture provided in Chapter 1. It elaborates four main themes. First, it deals with some of the primary sources of organisational culture. Second, the mechanisms by which cultures develop and are perpetuated are considered. Third, some of the methods used for discovering and researching organisational cultures are dealt with. Finally, several typologies of organisational cultures and two methods of ascertaining the strength of an organisation's culture are reviewed. This chapter completes the review of the general organisational culture literature begun by Chapter 1.

THE SOURCES OF ORGANISATIONAL CULTURE

The question 'From where does an organisation's culture originate?' has attracted considerable attention from scholars. There is a perhaps surprising degree of consensus that three of the most important sources of organisational culture are:

1 the *societal* or *national culture* within which an organisation is physically situated;
2 the vision, management style and personality of an organisation's *founder* or other *dominant leader*; and
3 the *type of business* an organisation conducts and the nature of its business environment.

To these three primary sources other authors have added a multiplicity of factors, such as an organisation's awareness and clarity of its mission, and the availability of various forms of technology. In fact, while the influences of national culture, dominant leaders and business activities are usually mentioned, every commentator seems to have his or her own unique list of factors that they consider to be the most significant sources of organisational culture, one of the more extensive of which (produced by Drennan, 1992) is provided in Exhibit 2.1. An important point to bear in mind is that all the factors described as sources of culture tend to be interrelated in fundamental ways. For example, leaders will be influenced by the broader social culture, and will in turn determine what sort of business to initiate and thus choose the nature of the business environment to be operated in. Furthermore, in the course of time it may well be that an organisation is itself able to exert influence over its business environment, and in the case of larger organisations to affect the community in which it is based. For example, the UK-based glass manufacturer Pilkington dominates its home town of St Helens, while IBM has had an enormous impact on the development of the IT industry worldwide. It is with these complexities and interdependencies in mind that the three primary sources of organisational culture identified above are examined here.

Exhibit 2.1
The sources of an organisation's culture

According to David Drennan the twelve key causal factors which shape a company's culture are:

1 Influence of a dominant leader
2 Company history and tradition
3 Technology, products and services
4 The industry and its competition
5 Customers
6 Company expectations
7 Information and control systems
8 Legislation and company environment
9 Procedures and policies
10 Rewards systems and measurement
11 Organisation and resources
12 Goals, values and beliefs

It is worth noting that many of what Drennan considers to be shapers of organisational culture have been interpreted as being integral parts of an organisation's culture by other commentators.

Source: adapted from Drennan (1992)

Societal and national culture

Although theorists agree that the broad social context in which an organisation subsists is a significant influence on its culture, many of the issues at stake here are far from clear cut. The best-known work in this field has been conducted by Geert Hofstede (1980), whose first book on the subject, *Culture's Consequences: International Differences in Work-related Values*, has been widely read and cited. In this and subsequent books Hofstede cautions that while his (and most other work) has focused on the importance of national culture, 'nations' are largely an invention of the twentieth century. The important point for us is that the boundaries between nations have in many instances been artificially and arbitrarily imposed on human societies, with the result that the homogeneity of many nations is quite low. The dissolution of countries such as the old Soviet Union and Yugoslavia is a vivid testament to the tenuous nature of some. Accordingly, we may legitimately ask whether we can in fact make meaningful distinctions between typical American, French, German or British organisations. Hofstede's response is that despite the heterogeneity of most nation states, there are nevertheless strong forces for integration (such as a dominant national language, common mass media, a national education system, army and political system) which bind a nation together. In practical terms, whatever reservations we might have concerning the validity of using national boundaries to examine cultural tendencies, nations are at least easily researchable.

With survey data drawn from employees of IBM worldwide, Hofstede (1991) has demonstrated that managers in different countries differ in the strength of their attitudes and values regarding various issues. He has used this information to argue that national cultures differ along five dimensions: *Power distance, individualism/collectivism, masculinity/femininity, uncertainty avoidance,* and *Confucian dynamism*. Further information is contained in Exhibit 2.2.

Power distance

Power distance is the extent to which the less powerful members of organisations within a country expect and accept that power is distributed unequally. In low power distance nations, inequalities among people will tend to be minimised, decentralisation of activities is more likely, subordinates expect to be consulted by superiors, and privileges and status symbols are less evident. Conversely, in high power distance nations, inequalities among people are considered desirable, there is greater reliance by the less powerful on those who hold power, centralisation is more normal, and subordinates are likely to be separated from their bosses by wide differentials in salary, privileges and status symbols.

Individualism/collectivism

Individualism/collectivism pertains to the extent to which individual independence or social cohesion dominate. In individualistic societies the ties between individuals are loose, and individuals are expected to look after themselves and possibly their immediate family. Here contracts with employers are based on mutual advantage, and hiring and promotion decisions are supposed to be based on skills and rules (see Exhibit 2.3). In collective societies people are integrated into strong, cohesive in-groups, which protect them in exchange for unquestioning loyalty. Here contracts with employers tend to be viewed in moral terms (like a family link), and hiring and promotion decisions take an employee's in-group into account.

Exhibit 2.2
Hofstede's analysis of national cultural differences

Power distance

High power distance countries		*Low power distance countries*	
Malaysia	Philippines	Austria	New Zealand
Guatemala	Mexico	Israel	Republic of Ireland
Panama	Venezuela	Denmark	Sweden

In general, Hofstede found that Latin American and Latin European countries (like France and Spain) had high power distance values, as did Asian and African countries. Low power distance was found to be a feature of the USA, the UK and its former colonies, and the non-Latin parts of Europe.

Individualism/collectivism

Individualist		*Collectivist*	
USA	Canada	Guatemala	Venezuela
Australia	Netherlands	Ecuador	Colombia
UK	New Zealand	Panama	Indonesia

Hofstede found that nearly all wealthy countries (Hong Kong and Singapore were two exceptions) scored highly on individualism, while nearly all poor countries were found to be more collectivist.

Masculinity/femininity

Masculine		*Feminine*	
Japan	Italy	Sweden	Denmark
Austria	Switzerland	Norway	Costa Rica
Venezuela	Mexico	Netherlands	Finland

The UK and West Germany were ranked equal ninth most masculine nations out of 53, with the USA in fifteenth place.

Uncertainty avoidance

High uncertainty avoidance		*Low uncertainty avoidance*	
Greece	Uruguay	Singapore	Sweden
Portugal	Belgium	Jamaica	Hong Kong
Guatemala	Japan	Denmark	UK

Hofstede found high uncertainty avoidance scores for Latin American, Latin European and Mediterranean countries, Japan and South Korea. The German-speaking countries (Austria, Germany and Switzerland) were medium–high. Except for Japan and South Korea all Asian countries scored medium–low, as did African and Anglo-Nordic countries plus the Netherlands.

Confucian/dynamism

Long-termist		*Short-termist*	
China	Japan	Pakistan	Canada
Hong Kong	South Korea	Nigeria	Zimbabwe
Taiwan	Brazil	Philippines	UK

Hofstede found that the USA tended towards being short-termist, while the Netherlands was the most long-termist European nation, ranked tenth out of twenty-three countries surveyed.

Source: adapted from Hofstede (1991)

Exhibit 2.3
Australian individualism: Foster & McKensie Pharmacy

According to Hofstede's findings Australia is a highly individualist nation. That this spirit of individualism pervades organisational life is illustrated by the following account of working life provided by a former shop assistant at Foster & McKensie Pharmacy.

'The Foster & McKensie Pharmacy is based in the city of Melbourne which is in the state of Victoria, Southern Australia. Melbourne is the second largest city in the country, and like many Australian cities is extremely culturally and racially diverse. Some of the most dominant minorities include Greeks, Turks, Italians, and Vietnamese. In fact, many of the more recent arrivals to Australia are still unable (or unwilling) to speak English, and the Foster & McKensie Pharmacy had a deliberate policy of employing shop assistants who were able to speak Greek and Turkish.'

'At the age of thirteen I realised that I needed to earn some money by doing part-time work in order to help me through school. I turned up at the Foster & McKensie Pharmacy every Saturday for four weeks asking for work, and eventually the shop manageress took me on. Over the course of the next five years it became apparent that certain behaviours were required, while others were not tolerated. These informal rules operated to keep all seven of us shop assistants under strict control. It was absolutely imperative that one showed up for work on time and wore what the manageress considered to be 'appropriate' clothing. While at work one had to look busy at all times as the manageress kept us under close surveillance. Everyone was acutely aware that they must not be the subject of a customer complaint, nor could one complain about the strict regime. Two shop assistants who ventured criticisms of the way in which the shop was run were promptly sacked. Sackings were a rather common place event at the Pharmacy, with those ladies unable to work fast enough being asked to leave at the end of their shift. Even competent employees who reached the age of 18 were not always kept on, because at this age Australian legislation dictates that they had to be paid more. The constant supply of labour (mostly the children of first generation immigrants) meant that there was never any problem about hiring new staff whenever they were required. This also meant that wages were very low, being in line with the national minimum wage. The result was a culture in which people came to work to earn money with few expectations of pleasure and no illusions about the caring nature of the owner/manager: hard work was traded for hard cash.'

Source: compiled from information supplied by Jasmine Georgiou

Masculinity/femininity

Masculinity/femininity refers to the degree to which social gender roles are clearly distinct. In high-masculinity societies, social gender roles are clearly distinct, with men supposed to be assertive, tough and focused on material success, and women supposed to be more modest, tender and concerned with the quality of life. At work managers are expected to be decisive and assertive, great emphasis is placed on competition among colleagues and high performance, disputes tend to be resolved by conflict, and the prevailing ethos is that one lives in order to work. In high femininity societies social gender roles overlap, with both men and women supposed to be modest, tender and concerned with the quality of work life. Here managers use intuition and strive for consensus, there is stress on equality, solidarity, and quality of work life, conflicts are resolved by compromise and negotiation, and the dominant idea is that one works in order to live.

Uncertainty avoidance

Uncertainty avoidance is defined as the extent to which the members of a culture feel threatened by uncertain or unknown situations. In weak uncertainty avoidance societies there is greater tolerance of ambiguous situations and unfamiliar risks, people are hard-working only when they need to be, precision and punctuality have to be learned, people are comfortable with deviant and innovative ideas and behaviour, and are motivated by achievement, and by esteem or belongingness. In strong uncertainty avoidance societies there is fear of ambiguous situations and unfamiliar risks, there is a feeling that time is money, there is an emotional need to be busy, precision and punctuality come naturally, novelty is resisted, and people are motivated by security, and by esteem or belongingness.

Confucian dynamism

Confucian dynamism refers to the degree to which long-termism or short-termism is the dominant orientation in life, and is linked to the Confucian conception of 'virtue' which Hofstede contrasts with a Western preoccupation with 'truth'. Short-term orientation societies have a high respect for traditions, emphasise the importance of social and status obligations, approve conspicuous consumption, demand quick results, and are concerned with 'truth'. Long-term orientation societies stress the adaptation of traditions to a modern context, place definite limits on respect for social and status obligations, are sparing with resources, stress perseverance, and are concerned with 'virtue'.

Hofstede's work on national cultural differences has had a major influence on how we think about the culture of organisations in different countries. For example, the results of Hofstede's research suggest that the culture of organisations in the UK will have a low power distance, be highly individualist, masculine, able to cope with uncertainty, and short-termist. By contrast, Hofstede's findings indicate that the culture of organisations in France and Spain will enforce greater psychological distance between employees and their managers, that Scandinavian countries will tend to accept the blurring of gender roles, and that organisations in China and Taiwan will be far more long-termist. This sort of information provides immensely valuable insights into the types of organisational cultures we can expect to find in different countries. Hofstede's conclusions also furnish us with a clear indication of the strength of the influence that national cultures exert over organisational cultures. It is, though, also important to note that a great deal of work by other researchers has also been undertaken in this field, one group of which have concerned themselves with business recipes, that is, sets of preferences for the conduct of economic activity. A sample of the sorts of findings that have emerged from theorists interested in national cultures in the form of business recipes in south-east Asia is contained in Exhibit 2.4.

Leadership and organisational culture

The importance of leadership as a source of organisational culture was commented on by Selznick as long ago as 1957. More recently, Davis (1984) has asserted that:

> If the leader is a great person, then inspiring ideas will permeate the corporation's culture. If the leader is mundane, then the guiding beliefs may well be uninspired. Strong beliefs make for strong cultures. The clearer the leader is about what he stands for, the more apparent will be the culture of that company. (Davis, 1984: 8)

It has, however, been Edgar Schein's (1985b) book *Organizational Culture and Leadership* which has been most responsible for the popularisation of the idea that a single influential individual, often the founder, can create organisational culture. Organisations do not form accidentally or spontaneously but are initiated by individuals (or groups) with specific goals. In the case of commercial organisations this usually involves a vision of how a group

Exhibit 2.4
Business recipes in south-east Asia

Some researchers interested in national cultures have focused their attention on business recipes. A business recipe is a set of preferences for the conduct of economic activity. Different business recipes dominate in different parts of the world, and are intimately linked with the legal and institutional framework that exists in a country. The results of business recipe research have cast fascinating light on the differences between nations' approaches to commercial organisation. Below is a summary of some of those findings as they relate to Japan, South Korea, Taiwan and Hong Kong.[1]

Japan
Japanese companies tend to form long-term strategic networks in which organisations work together on a collaborative basis, exchanging information and resources as necessary. This allows them to specialise in particular activities at lower risk levels than firms in Anglo-Saxon societies. When firms do extend into new industries there is a preference for separating them as distinct entities with their own access to financial resources once they are successful. Japanese businesses exhibit a bias for evolutionary growth strategies, and are reliant on high levels of employee commitment and flexibility for long-term success. Relationships between purchasers, suppliers and distributers tend to be more stable than in Chinese societies, and seem to involve greater levels of trust and, sometimes, reciprocal shareholding. The extent of co-ordination between Japanese economic organisations is truly impressive: long-term links with companies in other industries, 'presidents' club' meetings, the exchange of senior managerial personnel, and mutual support when under severe threat are all features of the commercial environment. The decision-making function of Japanese enterprises is less centralised than in Chinese and Korean firms, and this is linked to their collective authority system and strong separation of ownership from control. Japanese companies appear quite formal, with many written rules and procedures, though these do not necessarily govern organisational life. Finally, managers are expected to be close to their workforce, and are responsible for group morale and for facilitating group achievements.

Taiwan and Hong Kong
Taiwan and Hong Kong are typical Chinese business communities. Here, and indeed throughout south-east Asia, the primary unit of economic action in competitive markets is the Chinese family business. Like Japanese firms these tend to specialise on particular stages of production, which carries with it the risk of being committed to a declining industry and expertise. In order to offset this risk they remain small, and rely on elaborate networks of mutual obligations with employees, suppliers and agents. While these obligations are based on personal knowledge and reputations, they remain limited and highly flexible. Chinese family businesses are more opportunistic than Japanese firms and less exclusively tied to particular business partners. As with Korean businesses Chinese firms are generally owned and managed by the same people, with loyalties and obedience likewise focused on the individual owner rather than on the collective enterprise. While Chinese companies are less formal than Japanese organisations, Chinese managers are expected to reflect Confucian norms which dictate that they should demonstrate their moral superiority by being reserved, dignified and unemotional.

South Korea
In South Korea the economy is dominated by enormous family controlled conglomerates, or 'chaebol'. Korean chaebol are vertically integrated and centrally control a variety of functions and activities: that is, they are far less specialised than their Japanese and Chinese counterparts. Research suggests that they have successfully diversified into heavy industry, as well as newer industries such as construction and financial services. Although they appear disinclined to interconnect for economic reasons, they are liable to co-ordination by state agencies and political alliances. As with the Chinese managers, Korean bosses are highly directive, making little attempt to explain their decisions or justify their actions to their employees. Interestingly, there is a much higher labour turnover in Korean companies than in Japan or Taiwan, and loyalties here are much less emotional and intense than in Japan.

Source: adapted from Whitley (1990)

of people can create and successfully market a new product or service. During this early phase of an organisation's existence founders are in an extremely privileged position. They determine what mission is to be pursued and in what business context, they usually decide who is to be recruited and what rules, systems and procedures will be instigated, and have considerable powers of discretion over what constitutes acceptable patterns of behaviour in the workplace. In building their organisation founders tend to impose their beliefs and values about the nature of the world, organisations and human nature on other organisational participants. Henry Ford at the Ford Motor Company, Ken Olsen at Digital Equipment Company, and Gerard and Anton Philips at Philips are some of the most widely cited examples of founders whose personalities massively shaped the cultures of the organisations they created. While founders have the initial influence on their organisation's culture, if the organisation is successful it will outlast its progenitor. Other leaders may then have an opportunity to mould the organisation's culture according to their theories of what constitutes good organisational practice. A few of the many famous individuals who have attempted this include Lee Iacocca at General Motors, Sir John Harvey-Jones at ICI and John Scully at Apple Computers. For more information on the impact that leaders can have on organisational culture see Mini Case 5.1 and Chapter 5.

The nature of the business and the business environment

The nature of the activities an organisation undertakes and the particular operating environment in which it subsists may have a profound effect on its culture. According to Deal and Kennedy (1982: 13), the 'business environment is the single greatest influence in shaping a corporate culture'. The operational requirements of service organisations differ in fundamental ways from those of manufacturing organisations, organisations in the public sector tend to develop in markedly different ways from those in the private sector, and large organisations have a very different 'feel' compared with their smaller counterparts. Gordon (1985) has shown that utilities (such as electricity, gas and telephone companies) which have evolved in a relatively slow-changing environment tend to develop cultures which value stability, integration, clear communication, support from senior managers, fair compensation and opportunities for employees to grow. In contrast, dynamic-marketplace companies formed in highly competitive and changeable environments generally develop cultures which set ambitious goals and value innovative behaviour and individual initiative.[2] A vast range of factors are obviously in play here, and not all of them can be considered in detail. Typically, some of the more significant sources of an organisation's culture are its stakeholders, professional associations and strategic issues.

Stakeholders

Stakeholders are identifiable groups of individuals who have a stake or interest in the success of an organisation. They include customers, the Government, the public and shareholders.

Customers

Customers are an important stakeholder group for most organisations, and their power to influence organisational culture has been amply demonstrated in recent years by the increasing number of companies that have sought to improve the quality and reliability of

Mini Case 2.1

Leadership and organisational culture in the Bouygues Group

In 1952 Francis Bouygues founded the famous French construction company. Noted for his determined, dynamic and plain-speaking style Bouygues was a product of the prestigious Hautes Ecoles (the French equivalent of Oxbridge, Yale and Harvard). It is, however, his proud and charismatic character rather than his educational background which is usually said to be responsible for his creation of one of the largest construction firms in the world, and which has earned him the nickname *le roi du Beton/King Concrete*.

Having borrowed the start-up capital from his father, by 1956 he was able to start creating the first of many subsidiaries, which currently include companies involved in real estate, offshore oil platforms and television. One reason for this phenomenal expansion was that during the 1950s France's industrial growth rate was 50 per cent (compared with 15 per cent in the UK), and housing, schools, roads and hospitals, the Bouygues Group's principal concerns, were all high on the priority list. The result was not only that the organisation built some of the best-known Parisian landmarks, but that it grew into an 80 000 employee, worldwide conglomerate.

Accounting for Bouygues' rapid advancement, commentators have suggested that his personality, drive and characteristically French exploitation of the 'old boy network' all played a role. For example, the French Government's choice of Bouygues as the controlling stockholder when it privatised the television station TF1 in 1987 was rumoured to be an entirely political decision. Within the organisation Bouygues was described by his senior colleagues as 'despotic', 'a megalomaniac', a 'boss without scruples' and 'ruthless'. Indeed, he has been likened to a combination of Lee Iacocca, Donald Trump and Robert Maxwell. What this meant in practice was that he was firmly in control, and given to using rousing rhetoric and symbolism in order to create and sustain a vigorous corporate culture.

The development and management of culture was evidently a priority for Bouygues. In fact, all new recruits are soon subject to intensive enculturation processes, including a training programme which involves a presentation of the group's history, peppered with anecdotes from company folklore. Other channels for communicating cultural beliefs and values include a Charter which expounds twelve principles (such as teamwork, quality and success), which are familiarly known by employees as the twelve Commandments. These messages are taken up and reiterated by the numerous in-house magazines and bulletins, the largest of which, *Minorange*, is distributed to the home of every employee.

Bouygues has also sought to influence the culture of his organisation in more subtle ways. Thus managers are expected to dress stylishly (what the French call b.c.b.g./ *bon chic bon genre*), while the $200 000 000 head office was built in the style of a modern chateau and called 'Challenger'. The company not only has its own logo but its own colour, *minorange*, a reddish hue, and a privileged group of elite builders created by Francis himself in 1963 called Les Compagnons du Minorange. This grouping has been encouraged to develop its own values, such as craftsmanship and fraternal relations, distinctive clothing, its own magazine, and a special budget for ceremonies, professional awards and initiation rituals.

It should be recalled that construction work is a predominately male province, and that the typical Bouygues manager is French, male, around 35 years old, has a *baccalauréat*, and has been with the firm for five or more years. Interpersonal address was rather formal ('*vous*' being preferred to the more familiar '*tu*'), and it was said that Bouygues preferred his female staff not to wear trousers. This does not mean that the organisation is backward-looking in many important respects: training is better funded than in many firms, worker participation was encouraged through quality circles, and unions (despite their relative weakness in France) are recognised.

▶

With the culture of the organisation firmly in place, in 1989 Francis, then 67, decided to step down in favour of his youngest son, Martin. While certain differences in style (Martin is a far quieter man, and more democratic in a collegiate sense, than his father) and strategy (Bouygues is now even more highly diversified than before) are noticeable, the question is, to what degree is the organisation able to retain its original identity, and to what extent is this desirable?

Questions

1 What means of shaping culture did Bouygues employ?

2 Do you think that the culture of the Bouygues Group must inevitably change now that its founder and dominant leader has retired?

3 What steps can be taken to minimise the impact of the departure of a dominant leader on a culture that he or she has created?

Source: adapted from K. Meudell and T. Callen, 'King Concrete – an Analysis of the Bouygues Group', in Derek Adam-Smith and A. Peacock (eds) (1994)

their products and services (by creating a 'quality culture') in response to consumer demand. The Rank Xerox organisation is typical of those companies that have embraced the need to alter their culture to focus on quality, service and reliability issues in order to satisfy the requirements of their customers.

The Government

The Government has considerable power to affect the cultures of organisations within its territory, and often their overseas operations as well. In the UK, publicly owned organisations such as the NHS and the Post Office are highly regulated and subject to the whims of Government policy. Private organisations are also affected by the Government through adjustments to the legal framework, rulings on monopolies and mergers, and management of the economy. Perhaps the most stunning example of how the Government can reshape the culture of organisations in the UK was the Thatcher/Major Government's privatisation programme: privatised organisations like BT and the regional electricity companies have undergone (and are currently undergoing) dramatic cultural change as a result.

The public

The public in general can be an important source of an organisation's culture. In the UK the heightened levels of concern that women and ethnic minorities should be treated fairly in the workplace have led organisations like the retailer Littlewoods and Midland Bank to attempt to build an ethos of 'equality of opportunity for all' into their cultures. Another example is the strength of public opinion worldwide concerning the need to protect and maintain the environment, which has led to attempts by oil companies like Shell and Exxon to make these concerns their own, though not always with success.

Shareholders

Shareholders have surprisingly little influence on the cultural development of an organisation. Research by S.M. Davis (1985) suggests that the only two instances in which management pays serious attention to shareholders are when ownership is closely held by an individual or a family, or when management is afraid of a takeover. The influence of Richard Branson on the Virgin Group and in times past the Cadbury family on the sugar confectionery and chocolate company Cadbury are testament to the influence of

Mini Case 2.2

Shareholder influence at HomerLines

HomerLines is a publicly quoted Greek shipping company which has its base on a Mediterranean island. The organisation owns ten luxury ferries which it uses to transport passengers around the Mediterranean. The company's flagship is the largest ferry in Europe: it is twelve floors high, and able to accommodate more than 3500 people in considerable luxury. Its other ferries, while smaller, being able to accommodate only 2000 people, are no less luxurious. While the organisation was owned by approximately 5000 shareholders, one of these, Mr Papadopoulos, dominated. Papadopoulos was a self-made multimillionaire whose family was reputed to be among the most influential in the whole of Greece, and he took an active interest in how HomerLines was managed, even though he did not himself hold an executive position within the company.

To HomerLines employees Papadopoulos was a well-known figure who not only spent time at the docks watching the ferries preparing for their journeys, but frequently went with them as well. Whether on land or on board, however, his influence was all-pervasive. Such was Papadopoulos's authority that he was able to choose all the senior staff aboard a ship he took an interest in, including the captain, staff captain, chief engineer, chief steward and chief purser. Having chosen his crew and having decided to sail out with them, Papadopoulos would then dominate proceedings. It was he who decided everything from restaurant opening times to what music should be played in the bars – traditional folk music from the island where he was born and brought up.

Papadopoulos was, though, never the only shareholder aboard ship. The overwhelming majority of all employees at HomerLines were in fact small shareholders. This was as true of deckhands and stewards as it was of engineers and middle managers. Many of those who did not own stock in the company nevertheless came from families which did. One result was that everyone seemed to think that they were entitled to give advice (or even orders) to everyone else, even outside their nominal area of expertise. For example, it was not unknown for a senior engineer to proffer advice on how to run the on-board hotels facilities. Unsurprisingly, there were major problems of communication, co-ordination and control, not to mention corruption.

Three examples of the sorts of problem that occurred will suffice. First, on one occasion a ferry set sail with 600 salad bowls on board, packed into all the store rooms. Someone had obviously benefited from providing such a large order to the salad bowl manufacturers, but no one could be found who knew anything about it. Second, on another occasion a ferry was due to sail in two hours and had no clean linen aboard. All the linen cleaning services were performed by a single extremely unreliable company that never had a problem having its contract renewed: personal contacts, and an intricate system of favours owed, guaranteed it. Third, there was a general problem of motivation among the all-male crew, who had to leave their wives and families at home for long periods of time.

To conclude, it is evident that shareholder influence on HomerLines culture is broad and intense, though not always of a positive nature.

Questions

1 What problems do you think Mr Papadopoulos caused by interfering in the management of HomerLines?

2 Why do you think the fact that most employees were shareholders did not lead to greater enthusiasm and efficiency on HomerLines ferries?

3 If you were a consultant to HomerLines senior executives (based in a head office on an attractive Greek island) what advice would you offer them?

owner/managers. Threats of takeovers are important because these are in effect direct attacks on an organisation's culture which shareholders may either accept or reject. There are, however, some exceptions to this general rule, as Mini Case 2.2, focused on the Greek shipping company HomerLines, makes clear.

Professional associations

Many commentators have noticed that there are apparent similarities between organisations dominated by groups of similarly trained professionals. Health care organisations, teaching institutions and accountancy practices may not be completely homogeneous classes of organisation, but there are probably more cultural similarities between, say, two accountancy practices, than there are between an accountancy practice and a hospital. The idea is that professional associations like the British Medical Association (BMA), the Institute of Chartered Accountants (ICA) and the Association of University Teachers (AUT) often impose education and training requirements on their members, specify experience requirements, and publish codes of practice. The result is that it is possible to identify professional cultures. Furthermore, the beliefs and values promulgated by professional associations will be introduced into organisations by their members who are also members of professions. Even within a single organisation it is common to find clusters of similarly trained professionals: many large commercial organisations have a finance department peopled by accountants, a marketing department with trained marketeers, and a production department employing various sorts of engineer. In each instance it is likely that the cultures of these departments will be shaped, at least in part, by the professional culture of these groups. Professional associations, then, are an important source of an organisation's culture.

In a more general sense, it has been argued that managers as a group share in a professional culture (O'Toole, 1979). It has been suggested that this managerial culture in America enshrines values such as economic efficiency (the language of 'productivity', 'consumer sovereignty', 'optimisation' and 'least cost'); growth and profitability (the quest for higher turnover, bigger market shares and internationalisation); loyalty to the system (the manager must never question the appropriateness of, for instance, the prevailing forms of ownership and governance of the firm or the competitive structure of the industry); camaraderie (all interpersonal relations within the firm must be friendly and courteous, but not intimate). Other values, concerning security, power and stability, are also apparent, but this list provides a sufficient indication of the sorts of analyses produced by this approach. It should also be noted that this particular list of cultural values refers only to America, and that managerial cultures in, for example, China and Latin America, are likely to be rather different.

Strategic issues

According to Deal and Kennedy (1982) general classes of organisational culture can be distinguished based on two business strategic factors: degree of risk and the speed of feedback on decisions. The degree of risk an organisation faces depends on factors such as the number of potential suppliers and competitors, the relative scarcity of resources, the stability of the market, and so on. Some organisations, such as clothes retailers, face considerable uncertainty because of the degree of competition and the unpredictabilities of their market, while others, like the UK electricity supply companies, have a far more predictable business environment. In each of

Mini Case 2.3

The cultures of two university departments: cold fusion and social kinetics

This mini case illustrates that different organisations operating in essentially the same environment and providing the same service can, nevertheless, develop very different cultures. The two organisations discussed (the *department of cold fusion* and the *department of social kinetics*), are both science departments in the same British university. Universities in the UK currently face a variety of challenges, notably diminishing resources, increasing competition for students, the removal of lifetime employment for academic staff, and the introduction of quality and other control mechanisms into the working environment. These pressures were also acting on the two departments examined here.

The department of cold fusion

The department of cold fusion is a large, multisite department which was set up when the university was first founded. It employs 70 academic staff to teach 600 undergraduate and 150 postgraduate students. Respondents said that they were there to work, and that any extra contact with other members of the department was unnecessary and distracting. Few people claimed to have any close friends at work, preferring to describe others as 'colleagues' or 'close acquaintances'. Most respondents agreed that there was little room for 'sentiment' within the department, and this had interesting results. For example, working relations were said to be extremely professional and person-respecting. Romance was also not on anybody's agenda, with most respondents dismissive of the idea that a student–staff relationship would be appropriate. Staff–staff relationships, while not as heavily criticised, were considered unlikely to occur.

The extent of the psychological distance between individuals of different status was notable in the department of cold fusion. One secretary informed the researcher that her boss (a professor) always communicates through memos, even when he wants to communicate with his academic colleague in the adjacent office, and insists that she phone people and 'announce him' before he will take the phone himself. In fact the formal nature of the departmental culture was seen to hinder communication in such a way that uneasy tolerance characterised most working relationships. It was also noticeable that the female members of the department tended to occupy the more junior academic and secretarial/clerical positions, and one secretary commented that academics could be condescending towards secretaries. Interestingly, there was also little communication between the four different departmental sites and between the different research teams, who even sat together in their separate clusters at the annual Christmas party.

When quizzed about their attitudes towards intimacy most people claimed that it clouded judgements and detracted from one's ability to perform at an optimum level at work. Two of the women interviewed, both of whom had been sexually harassed in other university departments, felt far more comfortable about the department of cold fusion than they had in their previous departments. More negative evaluations of the department's culture were also made. Some argued that the culture hindered communication, and one person suggested that it encouraged 'back-stabbing'. One relatively new member of staff described the working environment as very strange, very competitive and intolerant: thus effective departmental operation and job satisfaction among employees to some extent seemed to be detrimentally affected by the prevailing culture.

The department of social kinetics

The department of social kinetics has only recently become a teaching and research centre in its own right, and currently employs 28 academic staff and 9 researchers to teach 160 postgraduate students. It is a single-site department with relatively clear lines of communication and far less emphasis on hierarchy than many larger departments. One respondent stated that the department was 'like a family' in which people could say what they felt without fear of repercussions. This did not mean

▶

that there were no disagreements, but that these were usually smoothed over at the various social events, parties and general out-of-work socialising, much of which did not observe hierarchy.

The most striking difference between the two departments was the extent to which romantic involvement was accepted in the department of social kinetics. Several staff–student liaisons were mentioned by respondents, including one that resulted in divorce. The prevailing view was that these did not unduly upset working relations within the department, and that people could be left to regulate their own lives. A few people were obviously unable to keep their personal lives sufficiently well regulated, and were castigated by other members of the department for their poor handling of social relations. For example, one individual admitted flirting all year with the result that this person had to fight off a co-worker at a departmental social event, while another had naively encouraged a member of staff's attentions to the extent that this person subsequently had difficulty in deterring this individual. Respondents

also named two events, one of which involved a serious assault, to which the police should arguably have been called.

While most respondents expressed positive attitudes towards the highly sexualised atmosphere of the department, there were obvious problems. The department of social kinetics was somewhat 'gossipy', with colleagues constantly fishing for personal information about each other which then spread quickly round the grapevine. There was also evidence of 'bitchiness' between certain individuals. It was also true that the norm of mutual respect sometimes slips: for example, secretaries consider that academics tend to undervalue their abilities. Furthermore, one individual suggested that the 'real' business of the department was conducted by the senior academics in the somewhat exclusive surroundings of the Staff Centre, which is quite separate from the department.

Question

1 How do you account for the cultural differences between the two departments?

Source: adapted from Brewis (1994)

these cases the demands on the organisations to be imaginative, innovative, flexible, customer-oriented, or health and safety conscious are different. These diverse functional requirements and constraints are likely to lead to the development of very different types of culture. Similarly, some organisations can anticipate very quick feedback on the quality of the decisions they take, while chemical and pharmaceutical companies such as ICI and Pfizer may have to wait years before the results of research into new products proves that a development programme was justified or not. Again, these strategic issues will almost certainly result in the evolution of radically different sorts of organisational culture. Further information on Deal and Kennedy's views concerning the link between strategy and culture is provided in the section on culture typologies later in this chapter.

While the influence of national culture and the nature of the business environment may be important, this does not mean that two similarly placed organisations performing the same sorts of activities will have any cultural commonalities. The vast array of environmental variables, the differential impact of dominant personalities, the unpredictable influences of organisational size, the buildings inhabited, and historical accident (among others), massively complicate issues of culture formation, making accurate prediction immensely difficult. This point is well illustrated in Mini Case 2.3, which contrasts some aspects of the cultures of two extremely dissimilar departments in the same UK university.

THE PERPETUATION OF ORGANISATIONAL CULTURE

The culture of a successful organisation tends to be transmitted to new recruits who join after the initial formation period. Three basic stages in the process by which a culture is perpetuated can be distinguished: preselection, socialisation and incorporation/rejection. These stages are illustrated in Fig. 2.1, while Mini Case 2.4 comments on these processes as they have been described in the Disneyland theme park.

Preselection

Even before individuals join an organisation they are likely to possess a considerable amount of information about its mission and work practices. Friends, relatives, newspaper articles, and annual reports and accounts are just some of the means by which individuals gain the information they need to judge whether they should apply for a job with an organisation. In effect individuals select and deselect themselves at this early stage. Potential recruits who aspire to become members of an organisation may make great efforts to learn about its history and culture, and even begin to subscribe to its espoused values. The result is that those who actually apply to join an organisation tend to be predisposed to accepting its culture. Merton (1957) has referred to this predisposition as *anticipatory socialisation*. Some organisations have sought to facilitate this process by providing intending applicants with a *realistic job preview*. This document is a detailed description of a job, the department in which it is based, and often the organisation as a whole. Research suggests that individuals exposed to a realistic job preview and who go on to take up positions within an organisation are more satisfied, have a lower turnover and are more easily socialised into the prevailing culture.

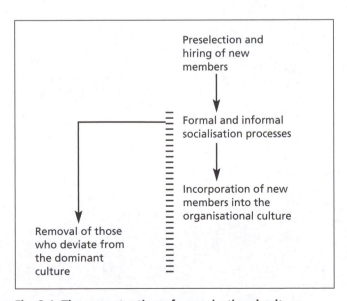

Fig. 2.1 The perpetuation of organisational culture

Mini Case 2.4

The perpetuation of organisational culture at Disneyland

First opened in 1955 in Anaheim, California, Disneyland has been a consistent moneymaker for Walt Disney Enterprises. Most of those who apply for work at Disneyland are aware that if accepted on to the payroll they will be expected to conform to the large number of rules that are supposed to guarantee that the theme park is the 'Happiest Place on Earth'. In fact, ride operators and other hourly paid employees are a well-screened and fairly homogeneous group: white males and females, generally in their early twenties, of above average height, without facial blemish, and radiating good health. When ethnic minorities are employed, apart from their colour they tend to be close copies of the standard Disneyland employee.

Once in paid employment new recruits are enrolled at the University of Disneyland where they undergo a forty-hour apprenticeship programme. In the classroom employees learn about the history and philosophy of Disneyland, and the regulations and procedures that govern work there. Some of the most important of these concern the use of language. For example, employees are generally on first name terms, customers must be referred to as 'guests', rides are called 'attractions' and Disneyland itself is a 'park' not an amusement centre. At work employees are encouraged to think of themselves as 'back-stage', 'on-stage' and 'staging' and their uniforms as 'costumes'. Classroom instruction also covers approved responses to probable questions ride operators will face from customers, and how to summon assistance when accidents (always called 'incidents') arise or particularly difficult 'guests' cannot be mollified. The curriculum includes the inculcation of particular Disneyland values like 'the customer is king' and 'everyone is a child at heart when at Disneyland'. Great emphasis is also placed on checklists of appearance standards that must be learned, and which ban the wearing of facial hair, fancy jewellery or more than very modest amounts of make-up. Motivation levels are hyped by inspirational films, and pep talks exhort employees to be happy and cheerful while 'on stage'. What is more, all relevant essential information is contained in a training manual, so no one can forget.

Informal socialisation mechanisms are equally well developed. New recruits soon learn that the job they are assigned to, the costume they are allocated and the area of the park in which they work determine their social status. Generally speaking the more highly skilled the work and glamorous the costume, the higher an individual's status. Employees also learn that there are strict limits to which the company line has to be taken seriously, and there is much satirical banter about the artificiality of Disneyland. Good performance on stage is, however, a necessity. Individuals soon realise that supervisors are not just there to help them, but to monitor and evaluate their performance: most old hands can be counted on to relate tales of employees who have been fired for taking too long a break, not wearing part of the official uniform or providing longer than usual rides. At the same time employees are taught by their peers how to get back at misbehaving 'guests' by tightening seat belts, slamming on the brakes unexpectedly, and drenching those standing on the banks of rivers. On the downside, although pranks are rarely played on newcomers, all are carefully scrutinised, and those deemed not to 'fit' are the subject of gossip and/or ostracism.

The formal and informal socialization procedures are not just fascinating to observe but commercially effective. Employees are generally willing to play the roles expected of them with good humour and kindly smiles, and this despite the fact that Disneyland does not pay well, the jobs require minimal intelligence and supervision is strict. Enculturation at Disneyland is thus a major feat of social engineering.

Questions

1 Why do you think the socialisation processes at work in Disneyland are so effective?

2 What lessons can other organisations learn from Disneyland's methods?

Source: adapted from Van Maanen (1991)

Socialisation

Once they have obtained admission to an organisation individuals become subject to both formal and informal socialisation processes. Organisational socialisation, sometimes termed *enculturation*, refers to those processes by which participants learn the culturally accepted beliefs, values and behaviours (and relinquish others that are not compatible with the culture), so that they are able to act as effective members of the group. While socialisation processes are usually most active for individuals who have recently joined an organisation, they are also associated with promotions, demotions and lateral movements of personnel across departmental boundaries. Organisations exhibit great diversity in the extent to which they consciously attempt to manage socialisation processes. Police forces, the armed services and some large corporations make extensive efforts to construct formal socialisation mechanisms, usually in the form of new employee orientation and induction courses, training programmes and mentoring systems. Most organisations, however, rely on informal socialisation processes, in which new recruits learn what is expected of them by trial and error under the guidance of their work colleagues.

When individuals first join an organisation they are faced with what appears to be considerable complexity and ambiguity. Part of the reason for this is that they are largely unaware of the shared experiences enjoyed by their colleagues and thus lack understanding and awareness of the norms, values, beliefs and assumptions that longer-serving employees take for granted. New recruits tend to seek to understand and make sense of their new environment by more or less careful observation and questioning. This learning process is often helped by organisational members who relate stories, jokes and anecdotes which can provide insights into what sorts of behaviours are acceptable, expected and desired. These informal socialisation processes are often more significant than an organisation's formal and official procedures, because they allow more relevant information to be transmitted in a more personal manner and by means that new recruits are more likely to remember. The length of time it takes individuals to become fully enculturated depends on their social and cognitive skills and abilities, the effectiveness of the organisation's formal and informal socialisation processes, and the relative complexity and opaqueness of the organisation's culture. An indication of the sorts of formal and informal processes at work is provided by Mini Case 2.4.

Formal socialisation processes are often termed *rites of passage*. The successful conclusion of these rites signals that an individual has undergone an important change in identity. Well-constructed rites of passage usually have three distinct phases. First, there are *separation rites*, which divorce individuals from their previous context and unfreeze them from the roles they have previously filled. Off-site testing and screening, possibly at specialist assessment centres, newcomer parties and entrance ceremonies of various kinds are all well-used examples. Second, there are *transition rites*, which reinforce rites of separation and the unlearning of previously held work norms. They frequently involve debasement experiences such as being refused entry to certain parts of a building, or not having a reserved car parking space, secretary or certain office equipment. This transitional or liminal state lasts until the individual experiences *rites of incorporation*. These may be more or less well defined, but always inform new recruits that they have been accepted and what their new responsibilities now are. Typical rites of incorporation include assigning individuals to their permanent departments after weeks or even months of temporary working arrangements, and formal induction ceremonies.

Organisational cultures vary greatly in terms of their *transparency/opaqueness* and *simplicity/complexity*. Both the transparency/opaqueness and simplicity/complexity dimensions of a culture refer to the extent to which it is easy for new recruits to 'read' and understand it, though for different reasons. Looking at the transparency/ opaqueness dimensions first, we can say that a transparent culture is one in which things are largely what they appear to be, the meaning of things is clear and new recruits are able to navigate their way around it relatively quickly. Conversely, an opaque culture is one in which the meaning of things and events is obscure, and requires considerable insight and shared experience to appreciate. Such cultures obviously pose far more problems for new employees. The relative transparency of a culture will depend on such factors as:

- the extent to which the various elements of a culture are tightly coupled (i.e. mutually supportive). For example, a culture in which people genuinely adhere to beliefs and values which they do not act on (for whatever reasons) is relatively more opaque than one in which there is tight coupling between various cultural elements; and
- the extent to which the actual culture corresponds with the culture as espoused by senior executives. As a general rule the closer the correspondence between the actual and espoused cultures, the more transparent an organisation's culture may be said to be.

In contrast, the simplicity/complexity dimension here refers to other aspects of a culture, namely:

- the number of artefacts, beliefs, assumptions and so forth. The greater the number of cultural items the greater the complexity;
- the diversity of cultural items. The greater the range of cultural items the more complex a culture may be said to be; and
- the number of embedded subcultures and their relation to the dominant culture. The larger the number of subcultures the more complex a culture is. This complexity will be even more extreme the larger the number of orthogonal and countercultures an organisation possesses.

These two dimensions of culture may be represented graphically as in Fig. 2.2. Examples of cultures that fit into each of the quadrants in Fig. 2.2 are not difficult to find. For instance, sports and social clubs are likely to possess simple/transparent cultures, small management consultancies will tend to have simple/opaque cultures, universities generally have complex/transparent cultures, and large multinationals like Digital and Shell often possess complex/opaque cultures. Simple/transparent cultures are the easiest organisations for new recruits to be socialised into, while complex/opaque cultures generally require the most time and effort for effective socialisation. The complex/transparent and simple/opaque cultures occupy a medial position in this framework. The important point for us is that the effective socialisation of new recruits is in part contingent on the nature of an organisation's culture.

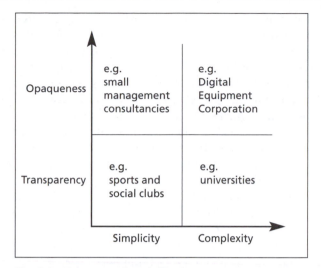

Fig. 2.2 Culture and socialisation

Incorporation/rejection

Continued subjection to organisational socialisation processes results in an individual being either incorporated or rejected. Full incorporation into an organisational culture is sometimes symbolised by a change in job title, for example, by deleting prefixes such as 'assistant', 'acting' or 'temporary'. Other indicators that the first phase of socialisation has officially come to an end can include being invited to a company dinner, being granted a reserved parking space, being given a permanent identification number or being sent an official memo from the boss. It should be recalled, however, that socialisation is an uncertain process. On the one hand it is possible to identify instances where individuals do not learn the culture of the host organisation. In these cases not only are the individuals likely to feel alienated and uncomfortable, but they may also be unproductive, disruptive and a source of countercultural activity. Such individuals are generally ultimately removed. On the other hand, if an organisation's socialisation mechanisms are particularly effective, employees may be 'oversocialised', leading to total conformity, and an inability to think and act creatively. David Kearns' removal of many 'company men' (whom he referred to as the 'Xeroids') from Xerox in the mid-1980s was a reaction against the dangers of conformity bred by overeffective socialisation. Finally, it is worth noting that most large organisations are complex conglomerations of interrelated cultures that may alter over time. Socialisation, then, is always likely to be an ongoing learning process for organisational participants.

DISCOVERING ORGANISATIONAL CULTURE

There are two basic approaches for examining an organisation's culture: first, the use of questionnaire survey techniques, and second, the conduct of interviews and direct observation. Questionnaire survey methods involve the use of lists of questions or statements about the organisation which employees have to evaluate. Ideally, these questionnaires should be circulated to a large and representative sample of employees. If the questionnaire has been well designed the results of the survey should then provide the researcher with a good overall impression of the prevailing beliefs, values and attitudes within the organisation. The main strength of these tools is that they yield quantitative information which can be used to make meaningful comparisons between departments within an organisation and between organisations. One basic problem with the questionnaire approach is that it does not collect vital information concerning the detail of stories, myths and legends, rites and rituals and other artefacts. Another difficulty with questionnaire survey methods is that they rely on the perceptions of employees who are probably largely unaware of their organisation's basic assumptions. A comprehensive analysis of an organisation's culture, therefore, is always likely to require a lot of additional data to be collected through detailed interviews with key employees and direct observation of the organisation's physical location, layout, artefacts and symbols by a researcher. The combined use of sophisticated questionnaire surveys and detailed interviews and observation may give great insight into an organisation's culture but is also extremely time-consuming and labour-intensive. Unsurprisingly, they are also quite rarely conducted.

Questionnaire survey techniques vary considerably, ranging from a few simple questions which provide basic information about a select number of aspects of an organisation to quite elaborate and sophisticated tools. A vast number of relatively simple questionnaires are currently employed by consultancies specialising in culture analyses. One interesting tool is reproduced as Exhibit 2.5. This questionnaire invites respondees to assess the state of their organisation's culture by answering questions in twelve categories. In each case the respondent has to decide whether a particular statement is definitely true, mostly true, mostly false, or definitely false. Only giving respondents four possible choices (rather than five) is a deliberate attempt to overcome the problem of what is known as 'central tendency bias', i.e. people's natural inclination not to make a real choice but to select a middle category. Those administering the questionnaire can treat each question as worthy of specific analysis, or they can group together all those questions in a category in order to get a general response. In order to get a good overview of an organisation's culture, a sufficient number of individuals at different levels in an organisation's hierarchy and in all departments and functions would have to fill in this questionnaire. The precise number of people required to undergo this exercise will, or course, vary with the size and complexity of the organisation, and complete accuracy can only be obtained if 100 per cent of employees take part. By matching the results against an agreed view of the desired state culture, senior managers can then gauge the need (or otherwise) for a change in the existing culture. This is, of course, particularly useful in culture change exercises (see Chapter 5).

Interviews and observation permit very different sorts of information to be collected from questionnaire surveys. It is recommended that as with the questionnaire surveys interviews should be conducted with a representative sample of employees. It is also probably advisable to interview respondents using a standard interview schedule (list of questions) but allow employees a fair amount of latitude in answering them. This semi-structured approach is more likely to be successful in encouraging people to disclose information concerning their culture than a more tightly structured interview format. Unstructured interviews in which respondents are encouraged to talk about their organisation with no fixed question set may be successful, but are likely to provide a lot of disjointed items of information that may be difficult to fit together into a coherent picture of the culture. Some ideas for questions to be included in a semistructured interview schedule are provided in Exhibit 2.6 (see p. 65).

Exhibit 2.5
Diagnosing organisational culture

No.	Orientation and statements	Definitely true	Mostly true	Mostly false	Definitely false
1	**Creativity and innovation orientation**				
1a	People here are generally imaginative in their approach	3	2	1	0
1b	Novel ideas are welcomed in this organisation	3	2	1	0
1c	Innovative people are valued and rewarded here	3	2	1	0
1d	People who lack creative minds are not tolerated by this organisation	3	2	1	0
1e	Most people have time to think through new ideas here	3	2	1	0
1f	People generally risk sharing their ideas because they are listened to and encouraged	3	2	1	0
1g	Good ideas are quickly adopted by the organisation	3	2	1	0
2	**Power and conflict orientation**				
2a	There is an atmosphere of trust in this organisation	0	1	2	3
2b	Important people here are always addressed as Sir or Madam, or by job title	3	2	1	0
2c	There is much criticism of policies and practices	3	2	1	0
2d	People here tend to manipulate situations for their own personal advantage	3	2	1	0
2e	There are cliques here which look after themselves	3	2	1	0
2f	Politics is a way of life for many people in this organisation	3	2	1	0
2g	Advancement is more a matter of who you know than what you know	3	2	1	0
3	**Information and communication orientation**				
3a	The organisation communicates effectively with staff	3	2	1	0
3b	Different departments generally transfer accurate work information on a timely basis	3	2	1	0
3c	Individuals tend to keep information to themselves	0	1	2	3
3d	The organisation has invested in reasonable IT systems	3	2	1	0
3e	Managers promote two-way dialogue with their subordinates	3	2	1	0
3f	Important information usually finds its way to those who need to know it	3	2	1	0
3g	Disruptive gossip and speculation are rife here	0	1	2	3

No.	Orientation and statements	Definitely true	Mostly true	Mostly false	Definitely false
4	**Rules orientation**				
4a	People are expected to report violations of the rules	3	2	1	0
4b	Work is well organised and progresses systematically over time	3	2	1	0
4c	Most people understand and obey the rules here	3	2	1	0
4d	This is a highly flexible organisation	0	1	2	3
4e	Policies and procedures change slowly here	3	2	1	0
4f	There is a lot of argument regarding the interpretation of rules in this organisation	0	1	2	3
4g	Systems of control over people's work are generally effective	3	2	1	0
5	**Learning orientation**				
5a	People in this organisation tend to learn from their mistakes	3	2	1	0
5b	When errors occur, the issues are discussed and learning takes place	3	2	1	0
5c	Organisational systems and policies generally encourage learning from experience	3	2	1	0
5d	When a department learns something of value to other departments, this learning is quickly communicated to them	3	2	1	0
5e	In this organisation the same old errors are repeated over and over again	0	1	2	3
5f	People here are too busy to learn effectively	0	1	2	3
5g	Managers here value a 'doing' rather than a 'learning' orientation among workers	0	1	2	3
6	**Individuality orientation**				
6a	People here are encouraged to express their own personalities in their work	3	2	1	0
6b	Mavericks are tolerated here	3	2	1	0
6c	People here are able to retain a sense of their own individuality	3	2	1	0
6d	There are few stereotypical 'company men' or 'company women' here	3	2	1	0
6e	The organisation encourages people to develop and mature	3	2	1	0
6f	People here are not criticised for their personal style	3	2	1	0
6g	In this organisation image is less important than substance	3	2	1	0

No.	Orientation and statements	Definitely true	Mostly true	Mostly false	Definitely false
7	**Co-operation orientation**				
7a	People here are generally helpful and considerate of others	3	2	1	0
7b	Formal rules and procedures encourage co-operation	3	2	1	0
7c	Most people here are good team players	3	2	1	0
7d	'Loners' do not tend to be promoted in this organisation	3	2	1	0
7e	People who work well in teams are usually rewarded	3	2	1	0
7f	'Lend a helping hand' is a good description of how this organisation works	3	2	1	0
7g	Everyone here has a strong sense of being in a team				
8	**Trust orientation**				
8a	People here are generally trusting of others in the organisation	3	2	1	0
8b	People here do not attempt to exploit others	3	2	1	0
8c	The rules here encourage mutuality	3	2	1	0
8d	Low-trust people find it difficult to survive in this organisation	3	2	1	0
8e	People here respect each other	3	2	1	0
8f	People here do not take credit for work accomplished by others	3	2	1	0
8g	Jealousy and envy dominate the work atmosphere here	0	1	2	3
9	**Conflict orientation**				
9a	There are a lot of petty conflicts here	3	2	1	0
9b	Departments tend to work together without rivalry	0	1	2	3
9c	Criticism is taken as a personal affront in this organisation	3	2	1	0
9d	People here are always trying to win an argument	3	2	1	0
9e	There are strong and cohesive subgroups here that look after themselves	3	2	1	0
9f	I have rarely experienced personal antagonism from others here	0	1	2	3
9g	Conflict in this organisation is generally more positive than negative	0	1	2	3
10	**Future orientation**				
10a	People here think and plan ahead	3	2	1	0

No.	Orientation and statements	Definitely true	Mostly true	Mostly false	Definitely false
10b	This organisation is firmly focused on the future	3	2	1	0
10c	Most people here are more interested in what will happen tomorrow than what happened yesterday	3	2	1	0
10d	The organisation's strategies for the future are well known by the workforce	3	2	1	0
10e	There are often lively discussions regarding where the organisation is heading	3	2	1	0
10f	People are appraised and valued in terms of their future potential	3	2	1	0
10g	People here generally take a long-term view on matters	3	2	1	0
11	**Loyalty and commitment orientation**				
11a	There are a lot of 'long servers' in this organisation	3	2	1	0
11b	Most people consider themselves to be loyal members of the organisation	3	2	1	0
11c	Few people are committed to a long-term career here	0	1	2	3
11d	This organisation is committed to its workforce	3	2	1	0
11e	Preferential treatment is given to long-serving employees	3	2	1	0
11f	I believe that my long-term future is with this organisation	3	2	1	0
11g	When the going gets tough the loyalty of the organisation to the workforce is questionable	0	1	2	3
12	**Work orientation**				
12a	People here generally enjoy their work	3	2	1	0
12b	People in this organisation are always willing to take a break	0	1	2	3
12c	People here live to work, rather than work to live	3	2	1	0
12d	Motivation is not a problem in this organisation	3	2	1	0
12e	Senior personnel work as hard (or harder) than those on other grades	3	2	1	0
12f	People here follow the maxim 'business before pleasure'	3	2	1	0
12g	Day-to-day activities do not require a sustained or intensive effort	0	1	2	3

Exhibit 2.6
Sample semistructured interview questions

Note, these questions will almost always require explanation by the interviewer before they can be adequately answered by the respondent.

1 What are the principal metaphors that people use to describe this organisation?
2 What physical impression do you think the organisation gives?
3 Does the organisation hold any ceremonies?
4 What are the main rites here?
5 What stories and legends do people tell here? What messages do you think these stories and legends convey?
6 Are there any corporate heroes in this organisation? In what ways are they symbols for the organisation?
7 Are there identifiable subcultures here? Where are they located? Are they in conflict or harmony with the dominant culture? What impact do they have?
8 How would you describe the culture of the organisation?
9 Do you think this organisation has a strong culture? Why?
10 Do you think you fit in with the dominant culture here? Why or why not?
11 How does the organisation deal with deviant individuals?
12 What was the last crisis faced by the organisation and how did it respond?

Deciphering a culture by interviewing participants in it is a difficult and unreliable process. It is difficult because much depends on the skills of the researcher to interpret what people say in a realistic and plausible way, and integrate this information into a valid picture of the organisation. This is a highly subjective activity, which means that two different researchers might collect the same data and yet still arrive at very different conclusions. As no interpretation of a culture can be proved to be 'right' or 'wrong' many commentators have suggested that the validity of an account of a culture should be judged according to the usefulness of the insights it generates. Discovering culture through interviews is an unreliable process because people's memories are not infallible, some people are mistaken in their recollection of things and events, and some people may be deliberately misleading or economical with the truth. The important point for us is that any interpretation of an organisational culture or subculture is just that, an interpretation, and not an account founded on objective truth.

TYPOLOGIES OF ORGANISATIONAL CULTURES

A large number of typologies or classifications of types of organisational cultures have been developed. These are useful because they provide broad overviews of the sorts of variations that exist between cultures. The typologies that have been evolved differ greatly in terms of their sophistication, the range of variables they take into consideration and their applicability across organisations. This section examines some of the best-known classification schemes, namely those devised by Harrison (1972) and modified by Handy (1978, 1985), Deal and Kennedy (1982), Quinn and McGrath (1985) and Scholz (1987).

The Harrison/Handy typology

In 1972 Harrison suggested that there are four main types of organisational culture, called *power*, *role*, *task* and *person*. Six years later in 1978 Handy reworked Harrison's ideas, describing the four cultures using simple pictograms and making reference to Greek mythology (see Fig. 2.3). This simple classification scheme has been extremely influential, and played a primary role in shaping the way in which culture scholars, students and practitioners have come to understand how organisations work.

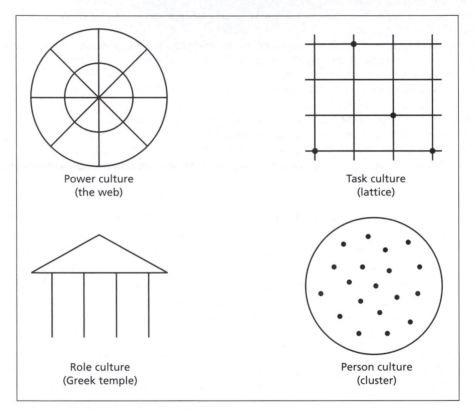

Fig. 2.3 Handy's four organisational cultures
Source: adapted from Handy (1985)

The power culture

A power culture has a single source of power from which rays of influence spread throughout the organisation. These rays are connected by functional and specialist strings which facilitate co-ordinated action. The structure of a power culture may thus be pictured as a web. In Handy's terminology this is a 'club' or 'Zeus' culture, Zeus being the omnipotent leader of the gods on Mount Olympus.

The internal organisation of a power culture is highly dependent on trust, empathy and personal communication for its effectiveness. There are few rules and little need for bureaucratic procedures, with control being exercised from the centre through the selection of key personnel and edict. Resource power and to a lesser extent charisma are the main bases for the exercise of authority here. For the most part individuals are encouraged to perform their tasks with few questions asked, though important decisions are likely to be made as a result of political manoeuvering. The greatest strength of power cultures is their ability to react quickly, but their success largely depends on the abilities of the person or people at the centre. Size can also be a problem, as the web can break if it is spread over too many activities and too great a geographic span. These cultures are often tough, abrasive and more interested in ends than the means used to attain them. Employees who are naturally political animals confident about the use of power, and unconcerned about taking risks or issues of job security will thrive in this environment. Failure to recruit appropriate personnel, however, may lead to low morale, high turnover in middle management positions, and decisive action to move in an inappropriate strategic direction.

The role culture

A role culture is a bureaucracy, the organising principles of which are logic and rationality. The strength of a role culture lies in its functions or specialities (finance, purchasing, production and so forth) which can be thought of as a series of pillars which are co-ordinated and controlled by a small group of senior executives (the pediment). The structure of a role culture may therefore be pictured as a Greek temple, and its associated god is Apollo, the god of reason.

Rules, procedures and job descriptions dominate the internal environment of a role culture, and promotion is based on the satisfactory performance of individuals in their jobs. Position power and to a lesser extent expert power are the main bases for the exercise of authority here. Role cultures are likely to be most successful in stable and predictable environments over which the organisation is able to exert some control or where product life spans are long. In those organisations where economies of scale are more important than the ability to adapt and technical expertise is more useful than product innovation the role culture will thrive. The civil service, the oil industry and retail banking are often cited as examples of role cultures. The main problem with role cultures is that they can be slow to recognise and react to change. For many individuals who value security and predictability these sorts of organisation are highly reassuring, while for those who are ambitious or power-oriented they can be extremely frustrating. A brief overview of a role culture is provided by Mini Case 2.5.

The task culture

A task culture is one in which power is somewhat diffuse, being based on expertise rather than position or charisma. This form of culture often develops in those organisations which can focus on specific jobs or projects to which teams may be assigned. Structurally the task culture may be thought of as a net or matrix, some strands of which are thicker than others, with power being located at its interstices. Originally, Handy ascribed the god 'Athena' to these sorts of organisations, but he later decided that no specific god was totally appropriate to this culture.

Task cultures focus on accomplishing the job in hand, and the internal organisation of such institutions centres on bringing together the appropriate people and resources to make the project successful. At its best this is a team culture in which

The Management Services Division of the Pakistan Cabinet Secretariat: a role culture

The Cabinet Secretariat is probably the most important part of the Pakistan Civil Service. It consists of four main divisions: Establishment, Women, Management Services and Cabinet. All four divisions are headed by a secretary (who is a senior civil servant) and a minister (who is a senior political figure). The Management Services Division (MSD) is responsible for the provision of consultancy services to all Federal Government organisations. Principally located in the capital city of Islamabad the MSD consists of 80 officers and 200 support staff. While there are two smaller offices (in Karachi and Lahore) which provide consultancy services in their local areas, the bulk of the work is conducted by staff in Islamabad. Here the 80 specialist officers are divided into seven teams, each of which is headed by a director general. Each team is composed of two subteams, both of which are headed by a director and staffed by deputy directors.

Work assignments are given to MSD by various Government offices and ministries. Typical assignments include studying how the estates office (responsible for Government housing facilities) can be reorganised, reviewing the activities of the Ministry of Culture and Tourism with a view to making suggestions concerning the relocation of functions, and conducting a management review at the Ministry of Health. In each case, once a study is complete the MSD's recommendations are passed on to a high-level committee (often chaired by the Prime Minister) for a final decision.

As part of Pakistan's civil service, MSD possesses a well-developed culture. Working life is governed by a large number of rules and procedures which are strictly enforced. Moreover, once a rule is formulated it is extremely difficult to have it abolished or modified, however inappropriate it may be. The most obvious examples are the rules concerning recruitment, which make it difficult to appoint staff even when everybody agrees that they are needed. Office hours are from 8.00 a.m. until 3.00 p.m., during which there is one long break in which lunch and afternoon prayers are combined. Two of the many control systems include the need for many signatures on documents authorising action, and (for junior and middle-ranking staff) the need to inform one's immediate superior whenever one leaves the office.

Within MSD, power is largely based on both position and expertise. The employees at MSD are probably the best-educated group within the whole of the civil service in Pakistan, with all the officers educated to first degree level and most in possession of a higher degree. Promotion is based both on length of service and merit as determined by one's immediate superior, whose decisions (elicited during an annual appraisal process) can have a major impact on an employee's career. This said, there is a considerable respect for peers at MSD, less psychological distance between superiors and subordinates than is normal in many bureaucracies, and a more collegiate atmosphere than is found elsewhere in the Pakistan civil service.

While MSD itself is an apolitical institution it is nevertheless subject to political pressures. For example, it is a not uncommon practice for the Ministries to organise a review by MSD and then attempt to influence its recommendations in order to obtain more staff and resources. MSD also faces a variety of operational problems, including severe resource constraints and the withholding of information by client organisations. What is more, despite the fact that there are numerous rules which have to be followed, senior civil servants sometimes exploit whatever flexibility there is for the advantage of their own department or section, adding some unpredictability to work patterns.

Question

1 Is MSD a pure role culture?

Source: compiled from information supplied by Mohammed Yaqoob work is the common enemy. Flexibility, adaptability, individual autonomy and mutual respect based on ability rather than age or status are the most important organising principles here. In those environments where the market is competitive, product life spans are short and constant innovation a necessity the task culture can be highly successful. Advertising agencies would seem to be a good example of this sort of culture. The problems with task cultures are, however, equally strong. Such organisations cannot easily maximise economies of scale, do not usually build up great depth of expertise and are heavily reliant on the quality of the people involved. Furthermore, when things go wrong and control needs to be exercised from the centre the task culture can quickly change into a role or power culture with either rules and procedures or political influence coming to dominate organisational life. In either case, morale tends to decline. Despite these potential difficulties the task culture is probably the most preferred form of organisation for middle and junior managers.

The person culture

A person culture develops when a group of people decide that it is in their own best interests to organise on a collective rather than an individual basis. This is often the case with barristers, doctors and architects who band together in order to share the costs of office space, equipment and secretarial assistance. Such organisations exist solely for the individuals who comprise it, and may be represented diagrammatically as a cluster in which no individual dominates. The god of the person culture is Dionysus, the god of the self-oriented individual.

In the person culture the individuals themselves decide on their own work allocation, with rules and co-ordinative mechanisms of minimal significance. Unlike other cultures in these organisations the individual has almost complete autonomy, influence is shared, and if power is to be exercised it is usually on the basis of expertise. While there are relatively few organisations that possess a person culture many individuals may be found with a preference for this form of organising. For example, university professors and technical specialists in R&D departments are often noted for their loose affiliations to the organisations they belong to.

The Deal and Kennedy typology

From their examination of hundreds of companies Deal and Kennedy (1982) claim to have identified four generic cultures: the *tough-guy, macho culture*, the *work-hard/play-hard culture*, the *bet-your-company culture* and the *process culture*. These cultures are determined by two factors in the marketplace: first, the degree of risk associated with the company's activities, and second, the speed at which the company and its employees receive feedback on their decisions and strategies. Deal and Kennedy recognise that no organisation will precisely fit any one of their four cultures and that some companies do not fit the model at all. Nevertheless they maintain that the framework is a useful first step in helping managers to identify the culture of their own organisations.

The tough-guy, macho culture

This is an organisation composed of individualists who are frequently called upon to take high risks and receive rapid feedback on the quality of their actions and decisions. As examples of this kind of culture Deal and Kennedy cite police departments, surgeons, management consulting firms and the entertainment industry. Tough-guy, macho cultures focus on speed and the short term and place enormous pressures on individuals, with the result that 'burn-out' is a common problem. These are risk-taking cultures in which those who succeed have to take a tough attitude towards their work and their colleagues. As a result internal competition, tension and conflict are normal. While these sorts of cultures can be highly successful in high-risk, quick-return environments they are unable to make long-term investments, tolerate temperamental personalities and breed superstition. Tough-guy, macho cultures are also unable to benefit from co-operative activity, tend to have a high turnover of staff, and thus often fail to develop a strong and cohesive culture.

The work-hard/play-hard culture

This is a low-risk, quick-feedback culture which emphasises fun and action. While sales organisations (such as real estate, computer companies and mass consumer companies like McDonald's) are typical work-hard/play-hard cultures so are many manufacturing organisations. In both cases the risks are generally small. No individual sale will severely damage a rep, and production systems have many checks and balances built into them to neutralise the occurrence of big risks. Similarly, both sales reps and production line operatives receive quick feedback on their performance. Such organisations tend to be highly dynamic, and sales organisations with work-hard/play-hard cultures are often customer-focused. Sales organisations also encourage games, rallies and competitions which keep morale up and momentum going. However, although work/play cultures are achievement cultures there may sometimes be a tendency for volume to displace quality, to concentrate on the present rather than the future, and when things go wrong to pursue 'quick-fix' solutions.

Bet-your-company culture

These cultures exist in environments where the risks are high and the feedback on actions and decisions takes a long time. Bet-your-company organisations include large aircraft manufacturers such as Boeing and oil companies like Shell. These vast firms invest millions in large-scale projects, the success or failure of which may take years to ascertain. Such organisations are invested with a sense of deliberateness which manifests itself in ritualised business meetings. Focused primarily on the future, decision making tends to be top-down, reflecting the hierarchical nature of bet-your-company cultures. The type of people who survive in these organisations respect authority and technical competence, are keen to act co-operatively with colleagues, and have the strength of character to deal with the high-pressure decisions required of them. Bet-your-company cultures are good at producing high-quality inventions and scientific breakthroughs, but their slow response times can also cause them problems.

The process culture

This is a low-risk and slow-feedback culture typified by banks, insurance companies and the civil service. Employees in process cultures work with little feedback on their activities with memos and reports seeming to disappear into a void. The lack of feedback means that employees tend to focus on how they do something rather than what they do. People in these cultures are often protective and cautious, keen to protect the system's integrity, and focused on technical perfection in the performance of their duties. Those who survive and thrive in these environments are orderly, punctual and attend to detail. Work activities are punctuated by long and rambling meetings about procedures and the possibilities for reorganisation. There is considerable emphasis on job titles and formality, reflecting the rigid nature of the hierarchy and the importance of position power. Process cultures are effective when dealing with a known and predictable environment, but are unable to react quickly and lack vision and creativity.

Quinn and McGrath's typology

Based on an analysis of the nature of the transactions associated with information exchange in organisations Quinn and McGrath (1985) have identified four generic cultures: the rational culture (*market*), the ideological culture (*adhocracy*), the consensual culture (*clan*) and the hierarchical culture (*hierarchy*). The intellectual basis of their typology is the notion that whenever an interaction between individuals or groups takes place valued things (such as facts, ideas and permission) are exchanged. These transactions or exchanges are important in organisations because they determine the status of individuals and groups, the power they are able to wield, and their degree of satisfaction with the status quo. Furthermore, the transactions will be governed by a set of rules or norms which reflect dominant belief/value clusters. Thus the nature of the transactions in an organisation provides a means for distinguishing between different sorts of cultures. An overview of Quinn and McGrath's typology is provided by Exhibit 2.7.

Scholz's typologies

In his attempt to understand the relationship between culture and strategy Scholz (1987) has identified three culture typologies. These describe what Scholz refers to as three different *dimensions* of culture, namely *evolution* (how cultures change over time), *internal* (how the internal circumstances of an organisation affect its culture) and *external* (how an organisation's environment affects its culture). The last of these, concerning the external-induced dimension, Scholz borrowed from Deal and Kennedy (see p. 68). For his evolution-induced typology Scholz turned to the literature on strategic management. From this he derived five primary culture types: *stable, reactive, anticipating, exploring* and *creative*. To these he ascribed a personality, time-orientation, risk-orientation, slogan and change-orientation. For his internal-induced dimension Scholz again sought to reformulate existing ideas about how organisations work, this time identifying three culture types *production, bureaucratic* and *professional*. These he distinguished by their degree of routineness, standardisation, skill requirements and variety of property rights. While none of the ideas contained in these typologies is new, the frameworks nevertheless provide another interesting perspective on organisational culture. Overviews of these typologies are provided by Figs. 2.4 and 2.5.

Exhibit 2.7
Typology of organisational cultures

The market
This is a rational culture designed to pursue objectives using productivity and efficiency as the primary criteria of performance. The 'boss' is firmly in charge of this culture, and competence is the basis of his or her authority. The style of leadership is directive and goal-oriented, decision making is decisive and the compliance of employees guaranteed by contractual agreement. Individuals are judged according to their tangible output and are encouraged to be achievement-oriented. According to McDonald and Gandz (1992) the salient values of market cultures are aggressiveness, diligence and initiative.

The adhocracy
This is an ideological culture which can support broad purposes as indicated by its favoured criteria of performance, namely external support, growth and resource acquisition. Authority is held on the basis of charisma and power is wielded by referring to values. In such organisations decisions are often taken as a result of intuition, leaders tend to be inventive and risk-oriented, and employee compliance is enforced by their commitment to organisational values. Individuals are evaluated according to the intensity of their effort and interested in growth rather than achievement. McDonald and Gandz (1992) suggest that these cultures are characterised by values such as adaptability, autonomy and creativity.

The clan
This is a consensual culture the organisational purpose of which is group maintenance, and which gauges performance in terms of whether or not it facilitates cohesion and morale. Authority is vested in those who are members of the organisation generally and the basis for the exercise of power is informal status. Decisions tend to be arrived at through participation and consensus and the dominant leadership style is one of concern and support. Employees comply with agreed decisions because they have shared in the process by which they were reached. Individuals are evaluated in terms of the quality of the relationships they enjoy with others and are expected to show loyalty to the organisation. For McDonald and Gandz (1992) the dominant values of a clan include courtesy, fairness, moral integrity and social equality.

The hierarchy
This is a hierarchical culture that exists to execute regulations while remaining stable and controlled. In these organisations authority is vested in the rules and power is exercised by those with technical knowledge. Decisions are made on the basis of factual analysis and leaders tend to be conservative and cautious. Here the compliance of employees is maintained by surveillance and control, and they are assessed against formally agreed criteria and are expected to value security. According to McDonald and Gandz (1992), some of the values associated with the hierarchy are formality, logic, obedience and orderliness.

Source: adapted from Quinn and McGrath (1985) and McDonald and Gandz (1992)

While these typologies may make interesting reading there are dangers associated with them. No organisation is likely to precisely fit any one category in any typology. The reality of organisations is just too complex to be captured in this way.

We should always remember that classifications of cultures present us with ideal types or models against which actual organisations can be compared and examined. The value of the typologies is that they present us with interesting ways to think about organisational cultures, what dimensions are important, why, and how they interact with each other to form a coherent social whole. Finally, it should be noted that only a small selection of the culture typologies that have been formulated by theorists have been presented here, and that many others, notably that by Wiener (1988), are also worthy of study.

Culture	Personality	Time-orientation	Risk-orientation	Slogan	Change-orientation
Stable	Introvert	Backward-looking	Risk averse	'Don't rock the boat'	No change accepted
Reactive	Introvert	Oriented to present	Accepts minimum risks	'Roll with the punches'	Minimal change accepted
Anticipating	Partially introvert, partially extrovert	Oriented to present	Accepts familiar risks	'Plan ahead'	Incremental change accepted
Exploring	Extrovert	Oriented to present and future	Operates on risk/ gain trade-off	'Be where the action is'	Accepts radical change
Creative	Extrovert	Oriented to future	Prefers unfamiliar risks	'Invent the future'	Seeks novel change

Fig. 2.4 The evolution-induced dimension

Source: adapted from Scholz (1987)

Culture type	Routineness	Standardisation	Skill requirements	Property rights
Production	High	High	Low	Weak
Bureaucratic	Medium	Medium	Medium	Derived from the position held in the hierarchy
Professional	Low	Low	High	Vested in the person by virtue of skills and knowledge possessed

Fig. 2.5 The internal-induced dimension

Source: adapted from Scholz (1987)

ASSESSING THE STRENGTH OF AN ORGANISATIONAL CULTURE

Organisational cultures can differ markedly in terms of their relative strength. According to Hampden-Turner (1990: 13) organisational culture tends to be especially strong in those situations where people need reassurance and certainty. Much of the interest in the strength of culture, however, derives from the supposed relationship between strong organisational cultures and good performance (see Chapter 6). This has led to various largely unsubstantiated claims that certain organisations possess a strong culture or need to strengthen a weak one. Organisations with so-called strong cultures tend to be described as having a certain style or other intangible differentiating factor like flair or atmosphere. While such general perceptions may be useful as first approximations, there are other and more reliable ways to evaluate the strength of an organisation's culture. For example, if the organisation is recognised not to have undergone any significant cultural change for a long period of time, then this might be taken as an indicator that the culture is strong. An alternative test occurs when a new CEO takes over an organisation. Continued cultural stability may not prove the strength of the culture (after all, the CEO might have been chosen on the grounds that he or she was culturally compatible), but it is often a good test of a culture's resilience. In addition, we can identify two quantitative approaches to measuring the strength of an organisation's culture. The first involves an examination of a range of a culture's artefacts and more superficial psychological traits, while the second focuses specifically on beliefs, values, attitudes and assumptions.

The artefactual approach

The examination of culture provided in Chapter 1 illustrated the many possible components of an organisation's culture. It should, though, be recalled that not all of these elements are necessarily present in any particular organisational culture. There are, for

Exhibit 2.8
Measuring the strength of an organisational culture: an artefactual approach

	Definitely true	Mostly true	Mostly false	Definitely false
1 There are many well-known organisation-specific stories here.	☐	☐	☐	☐
2 There are many well-known organisation-specific jokes here.	☐	☐	☐	☐
3 There is a well-developed organisation-specific vocabulary here.	☐	☐	☐	☐
4 The organisation has its own corporate heroes.	☐	☐	☐	☐
5 The organisation has its own way of doing things.	☐	☐	☐	☐
6 There are many rites and rituals here.	☐	☐	☐	☐
7 The organisation has a long and distinguished history.	☐	☐	☐	☐
8 People tend to work here for a long time.	☐	☐	☐	☐
9 The organisation is unique.	☐	☐	☐	☐
10 The organisation has its own mission statement.	☐	☐	☐	☐
11 Success here depends on fitting in to the organisation.	☐	☐	☐	☐
12 People here have a strong sense of being a member of a team.	☐	☐	☐	☐
13 There are strong traditions here.	☐	☐	☐	☐
14 People here would be proud of the fact that even outsiders know what the organisation stands for.	☐	☐	☐	☐
15 The organisation has it own philosophy.	☐	☐	☐	☐
16 The organisation attempts to recruit people who fit into its culture.	☐	☐	☐	☐

example, organisations which do not have easily identifiable heroes or commonly shared stories. In attempting to make an assessment of the strength of a culture we can ask certain questions of its composition. These questions can be employed in questionnaires (see Exhibit 2.8) which when completed by a representative sample of an organisation's employees yield considerable insight into the strength of a culture. This approach is limited in two respects: first, it relies on the perceptiveness of employees and their ability to make meaningful judgements about their organisation, and second, it tends to focus on the more easily identifiable aspects of culture, namely, artefacts and consciously held beliefs, values and attitudes. For those theorists who consider the essence of culture to be basic assumptions this approach to measuring culture strength is at best incomplete and at worst misguided and irrelevant.

The consensus/intensity approach

Payne (1990) has suggested that it is possible to gain an appreciation of the strength of an organisation's culture by plotting the *strength of consensus* among members against their *intensity* of feeling. Strength of consensus refers to the degree to which there is agreement on core beliefs, values, attitudes and assumptions. The greater the degree of consensus within an organisation the stronger its culture is said to be. The intensity variable is a little more complex, having two distinct components. First, *psychic depth*, and second, *range*. Psychic depth refers to how deeply felt and influential the culture is. A culture is categorised as strong if it determines basic assumptions, less strong if it shapes values and beliefs, and least powerful if it only influences attitudes. Range refers to the scope of assumptions, beliefs, values, attitudes and behaviours a culture influences. The idea is that stronger cultures will tend to affect a greater range of individuals' cognitive apparatus and behavioural dispositions than weaker cultures.

Figure 2.6 illustrates how these cultural co-ordinates might be used to examine the relative strength and weakness of organisational cultures. It suggests that organisations with weak socialisation practices that tend to employ people on a part-time basis such as supermarkets will usually develop cultures which are weak both in terms of consensus and intensity. On the other hand, there are organisations which often evolve high consensus but not deep feeling on a narrow range of activities. These high-consensus and low-intensity organisations include social and special activity clubs concerned with particular issues such as drama or a certain sport. Then there are the high-intensity but relatively low-consensus organisations such as the Church of England. Finally, it is possible to identify high-consensus and high-intensity organisations. In the commercial world the best exemplars of these strong cultures are those Japanese companies that employ people for life and provide a large range of other benefits. Very high-consensus/high-intensity organisations, however, are likely to be found in the form of special religious orders and elite military groups.

Interesting though this consensus/intensity approach is, it is not without its problems. The most important of these is designing research tools which can validly and reliably evaluate cultural consensus and intensity. Unless the subjective judgement of the researcher is to be relied upon, the only option would seem to be to employ some reformulated climate survey questionnaire, with all the difficulties associated with these methods (see pp. 59–60).

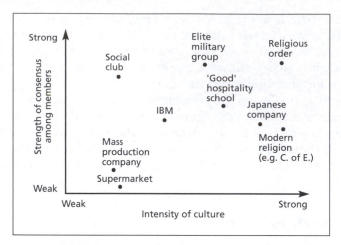

Fig. 2.6 Examples of strong and weak cultures
Source: adapted from Payne (1990)

SUMMARY AND CONCLUSIONS

In this chapter four main themes were elaborated.

1 The sources of organisational culture were considered. The influence of national cultures, the leaders of organisations and the nature of an organisation's business activities and business environment were all reviewed. It was suggested that the impact of national cultures on organisational cultures may be understood in terms of Hofstede's five dimensions and/or as containing business recipes which shape and constrain organisational forms. The importance of leaders (and especially founders) in making such vital decisions as the mission to be pursued, the business context to be operated in, who is to be recruited, and what rules, systems and procedures governing organisational life are to be instituted was then surveyed. Finally, the nature of the business and the business environment as a factor affecting organisational cultures was discussed in terms of a variety of stakeholders (customers, the Government, the public and shareholders), professional associations and various strategic issues.

2 The perpetuation of organisational cultures was reviewed. A model of cultural transmission was presented which illustrated how organisations preselect, socialise and incorporate/reject employees. It was argued that cultures vary greatly in terms of their transparency/opaqueness and simplicity/complexity, and that these factors determine how easy it is for new recruits to learn how to survive in the culture they have joined.

3 Some issues in the conduct of culture research were examined. The advantages and problems associated with both quantitative and qualitative methods were considered, and sample questions and questionnaires illustrated.

4 Four sets of the best known and most widely employed typologies for classifying organisational cultures were presented, namely those produced by Harrison/Handy, Deal and Kennedy, Quinn and McGrath, and Scholz. Two other means of gaining insight into an organisation's culture, this time by focusing on its supposed strength, one based on artefacts and the other on ideas of consensus and intensity, were also considered.

KEY CONCEPTS

National culture
Leadership
Type of business
Business environment
Power distance
Individualism/
    collectivism
Masculinity/femininity
Uncertainty avoidance
Confucian dynamism
Business recipes
Founders
Stakeholders
Customers
Government
Public
Shareholders
Professional associations

Strategy
Degree of risk
Speed of feedback
Trauma
Positive reinforcement
Preselection
Socialisation
Rites
Enculturation
Transparency/
    opaqueness
Simplicity/complexity
Incorporation/rejection
Questionnaire surveys
Ideology questionnaire
Interviews
Observation
Typologies of culture

Harrison/Handy
    typology
Power culture
Role culture
Task culture
Person culture
Deal and Kennedy
    typology
Tough-guy, macho
    culture
Work-hard/play-hard
    culture
Bet-your-company
    culture
Process culture
Scholz's typologies
Stable
Reactive

Anticipating
Exploring
Creative
Production
Bureaucratic
Professional
Quinn and McGrath's
    typology
Market
Adhocracy
Clan
Hierarchy
Culture strength
Artefactual approach
Consensus/intensity
    approach

QUESTIONS

1 What influence do national cultures have on organisational cultures?

2 Why are leaders (and especially founders) such important influences on an organisation's culture?

3 How important do you think the type of activities an organisation conducts and the nature of its environment are as influences on its culture? Illustrate your answer with reference to an organisation you know well.

4 With reference to an organisation you know well, discuss how its culture has developed over time.

5 Focusing on an organisation you know well, discuss its formal and informal socialisation mechanisms.

6 Which of the typologies discussed in this chapter do you find the most useful and relevant? Explain your answer.

7 What are the advantages and disadvantages associated with qualitative and quantitative approaches to researching organisational culture?

8 How would you go about assessing the strength of an organisational culture you know well?

EXPLORING ORGANISATIONAL CULTURE: OMEGA COLLEGE

Introduction

Omega College has its origins in the Omega Mechanics Institute, which was founded in the 1830s to promote 'general and liberal education for the workers of Omegaville'. An initial programme of evening lectures eventually gave way to regular evening classes, which ran four evenings a week and cost the attenders 2d. At the turn of the century the Mechanics Institute developed into a technical school with a formal curriculum emphasising the three Rs, technical education and science. Thirty years later the funds (nearly £80 000) were found by two local boroughs to begin construction of an educational establishment which was officially opened in 1936 as the Omega Technical College. According to the staff of Omega College the organisation can only be understood in this historical context, not least because the pattern of vocational and liberal education of those early evening classes was similar in kind to the educational programme offered in the

1990s. The forces for continuity were strong at Omega College: in 60 years there had been just four Principals, the first of whom served for more than 30 years. What is more, the then current Principal and his immediate predecessor were both long-serving Vice Principals before they eventually took up the most senior position in the college.

Omega College was one of the ten largest further education colleges in the UK, employing more than 400 full-time and some 500 part-time staff to teach approximately 6000 students. Formally, the college consisted of six academic divisions, each managed by a Head of School. Each Division consisted of between two and four departments, managed by Departmental Heads. Above the Heads of Schools were two Vice Principals and a Chief Administrative Officer who answered only to the Principal (see Fig. 2.7). In practice, however, all the senior management team reported to the Principal, who was the ultimate source of authority within the

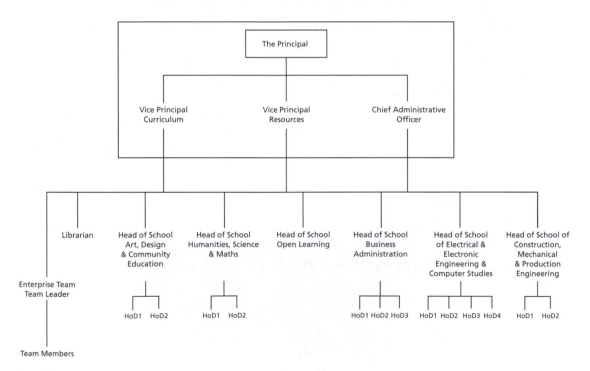

Fig. 2.7 Omega College of Technology

college. Thus despite paying homage to a traditional hierarchical management structure the power that individual senior managers were able to exert was fundamentally a function of their proximity to the Principal. In fact, the Vice Principals had no authority over the Heads of Schools, and many employees considered them to be politically and managerially impotent. Other significant members of the managerial group included those people responsible for marketing, R&D and personnel. All staff were expertly aware of the importance of invoking 'The Principal' in arguments to further their personal and School/Division interests, and the result was tremendous individual and institutionalised inertia.

The recent history

In the financial year 1980/81 the college overspent its budget by £400 000 (approximately 20 per cent of its total allocation), and this event sent shockwaves through the entire Omegaville education system. The main cause was that Chris, the Principal of the time, had run a relatively loose regime in which 'robber baron' Heads of Divisions ran their own internal affairs with few financial checks on them. The upshot of these events was that Chris was directed to attend before a full Local Education Committee where he pledged never to allow the college to overspend again. From then on there was a dramatic change in how the college operated, with the financial control system coming to dominate organisational life. Senior staff also noticed that the Principal was unwilling to delegate responsibility according to previously accepted tradition, that they were now treated with a degree of mistrust and suspicion, and that the exploration of alternative ideas and systems for ensuring that financial controls operated effectively was not pursued.

Perhaps the main beneficiary of the new order was the Chief Administrative Officer (CAO), who evolved into the arbiter of college rules and procedures, especially those governing finance. The reliance of the Principal on the CAO was enshrined in the recollections of long-serving employees, who reported a favourite saying of the Principal: 'if Sally (the CAO) is smiling, I'm happy – if she's not, I'm worried'. A decade later the then assistant to the CAO had herself become the CAO, and is deferred to as the authority on college rules and regulations even by the Principal himself. The power of the administra-tive hierarchy has thus been preserved, despite the fact that the college has increased in size by some 400 per cent since 1980 and that the old control systems are manifestly unable to cope with the volume of work. For example, as this research was being conducted in 1993 staff complained that they had to complete a four-part pro forma in order to request that a light bulb be replaced! The inevitable consequence was that the administrative system was treated with contempt by the teaching staff who referred to the CAO's office as the 'black hole' from which nothing emerged.

Organisational culture: the views of the teaching staff

Omega College is situated on the edge of a large industrial conurbation in the UK. The region has a distinctive (and, local people claim, unique) identity that is characterised by a strong sense of community. People here take pride in themselves as straight-talking, no-nonsense, down-to-earth folk who live according to traditional values. While the demise of the local heavy industries had had an impact on these community structures and beliefs, Omega College culture had been informed and imbued with the ethos of this earlier age.

The college consisted of an odd seven-sided 1930s red-brick building three floors high. The high-ceilinged rooms were linked by long narrow corridors. The academic departments were scattered seemingly haphazardly around the building, each with its own self-contained suite of rooms. The pattern of occupancy reflected patterns of power and historical ownership rights stretching back over the decades. A form of evolutionary progression was recognisable, with seasoned campaigners able to move into preferred office accommodation as the previous occupants moved on. Space and other small 'luxuries' were quite blatantly used to symbolise status and power. The Principal had the largest office, complete with *en suite* toilet facilities (for his personal use only) and a purpose-built garage. Heads of Departments had smaller offices and named parking spaces. Access to college rooms was strictly controlled by a key allocation mechanism that restricted the number of keys in circulation, in the case of many rooms to just one. The sheer size of the college, reinforced by its physical and managerial structures, meant that individuals and departments were effectively isolated from each other: 'one doesn't happen across people in their working environment, you have to make a point of looking them out, so most people keep themselves to themselves and get on with their work'.

The power of the Principal was immense (see Exhibit 2.9). While his formal powers were unquestioned, his actual influence was far more pervasive. For instance, discussions among staff members about any aspect of college policy were likely to centre on the likely views of the Principal: 'the Principal won't have it' or 'the Principal will stop it' being two of the most typical observations. The administrative staff (and especially the CAO) were particularly sensitive to the importance of the Principal, and appeared able to manipulate people's understandings of the Principal's views to enhance their own position. As one senior member of the teaching staff said: 'the important people are admin staff who are concerned only with sticking to rigid bureaucratic admin procedures, no matter how absurd they may be.' In order to survive and function effectively in this environment the teaching staff had evolved an alternative set of procedures for getting things done based on an informal network of collusion against the system, generally involving favours owed and returned. As one individual observed: 'the informal network of people helping one another is probably the mainstay of the college'. Unsurprisingly, the socialisation system for all new recruits involved intensive coaching on how these unofficial channels operated.

There was considerable discontent with this state of affairs among the senior academic staff, who thought that the mixture of centralised control and bureaucratic inefficiency had allowed people to avoid responsibility when things went wrong, encouraged a lack of strategic planning, and made the cultivating of politically useful relations a necessary evil:

> The influence of the Principal cannot be underestimated. He has developed an organisational culture which emphasises conflict rather than co-operation. There are many staff, myself included, who find Omega an extremely harsh working environment. There are small pockets of interesting and innovative development, but it's all so piecemeal!'

Many considered that the internal administrative problems of the college were affecting its ability to function as an educational institution. Teaching staff suggested

Exhibit 2.9
Principal power at Omega College

The Principal was at the centre of cultural life at Omega College, and an elaborate mythology had built up surrounding him. For example, all senior members of the college were able to recall the Principal's favourite story illustrating the importance of customer care, in which the Principal fondly recounted the time when as a student he attended an interview at UMIST, lost a scarf that was promptly returned to him, and hence decided to take his degree there. So numerous were the recitations of this story by the Principal that a departing Head of School was heard to say that one good thing about his new job was 'not having to listen to that bloody scarf story again'. More explicitly anti-Principal feelings were enshrined in another story, this time concerning the Principal's supposedly much inflated ego. It was said that a security officer attempting to help the Principal escape from a blocked car parking space mistakenly called him 'Mr' rather than 'Dr'. While the precise language used by the Principal to correct the unfortunate security officer did not emerge from this research it was clear that the Principal was most annoyed, a fact reported with glee by the storyteller. A final series of observations concerning the Principal involved how hard he was rumoured to work, though again it was uncertain that such comments were designed to be complimentary. Employees were more likely to claim that the Principal's workaholic mentality was linked to his refusal to delegate authority, which was a primary reason for the college's continuing managerial chaos.

An invitation to comment on the Principal:

> 'The Principal's management style is so appalling.' 'All expenditure is controlled by the Principal . . . he delegates responsibility, not power.'

> 'He employs people most likely to make changes . . . then wants to get rid of them so he doesn't have to change.' 'Uses people for their expertise and then is glad when they've left. . . .'

> 'After investing much time over a six month period in researching/planning for the implementation of a learning resource centre, the item was designated as item number five on the agenda – the Principal dismissed it with "Item 5 won't take five minutes", and responded to protests with "I'm the Chair of this bloody meeting".'

that while the college publicity material asserted that 'Customers and people are important' sometimes 'we appear to operate a college for its support mechanism (admin)'. In short, there was an enormous sense of frustration that the best possible service could not be provided to students. Few, however, were able to make any constructive suggestions as to what might be done to improve matters. Teaching staff at all levels claimed that they had 'responsibility without power', were just 'a cog in a large machine', and powerless in the face of 'petty rules' and an 'inflexible finance system'. The unanimity of opinion among the teaching staff was impressive, indicating that culturally this was a relatively homogeneous group. In those few instances where individuals had attempted to make progress against what they saw as an antiquated and dysfunctional organisational system, successes were hard to find: 'I have tried to undertake an operational planning exercise and have identified a number of issues. The major problem is that I have no power to carry out these plans, and continually hit barriers when I make suggestions for change.' Change, however, was being forced on Omega College, whether it was wanted or not.

Forces for change

During the 1980s the Government became increasingly alarmed by Audit Commission reports that millions of pounds were being wasted in Further Education. The 1988 Education Reform Act had little impact on Further Education (FE). The Further and Higher Education Act of 1992, though, marked a watershed in the history of FE. A new funding council, the Higher Education Funding Council (HEFC) was established to manage the funds provided to Local Education Authorities (LEAs) for post-16 education, with the explicit aim of revolutionising the management of FE. Specifically, the aim was to cut the 'fat' out of the system, to relate funding of institutions to their performance, and to increase participation in FE by 25 per cent in the first three years. In order to be incorporated into the new system FE colleges would now have to develop new corporate functions such as 'personnel' and 'estates management', and to manage themselves on a professional and strategic basis. An indication that the new funding council was going to take its

duties seriously came with 'directive 92/189', which requested FE colleges to prepare the following documentation:

- a mission statement;
- an educational needs analysis of the college's community;
- a three-year strategic overview;
- a sensitivity analysis; and
- an operating statement which for 1993/4 should identify those components of a college's strategic objectives which were to be put into effect in the forthcoming 16 months, how each component was to be delivered and where responsibility for its delivery lay, what resources were required, and what monitoring of progress and delivery there would be.

This information, together with detailed financial forecasts, was to be completed and returned to the HEFC by early 1993. Such demands came as a tremendous shock to the senior management at Omega College, who had little experience of planning, and tended to adopt 'a patchwork quilt approach to institutional development'. The immediate problem was that there were no mechanisms in place to accomplish these tasks. In the end a handful of senior managers got together and completed the documentation without reference to the real life of the college. Given the newness of the situation, and the decision by the HEFC to base the next year's funding using historical allocations as a guide, no serious damage was done to Omega. Nevertheless, it was clear to everyone that if Omega was going to prosper under the new rules things had to change, and fast.

Prospects for change

'I don't think strategically, I think incrementally – I'm a chemist. The success of this college has been founded in building by bits, building on what has already been achieved. Strategic planning would stifle this'.

(The Principal)

The senior managers among the academic staff at Omega not only recognised that change was needed, they claimed to welcome it with open arms:

I am genuinely enthusiastic about changes up to this point in time, and feel that the change rate has not been swift enough in many areas, i.e. promises have not been kept.

I am happy to accept these challenges . . . .

> 'I have no objection to managing change which can be seen to improve staff or student experiences . . . . I do feel resentment when asked to manage change masked by a cloak of 'this is good for students', when in fact we are simply implementing Government policy.

Few, though, were able to point to any significant changes that had actually occurred. Certainly, some individuals thought that they were being asked to work harder, take on more students and engage in more administrative duties. But when it came to making substantive and meaningful progress (however this was defined), the prevailing view was one of 'Change? What change?' As one Head of Division said, 'I have noticed no change in the last few years, nor do I expect any in the future'. Disillusionment with the college's ability to come to terms with the new educational environment had crystallised over the past year, with the gradual realisation that being accredited by the British Standards Institute (BSI) to BS 5750 had had little impact. While some maintained that BS 5750 had 'sharpened our focus', 'made us take stock of what we are doing' and 'begun to chip away at the established bad practice', the majority view was that BS 5750 'was never intended for use by education and it shows'.

There was, though, a less pessimistic view. Some suggested that there was evidence to suggest that the college was likely to be restructured, with the Schools being transformed into faculties, some Divisions amalgamated, and some new Divisions created. The basic thrust of the restructuring proposals was, however, to give those functions newly recognised as important (such as finance, marketing, estates and commercial development) a more formal standing. It was argued that the college had managed to formulate a mission statement: 'Serving the Community through High Quality Education and Training'. Here again the more optimistic view was difficult to sustain. There was much confusion concerning precisely what was meant by the mission statement (recruit more students? improve teaching quality? broaden the range of courses offered?), and most people thought that the current climate of cost cutting would inevitably result in a reduction in the quality of all the services the college offered. The view was expressed that the college had successfully started marketing itself overseas to foreign students, and that this was surely a positive thing. Others wondered whether this was the right moment to take on extra activities, and questioned whether the college had any distinctive competencies. Meanwhile, the time when more stringent demands were going to be made on Omega College was rapidly advancing.

Questions

1 How would you characterise the culture of Omega College? What are the most significant rites and symbols?

2 How confident are you that the college will successfully come to terms with the demands of the HEFC? Is there an unfreezing problem here? Explain your answer?

3 The senior and middle managers among the teaching staff claimed that they were powerless to initiate change. Do you think that this is a realistic appraisal of their potential?

4 Is Omega College more a prisoner of poor leadership than an inappropriate organisational culture?

5 A new Principal is appointed to Omega college who has no previous connections with the College. Her first move is to commission you (a team of management consultants) to provide short- and long-term recommendations as to how she should proceed. What recommendations would you make to her?

The data on which this case is based were collected by Mr D. J. McDougall, and the case study has been jointly written by Mr D. J. McDougall and Dr Andrew Brown

---

NOTES

1 For more information on business recipes in south-east Asia see Whitley (1992).

2 A more detailed review of Gordon's conclusions is provided in Chapter 6.

CHAPTER 3

Discovering issues in organisational culture

OBJECTIVES

To enable students to:

- learn about various types of subculture, how they form and their relation to the dominant organisational culture;

- familiarise themselves with the functions that culture has been said to play within organisations;

- explore the notion of identity and how it can be applied to assist our understanding of individuals and organisations;

- understand some of the principal issues in gender studies and why they are important to the culture perspective;

- become familiar with theories of organisational learning and relate them to theories of organisational culture;

- consider the phenomenon of groupthink, and how it can be both fostered and defended against by organisational cultures;

- discover the various ways in which ethical issues impinge on an organisational culture;

- identify postmodern approaches to organisation studies and their implications for the culture perspective.

INTRODUCTION

This chapter builds on the ideas and frameworks discussed in Chapters 1 and 2. It consists of eight principal sections. First, it deals with the issue of subcultures and subculture formation. Second, it reviews the functions that culture may play in organisations. Third, it discusses the notion of identity and its relationship to culture. Fourth, it focuses on issues of gender and culture. Fifth, it briefly reviews the literature on learning, and how cultures may facilitate and impede the processes by which organisations learn. Sixth, it considers Janis's (1972) notion of groupthink, and its relation to culture. Seventh, it analyses the linkages between organisational culture and ethical issues. Finally, postmodern approaches to understanding the importance of the culture concept are examined. This chapter completes the review of the general organisational culture literature. Together Chapters 1, 2 and 3 form the basis on which the next three chapters draw in their consideration of culture change, strategy and performance.

83

CULTURE, SUBCULTURE AND MULTICULTURALISM IN ORGANISATIONS

In most organisations most individuals are aware of a great many different subcultures. Some have argued that those national cultures which emphasise individualism and freedom of association will develop organisations with disproportionately large numbers of subcultures. However, it seems likely that any medium to large organisation anywhere in the world will be differentiated into subgroups of some kind. The point is that while it is often convenient to refer to organisations as if they possessed a single, homogeneous culture, this is rarely the case in practice. Organisations of any size contain many identifiable subcultures, the beliefs, values and assumptions of which may compete with the dominant culture. Gregory (1983: 365) has expressed this situation very well:

> the small-homogeneous-society metaphor is often inappropriate to those organisations that are large, internally differentiated, rapidly changing, and only command part-time commitment from members. Such organisations more nearly resemble the complex society of which they are a part. In large complex societies ... the robustness of any group as a culture is questionable ... Societies, and many organisations, can more correctly be viewed in terms of multiple, cross-cutting cultural contexts changing through time, rather than as stable, bounded, homogeneous cultures.

While very little research has yet been conducted, it seems plausible to suggest that subcultures do not just spring up within departments or functions. It is certainly possible for sets of shared values and beliefs to emerge within particular age cohorts in organisations, or according to hierarchical position. For example, it is an oft-quoted fact that managers are frequently more committed to their organisation than other employees (see Exhibit 3.1). The important point here is that within many (if not most) organisations, an array of nested, overlapping and sometimes competing cultures can be detected. What is more, the potential for conflict between them and between subcultures and a dominant organisational culture is considerable. Indeed, it was a central claim of Peters and Waterman (1982) that successful organisations tend to be those that have found ways of breaking down the barriers between subcultures and enforcing co-ordination and control.

One obvious question that needs to be addressed is why and how subcultures develop. Trice and Beyer (1993) have suggested four social conditions which promote the growth of subcultures. These are:

- *Differential interaction* The extent to which individuals associate with each other influences their likelihood of forming a subculture. Factors such as an organisation's size, structure, formal rules and so forth establish the frequency of interactions between individuals, with more interaction leading to the formation of more subcultures.
- *Shared experiences* Culture is a shared phenomenon that people develop over time in response to shared experiences, which engender agreed values and modes of behaviour, and which foster a similar outlook on the world. Working patterns which encourage people to engage in close co-ordination and communication and which encourage them to identify the same problems and share certain solutions and goals will be conducive to the formation of subcultures.

Exhibit 3.1
Non-managerial subcultures

The overwhelming majority of books and articles on organisational culture have been written from the standpoint of managers. T.R.V. Davis (1985) has convincingly argued that the study of organisation culture is incomplete without a thorough examination of the culture of employees with lower-level jobs. Moreover, there is good evidence to suggest that people in non-managerial positions often view their jobs and the experience of working very differently from those in more privileged positions. In other words, the non-managerial cadre of workers in organisations may often be considered a distinct subculture.

It is suggested that employees in non-managerial jobs do not accept their underprivileged status willingly. On the contrary, there is often an uneasy tension between the managers and the managed. A sense of resentment on the part of lower-level employees results from a perception that managers have all the power and prestige, superior pay and most of the privileges. The monotonous, routine and dull nature of many non-managerial jobs further heightens their feelings of injustice. The result is that these employees unite in a collective distrust of managers and identify with actions that alleviate boredom.

'Us' and 'them' attitudes may find expression in what UK employees refer to as *skiving*, that is, the deliberate evasion or avoidance of work. In practice, skiving means being somewhere else when work tasks are assigned, taking more time than is really necessary to perform jobs, and extending lunch times and coffee breaks. Skiving is often combined with covering up mistakes. When errors are made junior employees sometimes have to make a decision whether or not to inform supervisors. In these instances workers will often engage in deceptive behaviour in order to preserve the status quo or 'score points' against managers.

For some workers it is not the managers who are the main source of discontent but the nature of the work itself. In these cases employees may join together to avoid 'going nuts'. Those working on assembly lines, for example, have been found to develop their own unique language and set of rituals such as the giving and receiving of presents, which reduce the monotony and boredom of the work. In some instances, other departments are identified as the cause of unnecessary problems, and a vigorous warfare may be waged against them. Conflicts between production and quality control and sales and marketing are fairly common. What is more, it is frequently workers at lower levels that handle these conflicts on a day-to-day basis. Where these antagonisms arise individuals in the same department will tend to band together, sympathise with one another and swap war stories, giving everyone the feeling that they are not alone in having to deal with 'those idiots'.

In other situations it is the customers who provide the source of problems and difficulties that encourage lower-level subcultures to form. Junior employees from receptionists to bus drivers and sales people all have to interact continuously with outsiders, and bear the brunt of their criticisms and complaints. Such employees are likely to be characterised by cynicism and shared resentment of customers, who are thought of as dim, difficult and demanding. The machine-like behaviour of lower-level civil servants is a well-observed reaction to the sorts of customer-induced pressures from which managers are able to escape.

While the formation of distinct cultures at the bottom of organisations might seem inevitable, they can also be highly destructive:

> Managers and lower-level workers can fight instead of collaborate. Contempt for the work can result in destructive tactics, tardiness, absenteeism, and turnover, as well as reduced quality and lowered rates of productivity. Conflicts between departments can cause bottlenecks, annoying delays, and internal inefficiencies. Customer service can deteriorate, causing reduced sales, increased customer complaints, and loss of goodwill. (T.R.V. Davis, 1985: 170)

Question

1 What suggestions can you make for breaking down the barriers between managerial and worker subcultures?

Source: adapted from T.R.V. Davis (1985)

- *Similar personal characteristics* In those situations where people with similar characteristics (such as age, education and ethnicity) share the same social space, they are likely to form subcultures.
- *Cohesion* There are a whole range of factors that lead incipient groups to become subcultures. Features of groups such as perceived performance success, physical isolation from other groups and the experience of a crisis or threat can all lead to group cohesion.

Two particular types of subculture that deserve special mention are occupational subcultures and unions. In large internally differentiated organisations the professional training of accountants, lawyers, engineers, marketeers and so on plays a major role in shaping the nature of subcultures. Well-established occupations which claim exclusive rights to conduct certain tasks, sanction certain sorts of training and qualifications for their members, and are regulated by formal rules and codes of ethics are highly influential. They generally prescribe certain beliefs, values and behaviours for their members, often have their own specialist languages, and may even have identifiable rites, rituals, symbols and myths. Members of occupational subcultures are overwhelmingly likely to have their organisational allegiances tempered by the demands of their occupation, its training, rules and ethos. Similarly, in some organisations more employees will belong to a union (or professional association) than do not, and this affiliation may carry with it certain cultural requirements, such as the tendency to value collective action and/or a belief in the right to strike. Morgan (1986) has claimed that trade unions are foremost among all organisational subcultures, and argues that they may often be involved in an ideological struggle with the organisation for the loyalty and commitment of employees.

Looking at cultures more generally, Martin and Siehl (1983) have identified three distinct types of subculture, which they describe as enhancing, orthogonal and counterculture:

- *Enhancing subcultures* In these subcultures individuals adhere to the principal beliefs and values of the dominant culture more intensely than in the rest of the organisation. For example, in organisations with a lengthy history and stable employment pattern, there often develops a coterie of long-serving employees whose fierce commitment to the company culture contrasts with the weaker bonds felt by newer recruits.
- *Orthogonal subcultures* Here individuals subscribe to the core values and beliefs of the dominant organisational culture, while simultaneously accepting a separate and unconflicting belief/value set. For instance, employees working in an R&D department might both endorse their organisation's dominant culture and retain their own cultural identity as believers in the value of innovation, creativity and experimentation.
- *Countercultures* Countercultures present a direct challenge to the dominant culture of an organisation, and exist in an uneasy symbiotic relationship. This situation typically arises after a takeover or merger has occurred, in which case it is usual to see members of the dominant organisation attempting to expand the influence of their culture over the new subsidiary and its employees.

An illustration of subcultures in large, complex organisations is provided in Mini Case 3.1, which concerns General Motors. It is also worth noting here that the strength of an organisational culture is inextricably linked to the number and nature of subcultures it embraces (see Chapter 2).

General Motors

Martin and Siehl (1983) have illustrated how John DeLorean attempted to create a counterculture in opposition to the dominant culture at General Motors (GM). The methods DeLorean used are highly instructive, and provide great insight into the process of culture formation as well as the nature of subcultures.

GM culture

GM is a large US-based car manufacturer. Three of its most strictly observed belief/value clusters concerned respect for authority, conformity and loyalty. Each of these will be briefly considered. Deference to those in authority at GM was a central value, and was reflected in certain norms of behaviour. For example, subordinates were expected to meet their superiors from outside the area at the local airport, carry their bags, pay their hotel and meal bills, and drive them around. In fact, the higher the status of the superior, the larger the retinue that was obliged to wait at the airport: a chief engineer required at least one assistant engineer, while the chairman of the board would be met by literally dozens of senior people.

Invisibility through conformity was another key value. Ideal GM employees were supposed to fit in to the organisation without drawing attention to themselves in any way. This belief/value cluster was manifested in reprimands for employees who found themselves in the media, and in the dress code and decor of the organisation. GM's dress norms in the 1960s prescribed a dark suit, a light shirt and a muted tie, while the offices of GM buildings were all standardised and nondescript. Most importantly of all, the good GM worker had to be a team player ready to take part in the day-to-day rites and rituals of organisational life. Chief among these was the necessity to eat with colleagues at lunch times, generally on-site in a company dining room. Failure to comply with such norms of behaviour often led to individuals being described as 'poor team players', with its associated block on their promotion prospects.

The third core value was loyalty to one's boss and the company. This was most clearly illustrated in special ceremonies, such as retirement dinners. On these occasions glowing biographies of the retiree were expounded in long speeches which served to pledge continuing mutual respect, admiration and loyalty. So important was loyalty to GM's culture that the researchers could detect no organisational stories which cast the company in a negative light. There were also no stories concerning people who had left the firm only to return to the fold, because those who left were considered deserters and could not be welcomed back.

DeLorean's counterculture

DeLorean headed one division at GM for some years. During this time he behaved in ways which directly confronted the dominant culture, circulated stories which ridiculed certain core values, and attempted to alter various organisational artefacts. Helped by his senior position and charismatic personality, he succeeded in creating a counterculture.

DeLorean attacked the dominant culture by failing to meet his boss, Peter Estes, at the airport on one occasion. While Estes is reported to have flown into a rage and admonished DeLorean in unequivocal terms, DeLorean's lack of enthusiasm for deference to authority was clearly illustrated to his subordinates. DeLorean also enjoyed telling how a group of sales people preparing for a visit from an executive learned that he liked to have a refrigerator full of beer, sandwiches and fruit in his room. Accordingly, they rented a refrigerator and ordered food and beer. Unfortunately, the fridge proved to be too large to get through the door of the hotel suite they had lined up. As the hotel would not let them rip out the door and part of the adjoining wall they had to hire a crane to lift the fridge up, knock out a set of windows, and lower it through the gaping hole. The story obviously illustrates how a core cultural value can be taken to an unacceptable extreme, and DeLorean used it to ridicule a major feature of the then accepted GM culture.

DeLorean also opposed GM's emphasis on the need for employees to fit in and be good team players, a view he put into practice by changing the company's performance appraisal system: out went subjective criteria concerning how willing an employee was to conform, and in came more objective measures of performance. In addition, once head of the Chevrolet division he made radical decor changes, with bright carpets, restained panelling and modern furniture being brought in. Moreover, executives were empowered to decorate their own offices according to their individual tastes. DeLorean also role-modeled deviance in his personal appearance by wearing suits with a continental cut, off-white shirts and wider than normal ties. While his deviance was certainly carefully calibrated to remain within defined limits, it nevertheless tested the dominant culture's latitude of acceptance.

Finally, DeLorean opposed demands for unquestioning loyalty with a story concerning the Corvair. DeLorean told how the Corvair was initially seen as innovative and appealing by those in GM, and that it seemed to reflect the finest qualities of the company. However, the car suffered from serious design flaws. The rear engine was rumoured to be unsafe and there was evidence that the car was unstable at high speeds. Nevertheless, the car was launched and the inevitable deaths of motorists occurred. A 'Watergate mentality' took hold of the organisation, and attempts were made to buy and destroy evidence of owner complaints about the car. The resulting court cases, legal expenses and damage to GM's reputation were enumerated by the narrator. DeLorean then made his major point: groupthink based on misplaced loyalty to people and to the organisation could be extremely dangerous and costly.

Conclusions

While DeLorean was highly successful for a time his dissent finally led to his falling from grace within GM, and he left to found his own company. Countercultures, then, are not just hard to create but may be difficult for one person to sustain in the long term.

Questions

1 What were the dominant GM values that DeLorean attempted to counter?
2 How did DeLorean seek to create a counterculture?
3 Why was his success only fleeting?

Reprinted, by permission of the publisher, from *Organisational Dynamics*, autumn/1983 © 1983. American Management Association, New York. All rights reserved.

Source: adapted from Martin and Siehl (1983).

To conclude, the experience of individuals in organisations is thus, in general, a multicultural one. What is more, any given individual is likely to find that he or she is a member of a variety of different subcultures, and that these can make rather different demands on his or her values and behaviours. The situation is complicated still further by the possibility that individuals will, over time, move between different subcultures. While engineers are unlikely to become accountants, the human resource departments of many organisations are populated by individuals who have been moved from other parts of the organisation: in some organisations secretaries can join the ranks of the managers; in universities research students commonly become faculty members; and many workers slip in and out of union membership. The facts of multiculturalism and changing subcultural allegiances suggests that as students of culture we should focus our analyses both at the organisational and at a more micro level.

THE FUNCTIONS OF ORGANISATIONAL CULTURE

Most commentators tend to emphasise that culture is an asset. In this vein, a large number of functions have been attributed to organisational culture. For example, Hampden-Turner (1990: 11) has suggested that 'the culture of an organisation defines appropriate behaviour, bonds and motivates individuals and asserts solutions where there is ambiguity. It governs the way a company processes information, its internal relations and its values'. In more specific terms, the most significant functions of culture have been said to include: conflict reduction, co-ordination and control, the reduction of uncertainty, motivation and competitive advantage. However, some authors like Sathe (1985a, b) have argued that an organisation's culture can also be a liability. This is because shared beliefs, values and assumptions can interfere with the needs of the business and lead people to think and act in commercially and/or ethically inappropriate ways. With this caveat in mind, let us briefly review some of the more widely commented upon advantages of a culture.

Conflict reduction

Most culture theorists emphasise the important role that culture plays in fostering social cohesion. Culture has been described as the 'cement' or 'glue' that bonds an organisation together. A common culture promotes consistency of perception, problem definition, evaluation of issues and options, and preferences for action. Given that there are strong tendencies for organisations to be highly conflictual and antagonistic, culture is a useful force for integration and consensus. According to Schein (1985a) organisations need to evolve a consensus on two sets of issues: (1) those which help the group to survive in and adapt to the external environment, and (2) those which help an organisation to integrate its internal processes in order to survive and adapt. Some of the most significant problems of external adaptation and survival faced by organisations include developing consensus on its mission and strategy, its goals, the means by which those goals are to be achieved, the criteria used to measure how well the organisation is achieving its goals, and the appropriate corrective strategies that should be employed if the group is not meeting its goals. Concerning internal integration, individuals in organisations must reach consensus on how to communicate with each other, the bases for wielding power, the rules for conducting interpersonal relationships at work, how and why rewards are to be distributed, and how to deal with ambiguous and seemingly inexplicable situations.

Co-ordination and control

Largely because culture promotes consistency of outlook it also facilitates organisational processes of co-ordination and control. Culture in the form of stories and myths provides the agreed norms of behaviour or rules that enable individuals to reach agreement on how to organise in general and the process by which decisions should be reached in particular. Where a complex decision has to be taken organisational culture may even help narrow the range of options to be considered. The idea here is that some potential courses of action may be ruled out at the outset as being culturally incompatible (for example, they may be considered unethical) or having unacceptable countercultural consequences, such as a detrimental impact on the environment. Not only is culture a major force for co-ordination, but in the form of values, beliefs, attitudes and especially basic assumptions, culture is also a powerful means of control within organisations. Cultural preconceptions effectively delimit the extent to which employees are free to express their individuality in a way which is far more subtle and beguiling than an organisation's formal control systems, rules and procedures. The increasingly overt attempts by many organisations to mobilise their cultures for competitive advantage seems to illustrate a growing recognition of the power of culture to specify desired behaviour and enforce discipline.

Reduction of uncertainty

In the conduct of their work activities individuals and organisations face considerable uncertainty and complexity. At an individual level one of the functions of culture is in the transmission of learning or 'cultural knowledge' to new recruits. It is through the adoption of a coherent culture that members learn to perceive reality in a particular way, to make certain assumptions about what things are important, how things work and how to behave. The adoption of the cultural mindframe is an anxiety reducing device which simplifies the world, makes choices easier and rational action seem possible. Much the same is true at the level of the organisation. All organisations are confronted with overwhelming uncertainty, conflicts of interest and complexity. However, through a culture's myths, metaphors, stories and symbols an organisation is able to construct its own world. This is most usually a world in which complexity is much reduced, uncertainties are neutralised, and the organisation's ability to exert control over its own activities and engage in rational action is maximised. We should, however, always remember that culture is an enormously powerful means of influencing how we interpret the world, and naturally enough there are dangers associated with those cultures that perpetuate dysfunctional beliefs, values, attitudes and assumptions.

Motivation

Organisational culture can be an important source of motivation for employees, and thus a significant influence on the efficiency and effectiveness of organisations. Most organisations make strenuous attempts to motivate their employees by making use of rewards such as bonuses and promotions and the threat of punishments in the form of unwanted transfers, demotions and salary decrements, to name but a few. These extrinsic factors are effective up to a point, but are far more likely to have their desired effect when employees are also motivated by intrinsic factors. Intrinsic theories of motivation counsel that employees are motivated when they find their work meaningful and enjoyable, they identify their aims and objectives with those of the organisation, and they feel valued and secure. Organisational culture is obviously of great potential significance here. An appropriate and cohesive culture can offer employees a focus of identification and loyalty, foster beliefs and values that encourage employees to think of themselves as high performers doing worthwhile jobs, and promulgate stories, rites and ceremonies which create feelings of belonging.

Competitive advantage

It has been suggested that a strong organisational culture can be a source of competitive advantage. The argument is that because a strong culture promotes consistency, co-ordination and control, reduces uncertainty and enhances motivation, culture facilitates organisational effectiveness and therefore improves its chances of being successful in the marketplace. Most theorists, however, suggest that this is only a part of the picture. The point is that while there may often be a relationship between an organisation's culture and its performance, there is good evidence to indicate that the relationship is not always positive. In other words, weak cultures may be possessed by high performing companies and strong cultures may also be possessed by organisations with below average performance measures. Kotter and Heskett (1992), for example, have identified ten large and well known organisations (including Sears, Procter & Gamble and Goodyear) that have exceptionally strong cultures and relatively weak performance over the period 1977–1988 (see Chapter 6).

As was noted above writers on culture have tended to emphasise its positive implications for organisations, and indeed, in many cases these should not be underestimated. Not all organisational cultures are, though, necessarily functional. It is a common observation that many organisations are not performing to anything like their maximum potential, and large numbers of organisations decline and die every year. In these instances it seems reasonable to assume that a dysfunctional culture has played (and is playing) a role in thwarting organisational achievement. In short, it seems that there are cultures which feature beliefs, values and assumptions that promote conflict, undermine co-ordination and control, increase uncertainty and confusion, diminish employee motivation and reduce competitive advantage (see Chapter 6). What is clear is that culture has a pervasive influence on organisational life.

CULTURE AND IDENTITY

The concept of identity has attracted increasing attention in recent years, and has been linked to that of culture in two ways. First, some authors have chosen to describe groups and organisations, and indeed even professions and industries, as having identities, either instead of or in addition to cultures. Second, some theorists have suggested that the cultures of groups and organisations play a role in shaping the social identities of individuals. Here we will focus on two questions: (1) What is meant by 'organisational identity'? and (2) How does an organisation's culture influence the identities of organisational participants?

Organisational identity

An organisation's identity may be thought of as those cognitive traits and behavioural characteristics that participants attribute to their organisation. Organisational identity is often thought of as a narrower term than organisational culture, excluding many of the assumptions, symbols and rituals that participants do not consider as defining characteristics of their organisation. This may be because they do not recognise them as significant or, especially in the case of assumptions, are not aware of them at all. Identities can, of course, be attributed to organisations by third party observers, and these attributed identities may be much closer to what we understand as cultures. Keen to preserve a difference between culture and identity, some authors have argued that we should use the phrase 'external image' to refer to the identity an organisation chooses to project to the outside world. The external image of an organisation seems in many ways to be a near synonym for what we have previously described as an organisation's espoused culture (*see* Chapter 1, p. 31). The substantive difference is that while an organisation's espoused culture is projected internally as a control mechanism by senior managers as well as externally, the organisation's external image is the product of all members and is solely for external consumption.

The idea that organisations deliberately seek to project a particular identity or image to external constituencies is an important one for at least two reasons. In the first instance, it suggests that there may be instrumental value to an organisation in constructing a profile, that while it may have no relation to actual characteristics of the organisation, assists it in its attempt to pursue its mission. Alvesson and Berg (1992), for example, write of organisations that project images of service-mindedness, reliability, status and quality as part of their marketing efforts. Corporate identity, for the marketeer, is a strategic tool that is used to manipulate consumer perceptions of an organisation and its products. Second, it points to the danger that organisations face of coming to believe their own rhetoric. Morgan (1997: 259) has described the egocentrism of organisations which leads them to try 'to sustain unrealistic identities or to produce identities that ultimately destroy important elements of the contexts of which they are part'. Those firms which once produced watches and typewriters and which failed to take account of new digital and microprocessing technologies provide a salutary lesson in this respect. The same phenomenon has been described by Brown and Starkey (1994), who tell the story of a sugar confectionery company which defined itself as a manufacturing rather than a marketing concern, failed to systematically attend to its environment, with its attendant opportunities and threats, and was ultimately acquired by a competitor organisation.

Individual identity

It has been convincingly argued that our idea of self, or identity, is neither innate nor fixed, but rather develops in a continuous process. That is, we are creatures that have continually to realise ourselves and make sense of our place in a potentially chaotic world. The organisations and other groups to which we recognise allegiance will all play a role in shaping our conceptions of self. Thus the cultures and identities of the social groups of which we are members help us to define our individual identities. They provide cognitive, social and emotional frameworks that give us a sense of coherence, stability and belonging. Such memberships also allow us to develop favourable self-images that contribute to our general feelings of well-being and self-esteem. Where it is rewarding in these ways for us to identify with a particular group or organisation, our identification with that social group and our commitment to it are likely to be high. While memberships of some social categories are highly resistant to change (such as religious affiliation), others (such as work group) are more mobile. As we change organisations and join different groups, so our definitions of self can be expected to alter, though for the most part both subtly and gradually.

Some commentators have suggested that with the decline in the role of the church, work organisations have become increasingly influential in their impact on peoples' thinking and behaviour. Indeed, Bowles (1989) has hypothesised that work organisations are now the dominant creators of meaning for individuals. On the other hand, it has also been argued that the organisational culture perspective underestimates the role of individuals as self-governing agents (Golden, 1992). The crux of the argument is that writers on organisational culture have tended to emphasise the extent to which employee action is shaped and constrained by culture, forgetting that individuals are often highly critical and self-aware. For example, it is well known that employees are able to analyse and comment upon their situation in ways that often seem to challenge the existing status quo. Our understanding of culture, then, must be informed with the knowledge that individuals do challenge cultural guidelines. From her analysis Golden identified four strategies for individual action with respect to a dominant organisational culture: unequivocal adherence, strained adherence, secret non-adherence and overt non-adherence. Let us consider each of these in turn.

Unequivocal adherence

This refers to action which reinforces and directly corresponds with norms promulgated by the dominant culture. Individuals who employ this strategy are fully convinced of the efficacy of the culture to which they defer in framing their actions and decisions.

Strained adherence

This behaviour is consonant with cultural guidelines (and so may look like unequivocal adherence), but leads the individuals concerned to experience tension. Employees using this strategy are likely to have some reservations about the wisdom of certain cultural norms and proclivities. Perhaps the most common manifestations of strained adherence are the use of jokes and other forms of social comedy as the means for muting conflict and relieving frustrations.

Secret non-adherence

This consists of overt compliance with cultural norms but covert departure from them. Individuals employing this strategy wish to be seen (generally by senior managers) as conforming to the prescriptions of the dominant culture, but may sometimes act in ways which demonstrate their opposition, though usually only when it is safe to do so.

Open non-adherence

This behaviour involves departure from cultural norms in full view of others within the organisation. Employees using this strategy are sufficiently secure or uncaring that they will act in ways which directly challenge a dominant culture when it suits them.

While no organisation can continue to survive in the long term without some order and uniformity in action we should always recall that organisational culture is rarely a perfect control system. That is, unequivocal adherence is likely to be the exception rather than the rule. Individuals may often experience latitude and freedom in action when their personal codes of conduct conflict with those suggested by their organisation's culture. Furthermore, this potential for non-conformity is vital if a culture is to be able to adapt and change to meet altered circumstances.

CULTURE FOR ALL?

Most of this book assumes that organisations consist of educated professionals who are highly motivated to invest much of their time and energy in their work. Such people are ready and willing to join in their organisation's cultural life in order to survive and further their career ambitions. This perspective has similarities with McGregor's (1960) Theory Y, which suggests that individuals do not inherently dislike work, are intrinsically motivated, are able to exert self-control and seek responsibility. The extent to which this view can be taken as a general prescription of how individuals and organisations operate is, in some instances, highly questionable. Our assessment of the importance and influence of culture should be sensitive to the following four facts:

1   even the most enthusiastic of organisational participants give only a fraction of their time, energy and commitment to their place of work. Most people are members of a variety of different clubs and societies and often a union and/or a profession as well. Such people cannot be expected to adopt an organisational culture unquestioningly or wholeheartedly. At best, their acceptance will be diluted by the demands and constraints imposed on them by their other affiliations;

2   it is increasingly the case that employees are being engaged in part-time and often temporary employment. These people are far less likely to adopt the cultural mindset than full-time employees. Indeed, for some people the decision to be a part-time worker may well have been made to avoid being caught up in cultural control systems. In short, some people just do not like formal organisations, finding them oppressive and restrictive;

3   the 'hit and run' attitude of part-time and temporary workers is shared by large numbers of full-time employees (Barnatt, 1990). Large numbers of individuals perform relatively undemanding and unrewarding jobs solely for extrinsic rewards (mostly financial). These instrumentally oriented workers do not always see their work organisation as the centre of their existence, may feel a very loose attachment to it, and can even resent and rebel against a dominant culture. Such individuals may be better managed from a Theory X perspective, which assumes that people are lazy, extrinsically motivated, incapable of self-discipline and want security without responsibility;

4   organisations are becoming increasingly inclined to contract out non-core activities. For example, there are manufacturing organisations which subcontract all their marketing activities to advertising agencies rather than employ their own marketing staff. The same is true for many other support services such as cleaning, catering and data processing. As the staff employed in these contracted-out activities are members of separate organisations it is extremely difficult to make them feel part of the culture of the organisation which buys their services. The ultimate scenario is one in which an organisation exists in a sort of 'virtual reality' with all its functions contracted out. The virtual organisation would consist of a few key staff who co-ordinate the activities of substantial organisations in order to produce goods or provide a service. Even if this trend continues there are, of course, always likely to be substantial organisations, though the study of culture may become far more complex.

To sum up, not only are strong and cohesive organisational cultures not to everybody's taste, but in the future changing patterns of employment and changing organisational forms may make the identification and examination of particular cultures still more difficult. Some of the issues raised in this section are illustrated at AussieCo in Mini Case 3.2.

Culture for all at AussieCo.?

Introduction

AussieCo. was an Australian owned and operated producer of computer controlled high precision mechanical hardware. The company was located close to the city of Melbourne, where its 600 employees worked in three large inter-connected buildings. The owner established the organisation in 1962, and has retained full control throughout its expansion. Now acting as the chairman and chief executive most final decisions are made by him, though he is not involved in the daily running of the business. The executive director is the owner's nephew (who came to the organisation straight from university), while the key person in charge of day-to-day operations is the general manager.

AussieCo. had made its reputation on the basis of a single product which in 1980 dominated the market. Since this time, however, its share of the market dropped from 90% to 60% in the early 1990s. Furthermore, the company's attempts to diversify into other products have had only limited success, mainly due to the management's failure to understand the special situations in the markets concerned. In addition, senior managers were aware that while the company's machines sold for $AUS 9500 they should cost less than $AUS 1500 to make. Profitability was virtually nil. The quality of the final product was also suffering, and the company was losing its good name. Further problems were caused by the site installation staff, many of whom were unqualified, who damaged about 20% of stock.

Organisational culture

AussieCo. employed only migrant labour at the operative level, and these were mostly unqualified people with limited English. Even key personnel (programmers, engineers, technicians) were mainly of migrant origin or lacked formal qualifications. What is more, the system of finding jobs for family or friends (known in local parlance as 'mates') seemed prevalent. In the manufacturing process employees were subject to *efficiency measurements* (numerical targets) designed to ensure that they worked at a reasonable speed. This control system was the subject of ridicule by staff, who deliberately slowed down when efficiency measurements were calculated in order to avoid later harassment for not meeting daily standards. No rewards were given for the attainment of targets.

Staff at AussieCo. had little pride in the company. Operatives and long serving unqualified managers were constantly fearful of losing their jobs, while the technocrats had such a comfortable and easy life with good pay that few contemplated leaving. The owner's dictatorial attitude, ignorance of modern trends, memory loss and temper tantrums were also of increasing concern. What is more, anybody who tried to show him anything that was wrong with the company became his instant enemy. Poor communication between some departments and no communication at all between others meant that clusters of functions operated with an 'ivory tower' mentality.

A brief resume of a typical working day at AussieCo. provides a graphic insight into some of the organisation's problems. The working day for employees and lower management commenced at 7.30a.m. Most staff arrived frustrated from looking for a parking space or a 20 minute walk from the nearest station. Employees then rushed to punch time clocks. At 7.30 a.m. a bell rang and staff moved slowly to their positions. The female operatives on one production line were waiting for a supply of resistors. The stores computer showed a stock of 4700 pieces, but none could be located, and nor could any be ordered until the programme was corrected. A technician was sent out to purchase a week's supply of resistors from a local store (retail price $AUS 8) paid for by a supervisor.

Middle and senior managers arrived between 9.00 a.m. and 10.00 a.m. Assembly line workers held back production using any weak and vague excuse in the hope of being able to work overtime. This was possible because the production supervisor was a qualified carpet fitter with no knowledge of the day-to-day tasks of his subordinates. Meanwhile, in the programming department, a senior programmer had been told to prepare some programmes, work he is allowed to do at home. As he had done the same job a few years ago, however, he planned to take his wife on holiday to Queensland for five days.

Before lunch the owner announced that a big order had been received. The production manager complained that the order was from a company that did not pay for a shipment sent about a year ago, and was summarily ordered out of the chief executive's office. The production manager attempted to contact the administration manager in an attempt to prevent the order from being accepted, but he was unavailable as he was playing golf with the executive managing director. The general manager claimed that he had no idea what was going on and that the owner never told him anything. Lunch was then served in a staff canteen (for junior employees), an executive dining room (for senior managers) and a showroom (for sales staff).

After lunch the general manager walked around the building. Nobody knew why he did this as he never talked to anyone and few people other than senior managers knew who he was.

The workplace itself was cluttered and filthy, though filled with state-of-the-art machinery. The afternoon was punctuated with personnel problems. A process worker was sacked for complaining that he had to put handles on machines, which other workers had then to remove in order to assemble further parts. In the metalshop a new foreman discovered a man with no work; he had been forgotten since the fitting of a new welding automat. Part of the problem was that there was no personnel manager, the previous incumbent having been dismissed for sexual harassment two months ago. At 4.00 p.m. a bell rung and all the staff ran from the building. All, that is, except a select group of workers on the assembly line who had successfully played the overtime game, and who pulled out newspapers and coffee mugs.

Questions

1 'The culture and working practices of AussieCo. do not encourage individuals to identify positively with the organisation, and they do not derive self-esteem from their membership of it.'

(a) Is this true?
(b) If it is true, is it really a problem?
(c) If it is a problem, what can be done to improve matters?

Source: adapted from Jones and Gal (1994).

Gender

Gherardi (1995) relates how women working in an Italian bank had been treated over the past generation. At first, there were few of them, and they worked away from the public, hidden because it was thought that customers might experience discomfort talking about financial issues with women. Later, women were moved to the cash desks because it was considered that customers would appreciate a demure presence. More recently, the bank began to express an interest in promoting women to more senior levels, but only because there was a shortage of suitably qualified male personnel. What is more, the invitation to women to follow senior managerial career paths was dressed-up in language that suggested distrust of equality, contempt for women and reluctance to change.

This brief vignette is important for us because it helps us to focus on gender issues in organisational cultures, and especially how some cultures develop which systematically devalue everything associated with women. Many authors have argued that the study of organisations disregards gender issues, that organisations have traditionally and quite wrongly been depicted as genderless, and that this has led to a unidimensional view of organisations. The result is some bizarre conclusions in organisational research, such as Blauner's (1967) argument that male dissatisfaction is a valid expression of alienation from their working conditions, but that female discontent is the result of their weaker physical stamina and family commitments. Such highly prejudiced interpretations have stimulated feminist critiques of organisation studies, and these have found increasing support in recent years. Attempting to redress the balance some authors, such as Mills (1988) and Gherardi (1995), have suggested that a cultural approach to understanding gender issues is likely to yield considerable insights.

The first important point to note is that what happens in organisations is profoundly influenced by broader social rules of behaviour. A variety of authors have shown how organisations in the West reflect and reinforce popularly held images of women as low paid, lacking in authority, essentially domestic, illogical and fickle. These images incorporate a value structure which restricts the entry of women into the labour force, and limits their ability to succeed in organisations where they do gain entry. That a gender bias in favour of men prevails in other parts of the world has been demonstrated by Ouchi (1981), who has shown how large Japanese corporations gear their benefits to male employees. General trends at the level of national culture and society, however, still leave plenty of scope for variation between organisations.

Focusing at the organisational level, Gherardi (1995) has suggested that there are great differences in cultural orientation towards women. This is sometimes obvious in the architecture of an organisation's buildings, which may give the impression of strength and virility (masculinity) or care and intimacy (femininity). It may also be reflected in the language employed, which may be one of domination, battles, campaigns, conquests and power plays, or reflect a concern with care, needs and relationality. This said, Gherardi maintains that most organisations perpetuate broader social patterns of patriarchy in which women are depicted as subordinate and subservient. In short, while the upper echelons of hierarchy are occupied by men, women tend to be clustered at the bottom, and what is more, expected to be discreet (sometimes to the point of invisibility), generous, sensitive, nurturing and emotional. Such informal norms then make it difficult for women to aspire to more senior positions or compete with men.

It has been pointed out that there are gender differences between different types of organisation, and between different departments within organisations. The world of business is dominated by men, while professions such as the civil service, school teaching and nursing attract larger numbers of women, though even here senior positions are often held by men. In general, production departments are often more male, while personnel and administrative departments are more frequently staffed by women. There are, of course, exceptions to these very broad categorisations, and some authors have suggested that the real point to be made is that women tend to work in the less prestigious and powerful organisations and organisational departments. This argument is supported by research which shows that, for example, in the legal profession men dominate prestigious jobs in commercial and criminal case law, while women often do desk work and deal with matrimonial lawsuits (Podmore and Spender, 1986). Issues of gender and culture, then, are intimately connected with prevailing patterns of power.

Organisational culture, gender and career narratives

This mini case is based on a doctoral research programme concerned with the gendered construction of high-level careers in business and politics in Belgium, Britain and France. What follows is a summary of one interview and a tentative analysis that reveals much about how women construct their identities within organisational cultures.

The profile examined is of a personnel director for Europe in the Belgium office of a multinational company in the energy industry. She has a long service record with the company and has occupied her present position for approximately five years. The focus of the case is to consider what career histories, as told in the form of individual stories, can convey about organisational cultures. Underlying this is a belief that the way in which stories are told depends on the context of the experience, in this case the organisation in which the career has been pursued. Thus the way in which individuals talk about their careers tells us something about the organisational culture in which they work. In addition, their stories can tell us something about gender relations in organisational cultures.

The following extract is a summary of a single interview and is intended to illustrate some of the things that work histories can reveal about organisational cultures. The interviewee was asked to give an account of how she came to occupy her current position.

Mrs Personnel begins her story by saying that she was unable to find work in her field of study, the history of art. So she turned to the private sector and found a position in her current company. She explains this with reference to the opportunities created by certain organisational activities of the time, for example, large-scale advertising campaigns, which were a new development and required numerous personnel. After one year she applied for a job in personnel – in recruitment – commenting that the vacancy arose because the company was expanding its workforce. She had some internal training and, she says, she was self-taught. She gives almost no information between her first job in personnel (her second job in the company) and her current position, commenting only that she rose progressively, expanding the scope of her work,

until she replaced her boss as head of personnel for Belgium. This occurred at the moment that the company was celebrating the distribution of its products in Belgium. Since this time she has become head of personnel for Europe, which, she explains, came about as the company merged with another in the same industry and was then integrated into the European parent company. She says that this expansion of her responsibilities has not changed her work very much. She comments, "What progresses work is the way the company is managed."

I have chosen to explore here two elements of the way the personnel director talks about her career. First, the extent to which she presents it as the *intended* outcome of choices based on conscious long-term *strategies* as opposed to it being *contingent* or *unplanned*. We might expect that men would be more likely than wo men to pursue and/or present their careers as the outcome of rational decision making. Alternatively, it may be that women need to plan to achieve positions that men obtain without planning. In this case, the personnel manager describes herself as, in effect, *reacting* to newly created structural opportunities in the private sector generally, and in the company in particular, first in advertising, then in recruitment. This was initially the result of her not being able to find work in her chosen area.

Mrs Personnel then refers to herself as self-taught which is interesting. It may suggest a reactive approach, to the needs of the time, or a planned, instrumental approach oriented towards a future goal. It may be that her decisions were not strategically calculated, but an internalised sense of the organisational culture directed her in ways which were later rewarded. This may also be relevant for her relative silence on her progression within personnel. It suggests a taken-for-granted understanding of the inevitable career ladder she followed, such that it requires almost no description. All she says is that she expanded the scope of her work which does not tell us to what extent this was through her own initiative, that is strategic, or reactive and contingent. It is perhaps worth noting that her language is in the first person ('*I* expanded the scope of my work . . .') as a clue to the extent of her planning. Yet, overall, she stresses the structural changes in the organisation which both create opportunities and constrain individual strategies for long-term career planning, and her final remark re-emphasises the importance of company practices in shaping work.

This leads us to consider a second aspect of the story; whether Mrs Personnel says her career path has been partly *dependent* on other people or events, or as the result of her own *independent* achievements. In fact, she describes all of the moments of her career history in relation to a change or development in company practices. This is by no means inevitable. She could quite easily have talked about other life events, such as the birth of her children, or focused much more on how her career moves were rewards for her own achievements. Later, when prompted, she does talk of her debts to her boss and to her husband, but this is not how she first chooses to tell her story. This tells us something about her character, but also something of the culture of the organisation, for instance, that it emphasises collective rather than individual success.

It may also tell us something about gender relations within the organisation or more generally.

We might expect that contemporary ideas about masculinity and femininity would encourage men, more than women, to emphasise their own capacities and competencies rather than the people or events that have enabled them to succeed. We might expect also that a woman would consider herself to have been fortunate rather than smart in achieving such success. Alternatively, we could imagine that the achievement of such a high-level position requires the person to adopt certain kinds of behaviour, and even ways of thinking, which we can broadly characterise as masculine, such that we would find little difference between the stories of men and women in these positions.

Overall, we see that the ways in which people 'make sense' of their experience, in employment or more generally, are shaped by environmental factors. So, when they tell us about their working lives they also tell us about the cultures of the organisations in which they have lived them.

Questions

1 What general and specific lessons does this mini case teach us about gender relations and culture in organisations?

2 With reference to an organisation with which you are familiar, discuss how different individuals (men and women) would tell their career stories.

Source: This case was written by Dawn Lyon, Department of Social and Political Science, European University Institute, Florence, Italy.

Some theorists have suggested that organisations tend to use women to deal with particularly deviant or difficult external constituents and internal groups, because they are less threatening. The argument is that they are seen to lack authority themselves (i.e. to be exercising power vicariously on behalf of others), and can therefore effectively exercise control without exciting hostility and resentment. This exercise of control through sexuality and seduction is most obviously practised by women in, for example, the socialisation of new recruits, the maintaining of inter-organisational relationships with customers and suppliers, and by front-desk workers who interface with corporate visitors. In other words, sexuality can itself be thought of as a power resource, though in these instances it is one that is being exploited by the organisation for its own purposes rather than by women for themselves. The idea that women are systematically devalued, disempowered and manipulated by the cultures of some (possibly most) organisations is the central point of many feminist analyses (see Mini Case 3.3).

CULTURE AND LEARNING

'Organisational learning' is now a significant element of the organisational change and development literature. The idea that organisations are able to learn in ways analogous to those of individuals provides us with another way of understanding how and why organisations adapt to their environments. In an organisational context, learning has been described as 'a process in which people discover a problem, invent a solution to the problem, produce the solution, and evaluate the outcome, leading to the discovery of new problems' (Argyris, 1982: 38). Two basic types of learning are often distinguished: single-loop learning, which involves minor adjustments, replacements or refinements of response, and double-loop learning, which implies important changes in values and assumptions, making completely new responses possible. The importance of an organisation's culture to learning processes is not hard to discern: different cultures may assist or impede problem discovery, define the range of solutions that may be invented (or discovered) and produced, and influence the evaluation of outcomes and, subsequently, the perception of new problems. Here we will confine ourselves to the role of organisational culture in three fundamental questions: (1) How do organisations learn? (2) What are the barriers to learning? (3) How do organisations store (and retrieve) their learning?

How do organisations learn?

Organisations typically learn either through direct organisational experience or vicariously from the experience of other organisations. Learning from experience often involves trial-and-error experimentation with a range of different routines. Learning from others (competitors, customers, suppliers, professional organisations and so forth) generally involves a search procedure to discover potentially useful routines, and their subsequent imitation and incorporation. Learning from experience and from others is likely to be culture-sensitive, with cultures that encourage trial-and-error, search and mimetic behaviours associated with an increased capacity for organisational learning. Conversely, those cultures that do not promote these organisational behaviours may be less able to learn.

Both learning paths crucially depend on positive and negative *feedback*. People learn from the positive and negative feedback they receive about their actions, repeating what gains positive feedback (is successful) and giving up behaviour that receives negative feedback (is unsuccessful). For example, if an organisation works on the principle of always being first to the market with a new product, and that strategy succeeds, then the principle will be incorporated into the organisation's culture. As the validity of responses is being continually tested, so when the environment changes and previously successful strategies begin to fail, this will be recognised by the organisation and steps taken to alter the discredited policies.

The relationship between culture and learning is one of reciprocal interdependence. Not only is the rate at which organisations learn dependent on culture, but the culture of an organisation will be profoundly influenced by the rate, and content of, organisational learning. This view, championed by Edgar Schein, that organisational culture develops through complex interactive learning processes, has certain important implications. It means that for an organisation to develop a strong shared culture its members must have had opportunities for collective learning. In those organisations that have a high staff turnover, especially in senior positions, weaker, less integrated cultures may emerge. Conversely, organisations with a low staff turnover probably have a better chance of evolving a more cohesive culture, especially if their members have experienced a shared history of intensely felt events. It also suggests that cultures cannot be created by managerial fiat. If executives are able to impact on an organisation's culture their influence is likely to be felt in the long term, through the subtle manipulation of employees' work environment (see Chapter 5).

Barriers to organisational learning

The barriers to organisational learning are located at the individual and collective levels. At the individual level, cognitive limitations are highly significant. Evidence suggests that people are prone to selective perception, failing to notice some salient information and interpreting what they do detect in ways that reflect their own preconceptions. Individuals are well known to have rather limited short-term memory space, with the result that valuable data items can easily be forgotten. Psychologists have demonstrated that people are subject to a range of cognitive biases such as recency (over-attributing importance to more recently acquired information), and halo effects (allowing one positive feature to unduly affect our judgement). Studies show that we are imperfect statisticians, and that we often make systematic errors in recording events and making inferences. These cognitive limitations are most obviously exposed when individuals are faced with highly interconnected, fast-changing and complex environments, which overload people with what can seem to be ambiguous, confused and even contradictory messages. The implications of these phenomena for organisations, especially in terms of missed opportunities for organisational learning, can be profound.

At a collective level the influences of politics and culture are, perhaps, the most important potential inhibitors of organisational learning. Organisational politics can counteract and neutralise individuals' and groups' positive learning initiatives. The political influence of dominant coalitions can also be responsible for rejecting information, however valid, which does not suit their requirements, and refusing to pursue solutions to problems if such solutions threaten to undermine their authority. Organisational cultures can retard learning in any number of ways, some of which have already been described above. In addition to these, it is worth noting that cultures may prescribe reward and punishment systems that inadvertently paralyse individuals, specify ambiguous roles and tasks, making co-ordinated learning activity difficult, and fail to ensure that resources are distributed to learning-oriented individuals and groups. Cultures may also be responsible for promoting and protecting competency traps. This occurs where favourable performance with an inferior procedure leads an organisation to accumulate more experience with it. Under these conditions its replacement with a superior procedure is unlikely because the organisation cannot accumulate sufficient positive experience with the superior procedure to make it rewarding to use.

While organisational learning is assisted by positive and negative feedback, it is directly inhibited by *trauma*. Unlike trial-and-error behaviour, trauma does not involve an organisation in continually testing the validity of its responses. Many theorists have argued that people (individuals and groups) tend to act so as to reduce any work-related pain or anxiety they may experience. When an organisation is first formed there is likely to be considerable uncertainty as to whether it will survive and be successful. This uncertainty is extremely traumatic for those concerned, and the natural reaction of these individuals is to seek generally acceptable solutions to problems which both seem to work and make life more predictable. While the founder or other leader is often able to impose his or her preferred solutions on the organisation, they may also emerge as a result of group negotiation and consensus.

In addition to the traumas associated with starting a new organisation, most established organisations face occasional crises (real or perceived) at some time in their history. When such a crisis occurs the members develop ways to overcome their discomfort and reduce their anxiety. For example, a UK-based food manufacturer (Sugar Inc.) launched a new product called *Quirks*. The product failed, and the company inquest which followed diagnosed insufficient market research as the primary problem. Organisational members learned that in-depth market research was the way to avoid future trauma, the chief executive of the company started talking about Sugar Inc. as being marketing-led, and the organisation's next set of new products was subject to four separate research studies (see the Case study at the end of this chapter).

The major potential problem with the trauma-based learning mechanism is that once people have learned how to avoid a painful situation they tend to continue to employ the same heuristics and behaviour patterns. This habitual behaviour is a defence mechanism that people are unwilling to re-evaluate to see whether it is relevant or necessary. Part of the reason for this is that the learned response not only avoids the pain, but reduces anxiety, which is rewarding in itself. Trauma-based learning is thus very hard to undo. This means that when environmental change requires that an organisation modify its behaviour, the cultural modification needed may be very difficult to engineer.

Organisational memory

Memory may be defined as the faculty of retaining and recalling things past, and is normally associated with individuals. The idea that organisations have memories, indeed, that they must have some sort of memory capability in order to learn anything at all, is key to the literature on learning. Quite what form organisational memory takes, its distribution, modes of recall and accuracy, are, however, issues that fail to command consensus. Here we will follow Walsh and Ungson's (1991) suggestion that organisational memory consists in the shared interpretations of members, that allow knowledge of the past to be preserved even on the departure of key individuals. They propose that an organisation's memory is stored in six principal ways: (1) in the memories of individuals; (2) in culture, especially symbols, stories, myths and other artefacts; (3) in administrative systems and procedures such as selection and socialisation, and in rules; (4) in the structural roles that individuals perform; (5) in the physical structure of an organisation, its layout of offices and furniture; and (6) in external archives such as former employees, competitors and government regulatory bodies.

The important idea for us is that an organisation's culture constitutes an element of its memory, and is a repository of information that can be brought to bear on current problems and in the making of current decisions. While little empirical research has been conducted in this area, it is tempting to speculate that different cultures will vary enormously in terms of variables such as the ease with which stored information can be retrieved, and the accuracy of the retrieved information. Different cultures will thus be associated with different learning capacities as a consequence of their different qualities as memory devices.

CULTURE AND GROUPTHINK

Groupthink is a term coined by Irving Janis (1972) to describe the phenomenon where members of a group come to think and behave in similar ways. Groupthink consists of 'a collective pattern of defensive avoidance, lack of vigilance, unwarranted optimism, sloganistic thinking, suppression of worrisome defects, and reliance on shared rationalisations' (Janis, 1972: 399). It is most frequently associated with groups operating under pressure. The motivating force which generates groupthink is individual members' need for self-esteem. This implies that the greater the threat to members' self-esteem, the greater will be their tendency to engage in groupthink at the expense of critical thinking. This is because highly cohesive, concurrence-seeking groups provide a source of security for members, which reduces their anxiety and heightens their positive feelings about themselves and their worth.

Four particular characteristics of groupthink are worth noting. First, in circumstances of extreme crisis it is not unknown for groups to engage not just in collective panic, but violent acts of scapegoating. The scapegoating of organisational leaders associated with corporate failure and strike leaders who can conveniently be blamed for organisational problems are well-known examples. Second, groupthink is often associated with feelings of invulnerability, during which members may become euphoric about their capabilities and express boundless admiration for their leader. This happened to President Kennedy and his advisers in the decision-making processes leading to the Bay of Pigs disaster. Third, groupthink often leads to the making of rationalisations, that is, explanations based on stereotypes and ideological assumptions. A good example of this was the US Navy's reasoning that the Japanese would never attack Hawaii because this would cause a war which the USA would ultimately win. Fourth, groupthink can take the form of detachment or dissociation, in which members fail to take into account the consequences of their actions even where these violate their most cherished principles. An example of this was President Johnson's simultaneous espousal of humanitarian values and escalation of the Vietnam war, with all the appalling consequences this had for the Vietnamese people.

Groupthink is evidently a rather different concept than that of culture, in that it only refers to the shared cognitions/behaviours of relatively small and usually face-to-face groups. It also explicitly excludes all reference to group history and symbolism. It is, however, an important phenomenon for us. Some organisational cultures are more prone to groupthink than others, and given that its implications for organisational performance are likely to be profound, we need to be able to recognise and account for it. It suggests that organisational cultures which place extreme emphasis on conformity, allow individuals to work in small groups and in close proximity, and which have relatively few control mechanisms over such groups may well experience groupthink-related problems. Many management consultancy practices and advertising agencies, and all corporate boards, need to ensure that they take adequate measures (such as external monitors and regular reviews) to avoid groupthink.

CULTURE AND ETHICS

Ethical issues now occupy a prominent position on the agendas of many organisations. Pressure from the general public and mass media combined with the particular scrutiny of special interest groups keen to promote the interests of, for example, women, ethnic minorities, the disabled and the environment, has had its affect. Complementing this increased concern with the ethical stance of organisations, management education and development courses, notably MBAs, now often feature courses on business ethics, gender and environmental issues. The importance of culture to our understanding of how organisations deal with these new demands, the ethical choices that organisations in fact make, and their attempts to maintain legitimacy by projecting acceptable ethical stances externally, cannot easily be overestimated. In this section we consider three areas of culture–ethics overlap: (1) artefacts in the form of ethical codes; (2) how ethical choices are implied by values and assumptions; and (3) the linkages between ethics, organisational control mechanisms and individuality.

Ethical codes

While ethical codes may operate informally within some organisations, increasing numbers of corporations and public bodies are publishing their own formal codes of ethical conduct. In terms of Schein's model of culture these are identifiable as material organisational artefacts. Professional associations are particularly likely to have their own detailed codes of ethics, often stating that their members should put their clients' interests before those of their employing organisation. A code of ethics may be thought of as a set of moral principles or guidelines which govern behaviour and which enshrine a set of values and beliefs. Codes of ethics thus concern what is good and bad and right and wrong in organisational decision making, and often reflect attempts by senior managers to mould and manipulate the culture of their organisation. Perhaps the easiest way to promote an organisational code of ethics is to anchor it in some well known stories. Cadbury provides an excellent example of this. In Cadbury it is remembered that in the late nineteenth century Queen Victoria placed an order with the company to provide decorative tins of chocolate to all her soldiers fighting in South Africa. The order placed the company in a quandary because although the extra work was welcome, its owner was publicly opposed to the Anglo-Boer War. The dilemma was ultimately resolved by accepting the order, but carrying it out at cost. Cadbury therefore made no profit out of what was seen as an unjust war, the employees benefited from the additional work, and the soldiers received their royal present (Cadbury, 1987).

Values, assumptions and ethics

For Schein, organisational cultures vary along a continuum from the moralistic, which make decisions based on sets of principles, to the pragmatic, which make decisions based on their own experience of what works. The implication seems to be that some organisations can avoid making ethical choices, and this position is popularly entertained. Bate (1994: 286–7), for instance, asserts that 'the ethical dimension' can be 'missing' from cultures, leading to 'dirty tricks', 'paranoia' and single-loop learning.

However, it is suggested here that the values and assumptions of organisational cultures necessarily imply the adoption of moral positions and the making of ethical choices. That is, Schein's pragmatism and Bate's dirty tricks themselves reflect and incorporate ethical choices to act in particular ways and not to accept other principles for determining action. That we may find such choices repugnant does not mean that an ethical choice, of a sort, has not been made. The same general point has been made by scholars interested in ideologies. Of particular interest for us is Max Weber's illustration of how the Protestant work ethic, with values favouring individualism and hard work, laid the foundation for modern Western capitalism. His analysis shows how the adoption of particular values and assumptions, in particular that wealth is a sign of God's favour, dictates how people will resolve ethical dilemmas regarding how to live a good life, which for Calvinists meant exploiting natural resources to accumulate wealth. Evidently, the influence of a Protestant work ethic is still being felt today, and is an important determinant of many Western organisational cultures.

Ethics, control and individuality

Some authors have argued that organisational cultures exercise a third-order control function over individuals that is morally dubious. A third-order control mechanism is one which influences individuals' ways of thinking, generally without them realising that power has been exercised over them. This reading of organisational culture depicts it as a subtle but insidious way of manipulating people, of restricting their scope for individual expression and curtailing their freedom. Lewicki (1981), for example, refers to this covert manipulation as a form of organisational seduction, and argues that it potentially leads individuals to create a pseudo-world of order and simplicity. Kan (1989) suggests that culture may be viewed as an exploitative tool that legitimates existing power arrangements, and freezes relations of inequality and dominance in such a way as to present them as natural and immutable. While some theorists depict culture as a morally corrupt and corrupting influence on individuals, however, others such as Beyer and Trice (1993) have pointed to an alternative interpretation. They insist that cultures have some benefits for individuals, particularly by reducing their anxieties, and that this will always encourage individuals to form and join cultures. The implication is that because people are inevitably subject to the influence of some cultures (national, social, professional), and that all these exercise some influence on people, it is unfair to denigrate organisations as being particularly morally questionable. In addition, it is worth remembering that organisations vary tremendously in terms of the ethical codes incorporated into their values and assumptions, and most people would agree that, for example, the ethical stances of charities such as Friends of the Earth and Save the Children are less dubious than those of exploitative and acquisitive multinationals.

ORGANISATIONAL CULTURE AND POSTMODERNISM

Postmodern critiques of organisation studies seek to undermine the modernist assumptions that govern most of the work accomplished in this field. They question whether there are any universal, scientific principles which order human behaviour, and celebrate indeterminacy, heterogeneity and ambivalence (Martin, 1992). What follows is an extremely brief overview of some of the key elements of the postmodern critique, and some indications of its importance for those working in the field of organisational culture. It is in no way meant to be a complete or detailed account, for which students are recommended to refer to Hassard and Parker (1993) and Reed and Hughes (1992).

From a postmodern perspective notions of 'truth' and 'reality' do not refer to absolute positions, but effects which result from a reader's privileged reading of a text. For his or her work to be described as 'good research', an author has to present a text which the audience finds plausible and authoritative. In order to accomplish this the author must select an appropriate mode of representation. The mode of representation refers to the way in which a text is written, its use of examples, metaphor, metonymy, structuring of material, tone and other rhetorical devices. Those texts that a reader finds well written, coherent and verisimilitudinous he or she will most likely consider authoritative. The successful author is, therefore, the one who solves the problem of representation to produce texts to which their audience attributes authority. In representing their material texts assume and borrow from the conventions associated with their genre. These intertextual practices exert a profound influence over the production of texts, so much so that some theorists have suggested that later texts tend to re-work and re-represent the ideas of earlier texts without reference to an external world. For the ultimate postmodernist, then, all that exists is an endless production and consumption (critique) of texts.

Postmodernism is an important corpus of ideas for those interested in organisational studies in general and organisational culture in particular. Postmodern theory allows us to recognise at least three salient points:

1 *Organisational culture is an episode* 'Organisational culture' may be regarded as a historical and philosophical episode in organisation studies (Jeffcutt, 1994). This episode is one characterised by a high degree of 'dissensus' in terms of research approaches and epistemologies. Perhaps most striking is the contrast between those discourses that express a resurgent managerialism, and those that express a critical humanism. The important suggestion here, however, is rather that, being an episode, it will sooner or later come to an end. With time the discourse of organisation studies will alter, and as it refocuses the concepts and theories of organisation culture will figure less prominently.

2 *Organisational culture as legitimating device* That so many different authors conducting very different sorts of research work have chosen to describe themselves as focusing on issues of culture is itself significant. It indicates how successful a badge of authority the culture label has become for academics. In addition to scholarly authors keen to gain acceptance for their research, consultants attempting to gain and maintain their client base and organisational employees seeking to demonstrate their managerial acumen have equally found the culture concept a useful means of legitimating their ideas and actions. Organisational culture, then, is a rhetorical device deployed to legitimate, to inform and to persuade.

3 *Organisational culture as (a means of accessing?) critical insight* Numerous authors have suggested that by paying due attention to an organisation's culture more acute insight into that organisation's workings can be ascertained. A vast number of different books, journal papers, magazine and newspaper articles and television documentaries have all argued that organisational culture is the key to understanding what makes some organisations more successful than others. The postmodern perspective casts doubt on the validity of such claims. It suggests that what we term organisational culture is a combination of different themes and ideas that have been re-worked from older texts, rather than something radically new. It questions whether any theories, including those associated with organisational culture, can yield insights into organisations, because what counts as an insight is a subjective and contingent construction.

SUMMARY AND CONCLUSIONS

In this chapter seven main themes were elaborated.

1 It was suggested that organisations (especially larger organisations) rarely possess just one unitary and homogeneous culture. Rather, superimposed on the organisation-wide culture one is likely to find a patchwork quilt of related, overlapping and sometimes conflicting subcultures.

2 Some of the many functions that have been attributed to organisational cultures were described. The role that culture plays in conflict reduction, co-ordination and control, the reduction of uncertainty, motivation and competitive advantage were surveyed. Readers were then reminded that although most authors have tended to stress the positive implications of culture for organisations many organisations are characterised by cultures that are in some ways dysfunctional and damaging.

3 The idea that organisations have identities that they attempt to project into their environments was considered. The relationship between organisational culture and the individual was discussed. The argument that individuals derive part of their identity from the organisations to which they belong was reviewed. It was suggested that not every employee is a ready convert to his or her organisation's culture, that most people devote only a fraction of their time and energy to their place of work, and that the increasing use of temporary employees and the contracting-out of non-core activities are likely to complicate an already confused picture of how individuals relate to organisations. Four strategies for individual action within a culture (unequivocal adherence, strained adherence, secret non-adherence and open non-adherence) were then identified.

4 Issues of gender and sexuality as they link to organisational culture were discussed. It was argued that the place of women in organisations tends to reflect the position of women in society as a whole. In the West, while there is considerable variation between organisations in terms of their cultural attitudes towards women, most exhibit more masculine values. Indeed, women are often found in the less prestigious and powerful departments, tend to conduct more menial work, and are regularly deployed to exercise control without exciting resentment. It is important to analyse the role of women in organisational cultures not just because such analyses are fascinating in themselves, but because they provide useful information regarding patterns of power and deference.

5 The influence of organisational cultures on organisational learning was discussed. It was argued that culture affects the rate at which organisations learn, that some cultures actually impede organisational learning, and that cultures vary in their capacities to store and retrieve past learning. The concept of groupthink was introduced, and the tendency of some cultures to promote groupthink and thus prohibit learning discussed.

6 The increasing importance of ethical considerations in the development and analyses of organisational cultures was considered. It was suggested that ethical codes, which are types of corporate artefact, are being deliberately created by organisations and professional associations as control mechanisms. It was argued that in adopting particular beliefs and assumptions organisations necessarily make ethical choices. The idea that organisational cultures are themselves ethically dubious in that they operate as control mechanisms restricting individuality and individual freedom was discussed.

7 Finally, the body of ideas referred to as 'postmodernism' was very briefly sketched and applied to the culture perspective. This revealed that studies of organisational culture are likely to be a transient episode in the continuing history of organisation studies. It suggested that the label 'organisational culture' is important as a legitimating device for individuals keen to promote themselves and their work. It also invites us to consider whether the culture perspective is really different from other views on organisation, or just a re-grouping and re-labelling of old ideas.

KEY CONCEPTS

Subculture	Reduction of	Unequivocal	Double-loop learning
Enhancing subculture	uncertainty	adherence	Barriers to learning
Orthogonal subculture	Competitive	Strained adherence	Organisational
Counterculture	advantage	Secret non-adherence	memory
Conflict reduction		Open non-adherence	Groupthink
Co-ordination and	Organisational	Theory X and Theory Y	Ethics
control	identity	Gender	Postmodernism
Motivation	Individual identity	Single-loop learning	

QUESTIONS

1 Why do subcultures form in organisations? In what ways can subcultures relate to a dominant culture? Discuss with reference to an organisation that you know well.

2 What functions does culture play in organisations? Is an organisation's culture necessarily an asset? Exemplify your answer.

3 What is meant by the phrase 'organisational identity'? How does organisational identity differ from organisational culture?

4 Why is it that not all members of an organisation subscribe to its culture? What generic strategies for non-compliance are open to them?

5 Do you think it is true that most organisational cultures tend to systematically devalue and disempower women? Explain your answer. Suggest how those organisations which

do not treat women fairly might be re-engineered. Illustrate your answer with reference to organisations that you have worked for.

6   How does organisational culture influence the rate at which organisations learn?

7   Under what circumstances does groupthink usually occur? What are the main symptoms of groupthink? How can the dangers of groupthink be minimised?

8   Can organisations avoid making ethical choices? What does it mean to say that one culture is more ethical than another?

9   To what extent do you agree with the postmodern critique of organisational culture?

POLITICS, SYMBOLIC ACTION AND MYTH-MAKING AT BASSETT FOODS PLC

Bassett Foods plc consisted of five principal subsidiaries and a holdings board (see Case Study, p. 36). When the events related here took place, these had only recently been created (from one largely amorphous organisation) or acquired. The senior executives of all the subsidiaries (except in Geo Bassett) had been appointed within the past eighteen months, mostly from more junior posts within Bassett foods and expressed a deep-seated need and willingness to 'prove themselves' and, given the structure of the organisation, procedural necessity to justify their strategic intentions to holdings board members. Despite rescuing what had looked like a shipwreck of a business in the early 1980s, all the members of the GeoBassett holdings board still felt that they had to act with considerable caution after the excesses of the 1970s, and maintained an espoused philosophy of risk aversion. Indeed, the holdings board faced residual scepticism from shareholders and City institutions concerning the long-term prospects of the organisation, and open hostility from many senior managers in Bassett Food's largest subsidiary (Geo Bassett), who had lost power in the recent restructuring exercise. The project described here, therefore, provided a welcome opportunity for those involved to demonstrate their (and their organisation's) commercial acumen, both externally, to shareholders, other sugar confectionery companies and the City, and internally, to the senior executives in the subsidiaries and on the holdings board, and possibly also to the author of this case study.

On 29 April 1987 a large UK confectionery company, Candy Inc., offered Bassett Foods the opportunity to market and sell a wide range of its American products in the UK and Eire. The responsibility for investigating the potential of the product range was delegated by the chief executive of Bassett Foods to the development director, who was a senior member of the holdings board. After a lengthy internal debate within the holdings board it was decided to pursue the project through one of Bassett Food's principal subsidiaries, ABW, which the development director had helped to create. On the face of it this was a remarkable decision: ABW was not only very new but very small, composed of mostly inexperienced senior executives, lacked a well-developed cadre of middle managers, and had only one trained specialist in marketing, and almost no one experienced in large-scale project management or new product development. All this expertise and experience was, however, available in Geo Bassett. When quizzed, the development director provided an explanation that indicates the extent to which the dictates of 'rational' decision making as espoused by classical theory may be overwhelmed by cultural and political considerations:

> In a world without anything else affecting you you would naturally go to GeoBassett .... One aspect of it was that we had taken a bit of flack from GeoBassett, having split ABW off in the first place, which all of the wise owls down there thought was a totally wrong thing to do. We thought it would be rather a nice thing if ABW could succeed with this project.... We're a bit evil really, we play one off against the other.

This is not the whole story. At other times the development director and other members of the holdings board maintained that it was a perceived strategic need to make ABW less dependent on Geo Bassett as a market, and Bassett Foods as an organisation less dependent on Geo Bassett for its profitability, that was the impetus behind the decision. While such a strategy appeared reasonable given the nature of the organisation and its markets, the possibility that strategic planning was being driven by personal antagonisms and political intent cannot be ignored. In other words, it is conceivable that the language of rational strategic planning was being employed by members of the holdings board as a facade to mask the expression of personal and political prejudices which favoured ABW over Geo Bassett.

While the development director initially had sole responsibility for the project, he very quickly devolved many of the day-to-day operational decisions to the managing director of ABW, together with his sales director and marketing manager. These four individuals effectively controlled and shaped the evolution of the project within Bassett Foods. Together they formed a tight-knit team which kept information to itself, disclosing only what they wanted others to know when they wanted them to know it. At the outset they developed a plan to launch a family of products that would expose the organisation to the minimum possible risk. As the development director said at the time, 'On a major project, minimising risk is vital'. The launch of a family of products was deemed necessary because any single product might fail. Furthermore, it needed to be determined that the products would be purchased by teenagers and by adults on behalf of children as well as by children themselves because ABW's sales force could not adequately service confectioners, tobacconists and newsagents (CTNs), through which pure child self-purchase products had to be sold: the risk could not be tolerated. Most important of all was the realisation that buying in the products from America was going to be extremely expensive, so much so that Bassett Food's margin of profit on the goods they would sell in the UK would be too small to justify full marketing support. In response to this finding the development director devised a two-phase plan whereby the products would be purchased from the US in the first year of operation and provided with test market support at a small loss to Bassett Foods. Assuming this phase of the project was a success, capital expenditure would then be authorised (for manufacturing equipment and warehouse facilities) incrementally in order of profitability by product and by actual expansion of sales volume, rather than estimates. In this way the risks associated with the purchase of expensive capital equipment would be minimised, and the option of providing full marketing support at a later date left open.

Politics and symbolic action

In order to secure funding for the project from the holdings board, the development director and his three colleagues from ABW needed to provide evidence that the products could be profitably marketed in the UK. Their response was to commission product market research. While it was known that the products were successful in the United States, the expenditure was justified as a means of reducing uncertainty and therefore risk. The results, presented to the team on 28 July 1987, were the antithesis of their expectations, and the information was both repudiated by them and subsequently withheld from other members of ABW and the holdings board. As the development director later admitted:

> Projects are very easily killed. One could have easily killed this project stone dead by presenting this [market research] report to the holdings board – it would perhaps have killed it stone dead.

The espoused grounds for rejecting the results were threefold: that whatever the market research suggested, the product range was 'exciting' and 'impressive', that new products of any kind are 'extremely rare' in sugar confectionery and cannot be discarded out of hand, and that the research only reflected 'one woman's view'. The fact that the research had been conducted by a woman seemed to be significant for the three male members of the team, who were the more easily able to convince themselves that the research findings were dubious. The marketing manager, the only female member of the team, shared the view that the research was too confused to provide reliable information on which to pass judgement on the product range. In response to other questions, however, respondents revealed more compelling strategic reasons why they were unwilling to accept the findings of the research:

> Therefore, strategically, at the end of the first year of ABW trading we were in a position to clearly identify and state that we had a need for a flagship brand ... We were crying out for something and we didn't really have the in-house facilities in research terms or laboratory product development terms to come up with the answer (*Managing Director*).

Thus despite the fact that the research had confounded all the team's initial assumptions, it was a relatively easy decision for them to commission a second market research report from a different agency. This research confirmed the findings of the first report, but concluded that one product (which we will refer to by the pseudonym 'Beta') did seem to possess enormous potential in the UK. The positive aspects of the report caused considerable excitement, and were highlighted to the holdings board. The report was extremely influential, and its conclusions had a major impact on the development of the project:

> this was the first official feedback we had that our wildest hopes were looking slightly more than instincts, gut feel – albeit professional instincts and professional gut feel. It was the first feedback I think I'm right in saying from a professional research team (*Managing Director*).

> [It was on the basis of the report] that the decision to go ahead was made, and on that it was Beta only, and on that we fought for a 20p price point (*Marketing Manager*).

The fact that the product was of the child self-purchase type, that it did not appeal to teenagers and that therefore ABW would find it difficult to distribute and sell, was conveniently forgotten. This selective use of information suggests that while the conclusions of the two phases of market research did have a substantive influence on the project, it was also employed as a symbolic device. In subjecting the product range to market research the team was not merely concerned to obtain valuable information: the tests also constituted rites of passage for the project. So long as the project remained essentially intact, alterations to the number of products launched were more than acceptable, they constituted a form of 'customisation' from the American to the British market which established the team's authority and expertise. The market research was important for the legitimacy it conferred on the project, which was a *sine qua non* for the holdings board sanctioning the large expenditure required to take it further: whatever subsequently occurred, the organisation could always point out to its critics that market research had been commissioned which justified the action taken. In sum, the market research could be presented both internally and to the outside world as evidence that the risks involved were both known and acceptable: the fact that research had been commissioned was in some respects more important than the results themselves. That the inherent risks associated with the project were greater now that only a single product was to be launched, that the market it was aimed at was significantly smaller than first thought and that distribution and sales problems were anticipated, were ignored.

The events described illustrate the attempts of the team to construct a frame of reference that supported their preference for the project to be continued in the face of equivocal and even damaging evidence. Crucial to their efforts to render their interpretation of information and events dominant was reference to the notion of ABW's 'strategic need'. Their argument that the strategic position and needs of ABW for a flagship brand demanded that the project be pursued might have some validity (though not the logical connection that sometimes seemed to be implied), but it was also a convenient means of furthering the self-interested goals of the group. In short, the putative strategic necessity for a branded product was apparently being deliberately employed as a vehicle for promoting the personal agendas of the team members: the emotive appeal of the message of 'strategic need' was being

used as a rallying cry in order to position the project as strategically compelling, and this was a means of masking political intent. That such a theme struck a chord with the members of the holdings board was fortuitous. In fact, the recourse to market research may be interpreted as a ritualistic response that was the overt expression of tensions concerning underlying power relations between members of the team and the holdings board. On this reading of events the commissioning of product market research constituted symbolic rites of risk minimisation, which hid the true extent to which risk was actually being incurred, and led members of the holdings board to overlook the substantive risk implications of the venture.

The team's efforts to legitimate their interpretation of events and desired course of action was an exercise in power. They were successful largely because they controlled access to that information (product market research data) which could influence perceptions and evaluations of critical organisational uncertainty: there is much evidence to suggest that under these conditions the shrewd tactical use of information is often effective. By withholding and filtering the more negative conclusions of the first market research report, and using carefully worded reports and well-planned presentations which focused attention specifically on the positive findings of the second report, the team manipulated holdings board members' understandings of what were detailed and complex research results. The members of the holdings board were disadvantaged not only in that they had no direct access to the marketing agency or the market reports, but also by the time demands made on them by other large-scale projects, and most importantly by the trust they placed in the development director to act as an 'objective' arbiter and critic. It is interesting to note that in these circumstances the control members of the holdings board exercised over the formal agenda of ABW's executive board meetings, their unlimited authority to sanction and prohibit expenditure, and unquestioned position power merely served as constraints in a context in which power was exerted over them.

Myth making

The team's success in structuring the understandings of the holdings board members was intimately tied to the trust and confidence Bassett Food's most senior executives placed in them. The holdings board's willingness to rely on the team can be traced to the team members' ability to present their actions as rational, justified and legitimate. They managed this by skilfully portraying their activities as conforming to the prevailing organisational view of what constituted commercial 'best practice'. According to this view good decision making and project management should be founded on high quality and undisputed information from which rational and indisputably correct courses of action would naturally emerge. One rationale for this view, provided by the respondents themselves, was that such an approach led to the maximum reduction of uncertainty and therefore to the minimisation of risk. The team also seems to have felt a need to convince themselves that the project had been (and was being) systematically planned and professionally conducted, perhaps in order to preserve individuals' self-esteem, and certainly to facilitate group cohesion. The myth that the project had been conducted in an objective, rational and apolitical manner in which the dictates of commercial logic had dominated over individual and group self-interests was thus both psychologically and sociologically compelling for members of the team and the holdings board alike:

> As a project it's undoubtedly been more closely evaluated, with more professional assistance and more deep thought over a greater period of time than any other project that we have ever tackled (*Managing Director, ABW*).

> I think taking it as a one-off project, analysing it from start to finish, I think you would be hard-pressed really to find a better and more systematic review of the product, potential of it and putting it actually together (*Company solicitor and holdings board member*).

> I think it's probably one of the most professional pre-sales we've ever done, and professional launches that I've ever been involved in. We got it right (*Sales Director, ABW*).

It has been suggested that every datum becomes meaningful only when there is a relatum. In this case the relatum against which the members of the holdings board and the team compared this project was a similar-type project (here called 'Epsilon') that had been conducted some years previously. Epsilon was considered to have been an unmitigated disaster, with severe financial implications, and occupied a special place in the folklore of Bassett Foods as the archetype of mismanagement and poor commercial judgement. The members of the team made persistent comparisons between the current and historical projects across almost all dimensions of activity – sales, marketing and finance – in their day-to-day work interactions. The members of the holdings board were also acutely aware of what were perceived to have been major errors of judgement associated with the Epsilon project (some of them, notably the chief executive and development director, had been involved), and the memories of the Epsilon project were significant features of the cultural milieu which shaped project Beta:

> A few weeks ago [the MD] asked me the question, 'OK, Steve you've been selling the product 6–8 weeks. What's your feeling apropos of where you were when you were doing the Epsilon thing? Rate it on a scale for me.' So I said 'probably Epsilon something like 3 out of 10, and Beta 10 out of 10 – or 11' (*Sales Director, ABW*).

> A lot of stuff was learned from Epsilon. That had been launched on a margin that was not high enough to support the marketing costs (*Development Director, holdings board member*).

It is evident that employees' decisions about how to act were being influenced by their memories of their (and others) past actions and events, and that these considerations combined to form a matrix of constraints which limited actors' perceptions about the responses that were desirable and appropriate in this situation. The deep structures of power within Bassett Foods had been informed by the influence of the Epsilon episode, which had affected the preconscious basic assumptions about what were and what were not appropriate and legitimate actions.

Thus the memories of the failed Epsilon project provoked a series of apparently rational commercial actions by the team, and this procedural rationality was the key to the holdings board agreeing to sanction the relatively large amounts of expenditure required to see the project to a conclusion. The close attention paid by the members of the team and the holdings board to what they considered to be procedurally rational actions was the source of the myth that the project had in fact been rationally conducted even according to their own criteria. That this was not the case was well documented by the research. Interestingly, the same individuals could, often in the same interview, both uphold the myth and offer striking evidence that it had no empirical justification.

Many respondents volunteered their knowledge that the project had been more costly than initially anticipated, that projected profitability was declining, that expenditure on a new factory had been sanctioned without the true level of sales being known, and that a regional TV test had been cancelled so that the value of the £1 million TV advertising campaign could not be properly evaluated. In short, decisions had been taken out of sequence and important information discounted, ignored or not sought: the facade of risk minimisation was preserved by the myth, which was more powerful than the experience of events themselves.

Epilogue

Beta was launched using product purchased from America, and immediately exceeded even the most optimistic projections of the team. Despite placing new orders for Beta in the USA, ABW were soon having to ration the amount they could sell to any one shop in an effort not to upset retailers. While some commentators in the sugar confectionery industry warned that Beta was likely to prove a fad product with a short lifecycle, the team were euphoric. Meanwhile a new factory facility with special equipment to produce Beta was being erected adjacent to ABW's main complex. Disaster then struck. Glass was discovered in a packet of Beta and the product had to be withdrawn. Foul play was sus-pected. Before this problem could be resolved Bassett Foods became the target of a hostile takeover bid. This bid was fought off with the help of Cadbury, who, acting as a white knight, took over Bassett Foods. A clause in the original contract with Candy Inc. stated that if Bassett was acquired then all rights to Beta were forfeit. Beta has never yet been relaunched in the UK.

Questions

1 Were the team prone to groupthink? Explain your answer.

2 What role did trauma-based learning play in determining the course of the project?

3 Why were the findings of the first market research not accepted by the team? How reasonable were their objections?

4 How important were (a) ritualised behaviour, (b) symbolic action and (c) myth-making in the conduct of the project?

5 To what extent does the fact that Beta was successful in the marketplace justify the actions and thought processes of the team?

6 Is this case in any way representative of how new product developments are conducted in organisations generally? Comment using your own experience.

CHAPTER 4

Understanding organisational culture change

OBJECTIVES

To enable students to:

- understanding the central issues in modelling culture change;
- become familiar with five models for understanding culture change;
- appreciate the advantages and problems associated with each model;
- consider the key common factors shared by the models;
- learn that the nature of an organisation's culture is an important influence on its propensity for change;
- consider the value of the models for us in our attempts to understand the process of culture change.

INTRODUCTION

This chapter is specifically focused on the models that scholars have developed in their attempts to understand culture change. How and why organisational culture change occurs is an extremely important issue because a thorough understanding of these processes seems likely to be a key to improving organisational performance and effectiveness. This chapter has four main sections. First, some general issues concerning the culture change literature are reviewed. Second, five of the most interesting and coherent models of culture change are examined in some detail. Third, from this overview of the models a number of common themes (crises, leadership, success and learning) are identified and commented upon. Finally, it is suggested that the models require considerable refinement before they can become really useful, and that they most especially need to be sensitive to different culture types. This chapter provides a broad understanding of culture change which the next two chapters draw on in their consideration of the practical means of accomplishing culture change, the formulation of strategy, and organisational performance.

ISSUES IN UNDERSTANDING CULTURE CHANGE

A large number of models for understanding organisational culture change have been formulated. As with definitions of organisational culture none of these has as yet achieved wide acceptance as the definitive means of modelling culture change. This state of affairs is testament to the relatively early stage of intellectual development of culture theory. It also reflects the lack of certainty and understanding of how organisations change that afflicts organisation studies in general. Part of the problem in coming to a reasonable understanding of how cultures change is that the term change has itself come to mean a variety of different things. Depending on the context organisational change can now mean everything from a major upheaval to a minor disruption in normal routine. To complicate matters still further authors are often unclear how their use of synonyms and near synonyms such as *evolution*, *adaptation* and *re-learning* relate to more general notions of change. In examining models of culture change problems relating to how culture should be defined, ambiguity concerning the scale of change being modelled, questions relating to the locus of change, and uncertainty relating to the timescale over which changes are supposed to be occurring will arise, and therefore require brief consideration at the outset.

Definitions

As we saw in Chapter 1 when different authors write about culture change they do not always have the same notion of culture in mind. This can have profound implications for the conclusions that the authors draw concerning the possibility and ease of changing an organisational culture. For example, Kilmann (1984) chooses to identify *norms* as the essence of culture whereas Lundberg (1985) locates culture at the *assumptions* level. The result is that for Kilmann culture change is a far simpler process than for Lundberg, because norms are generally easier to alter than assumptions. In order to minimise confusion arising from the different use of terms the models of culture change presented in this chapter have been chosen because they define culture in very similar ways, that is, as deeply held beliefs and values or as assumptions.

Scale of change

Models of culture change differ in terms of the scale of change to which they are relevant. A distinction is usually made between small-scale changes (often called *incremental* or *first order*) and large-scale change (sometimes called *radical* or *second order* change). Reality is of course far more complicated than this simple distinction suggests, with a succession of small alterations often leading to large-scale change. What is more, one person's idea of a small change can fit someone else's view of a large change. Despite these difficulties, when we are examining a model of culture change it is obviously vital that we know whether it principally refers to change on an incremental or radical scale. In this chapter all the models refer to large-scale culture change with the exception of Gagliardi's (1986) model, which is formulated to account for incremental change.

Locus of change

When we talk about change in organisations there is plenty of scope for confusion over the precise location in which change is supposed to occur. For example, change may be identified at the level of an entire nation, an industry, or a market segment, an organisation as a whole, or a single department. Similarly, in the case of larger organisations one or a few regions might experience radical change while others undergo only incremental change. In some instances we may even speak of individual employees changing while the organisation as a whole remains fairly constant. All the models of culture change reviewed in this chapter are fundamentally concerned with change at the level of the organisation, though many of the principles they espouse are applicable at other levels.

Nature of change

Some commentators, notably Sathe (1985a, b), have suggested that there is an important distinction to be made between behavioural change and cognitive change. It is argued that when an organisation embarks on a change programme there are three basic outcomes. First, there can be change at the level of individuals' cognitions (for example, beliefs and values) with no complementary change in their behaviour. This can occur when individuals intellectually agree that, for instance, new working practices are a good idea, but find it difficult to adopt them because of ingrained habits or because they lack the relevant knowledge and skills to put them into effect. Second, change at the behavioural level may not be matched by change at the cognitive level. This is possible when, for instance, compliance with new organisational rules and procedures is enforced by the threat of reprimand, demotion or firing rather than employee enthusiasm. Third, there can be change at both the behavioural and cognitive levels. This is almost certainly the most permanent form of change as people both genuinely believe and value their new way of doing things, thus making the new order both self-sustaining and mutually reinforcing.

Timescales

Organisational changes occur over time and it might be expected that models of culture change would provide some indication of timescales. However, of the models surveyed in this chapter only that proposed by Schein (1985b) pays much attention to the time variable, and then only in the context of a simple life-cycle framework. The consequence is that when we read these models we do not know whether the events and processes they predict are supposed to occur over days, weeks, months or years. On the face of it this would seem to be a considerable weakness which again reflects a lack of understanding of how cultures function in organisations. While this is in part true, it is likely that similar-type processes can occur at different speeds in different organisations depending on a whole range of organisational variables. In other words, it is arguable that the sheer complexity of organisations and the process of organisational change make the specification of definite time-scales impossible. Some commentators, however, have interpreted this as a failing which reflects a more general neglect of history in the culture literature (Rowlinson and Hassard, 1993).

With these points in mind let us now proceed to examine five models for understanding culture change. These models have been chosen because they provide a fairly representative sample of the different approaches that have been taken by academics specialist in this field. All the frameworks are of relatively recent origin, have been widely publicised, and have exercised influence over the intellectual development of organisational culture studies. The following models are elaborated:

- *Lundberg's model*, which is based on earlier learning-cycle models of organisational change, and is notable for its attention to external environmental factors as well as the internal characteristics of organisations.
- *Dyer's model*, which posits that the perception of a crisis in conjunction with a leadership change are required in order for culture change to occur.
- *Schein's model*, which is based on a simple life-cycle framework, and which posits that different culture change mechanisms are associated with different stages in an organisation's development.
- *Gagliardi's model*, which suggests that only incremental culture change can properly be described as a form of organisational change.
- *A composite model*, based on the ideas of Lewin, Beyer and Trice, and Isabella, which provides some insights into the microprocesses of culture change.

MODELS FOR UNDERSTANDING CULTURE CHANGE

Lundberg's model

Lundberg (1985) has formulated a sophisticated model for understanding culture change in organisations. In essence, Lundberg's model is a much elaborated learning cycle. The basic notion is that a culture experiences some form of organisational predicament which prompts surprise. This surprise (which may be either pleasing or unpleasing), when combined with sufficient concern, prompts inquiry. The process of inquiry may then lead to the discovery of previously unknown phenomena. Cultural change thus becomes possible. While the modus operandi of Lundberg's model is relatively straightforward its sheer breadth of coverage is so great that the reader is advised to read the following description of it in conjunction with Mini Case 4.1, which illustrates the principal phases of the model with reference to Ciba-Geigy. Let us now consider this model (illustrated in Fig. 4.1) in more detail.

The starting point for Lundberg's framework is an organisational culture, which in large, differentiated organisations is likely to include multiple subcultures. Lundberg suggests that in order for cultural change to occur the requisite external and internal circumstances must exist. Two *external enabling conditions* are theorised to facilitate culture change. First, *domain forgiveness*, which refers to the degree of threat to an organisation posed by, among other things, competition, the relative scarcity or abundance of resources and the relative stability or instability of the environment. The intent of Lundberg's model seems to be that the more forgiving the environment is the more likely that change will occur because the less risky it is perceived to be. The second external enabling condition is *organisation–domain* congruence. If the degree of congruence between an organisation and its domains is too little or too great then

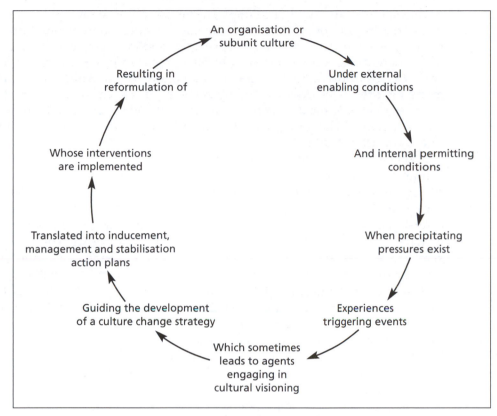

Fig. 4.1 The organisational learning cycle of culture change
Source: reproduction with permission from Lundberg (1985)

change may seem overly threatening or unnecessary. Change is more likely when the degree of congruence is perceived to be relatively modest.

In addition, Lundberg identifies four *internal permitting conditions* that allow change. These are: first, sufficient change resources, such as money and managerial time and energy; second, system readiness, which is a collective sense that people are willing to change; third, the existence of co-ordinative and integrative mechanisms that facilitate communication and control; and fourth, a relatively stable leadership team with enough strategic awareness, vision, power resources and communication skills to guide the cultural transition. Lundberg then postulates that if organisations face certain *precipitating pressures* then organisational members are more likely to change. He recognises four types of pressure. These are: first, atypical performance demands (such as to be more productive); second, stakeholder pressures (which might come from the public, the Government, unions and so forth); third, pressures resulting from organisational growth or decrement; and fourth, the perception of a crisis (for example, resource deprivation).

Lundberg's model requires one further condition before cultural change can be initiated, namely, the occurrence of a *triggering event*. A triggering event is a stimulus that leads to the release of the tensions built up by the precipitating pressures. Five classes of triggering event are described: environmental calamities (such as a recession), environmental opportunities (for example, technological breakthroughs), internal revolutions (the imposition of a new management team), external revolutions (such as nationalisation or other restrictive legislation) and managerial crises (the committing of a serious blunder by senior executives). In those instances where the trigger event comes as a surprise to the leadership of an organisation, which puts it in a predicament, the executives may respond by engaging in a process of inquiry. This process involves rendering the dominant culture explicit and sketching out a new and preferable alternative. The descriptive shaping of a new organisational culture Lundberg refers to as *cultural visioning*.

While the creation of a new cultural vision is a necessary step towards the establishment of a new order, its success depends on it being translated into a *culture change strategy* implemented through *action plans*. The overall strategy should determine three things: the *pace of change* (will it be swift or slow?), the *scope of change* (how much change will occur?) and the *time span* over which the change will take place. With the general strategy formulated, three forms of action planning are required. First, *inducement action plans* that heighten system readiness for change and counter resistance must be devised. Second, *management action plans* that enable people to redefine the culture should be implemented. Finally, *stabilisation action plans* that institutionalise the changes and ensure that they persist over time must be established. These plans may well involve discrediting dominant myths and stories, reconstructing the organisation's history and creating new desirable metaphors. They may also include bringing in external consultants, the devising of new slogans and logos, the refashioning of training programmes and the changing of the criteria for personnel recruitment and selection, among others.

Lundberg is notably (and understandably) vague about the specifics of managing culture change. He does, however, emphasise two points. First, successful cultural intervention requires that all levels of a culture from artefacts to assumptions are tackled. Second, it is likely that continuous, repeated, multiple interventions will have more chance of success than single short-run efforts. To sum up, Lundberg's model of culture change suggests that its feasibility depends on a large number of sets of appropriate internal and external circumstances, the conjunction of which would seem to be quite rare. As Lundberg asserts:

> The complexity of the phenomena of organizational culture, the inherent difficulty of impacting deep levels of cultural meaning, the vision required for designing and sequencing the multiple interventions needed suggests that managing culture change is not often likely, even if it is possible ... Yet organizational culture change does happen. (Lundberg, 1985: 183).

Evaluation

Lundberg's model is an intellectually coherent and internally consistent framework that can be successfully employed to explain at least some instances of organisational change, as we have seen with the case of Ciba-Geigy. Lundberg also deserves credit for explicitly recognising that organisational cultures can be highly differentiated and include multiple subcultures, which makes the actual conduct of culture change analyses extremely complex. That the model takes external as well as internal factors into account is another plus point, as there is considerable evidence that much radical organisational change occurs in response to environmental stimuli. Two further

Culture change at Ciba-Geigy

The process of culture change currently being undergone by Ciba-Geigy provides us with a good opportunity to illustrate the power of Lundberg's model. Ciba-Geigy is Switzerland's largest chemical and pharmaceutical group, and employs approximately 90 000 people worldwide. The Group is extremely financially strong, and in 1991 Group profits rose by 24 per cent and cash flow increased by 17 per cent despite difficult trading conditions. However, rather than take these figures as evidence of the Group's good health Heini Lippuner, the chairman of the executive committee of Ciba-Geigy, decided to embark on a major culture change strategy.

External enabling conditions

From the mid-1980s onwards Ciba-Geigy recognised a growing rift between its culture and the world around it, which it interpreted as a decline in organisation–environment congruence. Specifically, there was a realisation that while the organisation was intent on pursuing economic goals the public were becoming more interested in the environment and employees were coming to value self-fulfilment, fairness and a sense of cultural identity.

Internal permitting conditions

Fortunately, all of Lundberg's internal permitting conditions were met by Ciba-Geigy. A strong financial performance in recent times meant that there were sufficient change resources. Discontent among many younger employees with how the organisation was run meant that there was a collective willingness to change that could be exploited by a senior executive team convinced by the need to evolve and reform. Moreover, as Ciba-Geigy was an established company it did not lack the formal integrative and co-ordinative mechanisms required to facilitate change, though many more had to be developed *ad hoc* to deal with the extra demands made by the programme of change. Finally, Heini Lippuner, who acts as the organisation's president and chief operating officer, was sufficiently motivated to play a key role in the change process.

Precipitating pressures

The main precipitating pressure came from one particular stakeholder group, namely, the public. As Lippuner later stated: 'The values of the public were no longer those at the basis of industry . . . . They had begun to question whether it was right simply to continue on a path of more roads, more cars, more luxury, more affluence – and somehow we hadn't taken account of that up to that time.' An added pressure was largely internally induced, that is, the perceived need to perform in order to grow at least at the same rate as other leading organisations in the field. By 1988 it was apparent that the 1980s boom would eventually come to an end, and casting a critical eye over their organisation senior executives began to realise that they had become bureaucratic and complacent.

Trigger events

Undoubtedly the crucial catalyst behind the group's decision to overhaul its culture was an environmental disaster involving the leakage of 30 tonnes of toxic compounds into the Rhine. The public outcry was enormous, and even though it was another company (Sandoz) not Ciba-Geigy that was responsible, it was clear to everyone that all companies in the industry were threatened as a result.

Cultural visioning

Against this background of events a massive programme of strategic, structural and culture change was developed called *Vision 2000*. The documentation for this project included a large number of commitments to the environment and to the organisation's employees. For instance, it was stated that the organisation would, over time, attempt to reduce its impact on the environment and take notice of the personal concerns of employees. With specific regard to culture the documentation suggested that Ciba-Geigy would act according to certain principles of leadership and teamwork which would contribute 'to a corporate culture in which we are challenged, can develop personally, and are able to give our best'.

▶

Culture change strategy

The details of how the vision was to be implemented were worked out and set down in a 'strategic direction plan', the main objective of which was to give employees a sense of identification with the company's goals, and a sense that those goals would be compatible with their own ethics. A separate document, called the 'Master Plan for Transformation', contained more specific information, especially pertaining to the reshaping of the business portfolio and the divisional strategies. The overarching strategy which informed structural and portfolio changes was one of *directed autonomy*. First formulated by Robert Waterman in his book *The Renewal Factor*, directed autonomy refers to a situation in which employees are encouraged to act on their own initiative within a framework imposed by the organisation. As the culture change strategy was formulated it was translated into action plans.

Implementation

Since the inception of Vision 2000 a vast number of significant changes have been implemented at Ciba-Geigy. At the portfolio level the organisation disposed of its photographic film business. In terms of organisational structure Ciba-Geigy reorganised from eight divisions into fourteen divisions. In addition, the divisions were made responsible for their performance and results, breaking the stranglehold of the centre and making the new philosophy of decentralisation and autonomy a reality. To develop the leadership and entrepreneurial qualities desired a large number of in-house training programmes and management seminars have been conducted. This is not to say that everything has always run smoothly. The programme of radical change has come up against resistance and suspicion from middle managers who feel threatened by the new demands being made upon them, and some of the most intransigent of these people have had to be removed.

Culture change?

While Lippuner is realistic enough to know that the sort of cultural transformation he is seeking will take years (he claims between three and five), some degree of success is already apparent. Total quality including service quality is now a group strategic objective, partnership relations with customers are now developing so that co-operation on new product development is possible, and financial indicators such as return on investment and net cash flow are healthy. Real culture change is, however, still difficult to detect. As Lippuner himself has said: 'What we would like to see is a lot more taking of personal responsibility and initiative. I fear that it's a typically Swiss trait – and one enhanced by the organisation we had in the past – to make doubly, trebly, four times sure that you don't make a mistake, that you get all the signatures before you go into action . . . We are maybe halfway down the road to transformation.'

Questions

1 Is Ciba-Geigy experiencing a serious attempt at culture change?

2 Has Ciba-Geigy undergone culture change?

3 How convincing an illustration of Lundberg's model is this account of change management at Ciba-Geigy?

4 What learning points are there here for other organisations attempting culture change?

5 How useful do you think Lundberg's model is for understanding culture change?

Source: adapted from *Long Range Planning*, Vol. 26. No. 1, Kennedy, C., 'Changing the Company Culture at Ciba-Geigy', pp. 18–27, © 1993, with permission from Elsevier Science.

strengths of Lundberg's work are first, its embracing of the need to alter not just artefacts but basic assumptions as well if culture change is to occur, and second, its specification that continued and multiple interventions over a substantial period of time are often necessary in order to induce cultural revolution.

Lundberg's model is, however, far from perfect. It presents us with a checklist of factors to be taken into account rather than a detailed analysis of the process of culture change. There is, for instance, little indication given on how different factors impact on each other, as surely they must: just how do domain forgiveness and organisation–domain congruence relate to each other? There is also little indication given concerning the detail of how different factors operate to induce or prevent culture change. Thus one is left to ponder what degree of organisation–domain congruence is required in order to facilitate culture change, and how one is supposed to recognise it in any given instance. Similarly, one may question whether culture change can occur if only three of the four internal permitting conditions are present or whether triggering events can occur without a build-up of precipitating pressures, both of which seem likely. Furthermore, while Lundberg asserts that a relatively stable leadership team is required to effect culture change, other commentators have suggested that it is only with a change in leadership that culture change can possibly occur (see, for example, Dyer's model). To conclude, Lundberg's model sacrifices detail and specificity for generalisability and simplicity. The result is an interesting but inherently limited and approximate view of just some of the organisational processes that precede and promote culture change.

Dyer's cycle of cultural evolution

As with Lundberg's learning cycle Dyer's (1985) framework has been formulated to model large-scale cultural transformations rather than incremental change. Derived from case histories of five large American companies (General Motors, Levi Strauss, National Cash Register, the Balfour Company, and the Brown Corporation[1]) Dyer's cycle of cultural evolution is based on a sophisticated understanding of culture as consisting of four levels: artefacts, perspectives (which have been referred to in this book – see Chapter 1 – as rules and norms), values and assumptions. The workings of this model are illustrated in Mini Case 4.2, which concerns culture change at Nissan. While Dyer presents his model as a series of sequentially ordered stages he explicitly recognises that it is possible for these stages to overlap or indeed to occur simultaneously. An overview of Dyer's six-phase framework is provided by Fig. 4.2.

1   In the first stage of the process the leadership's abilities and the current practices of the organisation are called into question. The idea is that some sort of triggering event occurs which creates the perception of a crisis that members of the organisation consider cannot be solved using traditional methods. Organisational participants therefore engage in a search for alternative solutions to the crisis. Dyer's research suggested that environmental shock in the form of a depression or recession is the typical cause of this period of questioning. For example, it is argued that Levi Strauss started the process of culture change when its European division lost $12 million.

2   The perception of a crisis leads to a breakdown in what Dyer terms the pattern-maintenance symbols, beliefs and structures. These are the means by which a culture is sustained, and in order for a new culture to be created they must first be altered. Pattern-maintenance symbols, beliefs and structures can include dominant leaders, reward systems, and all system-supportive beliefs. With their destruction the old cultural order may be threatened. For instance, at NCR the culture created around the egocentric and eccentric personality of the president, John Patterson, was subject to change only with Patterson's declining health, which led to a deterioration in the mechanisms of pattern-maintenance associated with him.

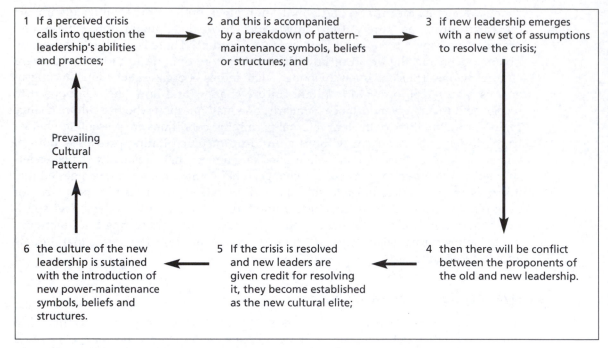

Fig. 4.2 The cycle of cultural evolution in organisations
Source: reproduction with permission from Dyer (1985)

3   The breakdown of an organisation's power-sustaining symbols, beliefs and structures is, however, only a necessary and not a sufficient condition for culture change.
What is also required is the promulgation of some alternative set of artefacts, values
and assumptions. In all the organisations surveyed by Dyer a cultural alternative was
provided by a new leader or leadership team. For example, at General Motors in the
1920s the culture began to change when Alfred Sloan took over from William Durant.

4   With the arrival of a new leader comes a period of conflict between supporters of
the old and proponents of the new cultures. The successful imposition of a new cultural order seems to require that those employees who are unable to accept the change
must leave voluntarily, be fired or be transferred to positions where they exercise no
influence. This demotion of what may often be a large number of individuals may
result in their attempting to sabotage the new regime. It is partly for this reason that
these periods of conflict often tend to be managed quickly, though, as Dyer notes, they
can drag on for years.

5   The next stage in Dyer's cycle of cultural evolution calls for the new leadership
elite to overcome the conflicts and resentments caused by their new practices. Two
conditions must be met in order to achieve this. First, the crisis must appear to have
been resolved, so that the tension and anxiety associated with the uncertainties it generated are ameliorated. Second, the new leader must be given the credit for solving the
crisis situation. This occurred at Levi Strauss in the mid-1970s, where the new leader
Robert Grohman was credited with having increased sales by more than one-third to

$987.6 million, the largest increase both in dollars and as a percentage in the history of the corporation. The attribution of success to a particular leader or leadership team increases that individual's or group's power to then implement further changes to an organisation's culture and eliminate rivals.

6   In order to stabilise the organisation and institutionalise the new culture the leadership begins to create new pattern-maintenance symbols, beliefs and structures. This means, among other things, recruiting and selecting people supportive of the new culture, weeding out any residual non-conformists, making sure that everyone is aware of the leadership's success, discrediting the old leaders, and restructuring the ownership of the organisation through stock options. One of the most interesting elements of this process is reinterpreting the past history of the organisation to suit the new leaders. This frequently means criticising the old leadership team as having 'failed', being 'unprofessional' or 'not tough enough'. In the words of George Orwell in his book *1984* (1949: 32), 'who controls the past controls the future, [and] who controls the present controls the past'.

Dyer's cycle of cultural evolution presents us with a relatively simple framework for understanding some of the mechanisms which promote culture change in organisations. The key to Dyer's model is its supposition that a crisis in concert with a leadership change is required in order for large-scale cultural adaptation. Thus organisations may face many crises and undergo a number of leadership changes without the occurrence of culture change. Indeed, crises may cohere an organisation and strengthen its cultural resolve, while new leaders may be chosen on the basis of their compatibility with the existing culture and likelihood of strengthening already established beliefs. Only when a crisis and a change in leadership occur fairly simultaneously is substantial culture change possible. Like so many other models of cultural adaptation and change, then, Dyer's framework is heavily dependent on the concept of *leadership*:

> According to the model of change described here, the most important decision in culture change concerns the selection of a new leader inasmuch as a new leader who enters an organisation during a period of crisis has unique opportunities to transform the organisation's culture by bringing and embedding new artifacts, perspectives, values, and assumptions into the organization. Leaders do indeed appear to be the creators and transmitters of culture. (Dyer, 1985: 223)

Evaluation

Dyer's model has many obvious similarities with that proposed by Lundberg, not least of which is that it is formulated as a continuous cycle and focused on the macro aspects of organisational change. Based on empirical research conducted at five companies we can be confident that it is applicable to a substantial number of instances of culture change. The sophisticated appreciation of culture on which the model is based is also reassuring, as is the recognition that the six phases identified need not be distinct and may overlap and occur simultaneously. Furthermore, the two pivots of the model – leadership change and the perception of a crisis – are fairly easily identifiable in other instances of organisational change, making Dyer's model testable in a way that more theoretical models are not.

125

Culture change at Nissan

The story of culture change at Nissan provides us with an opportunity to illustrate the value of Dyer's cycle of cultural evolution. Nissan is one of the world's leading manufacturers of automobiles with approximately 6 per cent of the global market. While it is domiciled in Japan it has extensive overseas operations in both the UK and USA by means of which it hopes to overcome any potential difficulties caused by increased protectionism in the European and American markets.

A perceived crisis

Throughout the early 1980s the perception that Nissan was in crisis began to take hold of the organisation. The main causes of this perception were economic. A slow-down in demand in Japan resulted in declining sales. This was accompanied by a fall in Nissan's domestic market share from around 30 per cent to less than 24 per cent in 1987. Commentators both within and outside the organisation were quick to criticise Nissan for directing all of its attention overseas while ignoring its home market. In addition, because of the large investments overseas the company's profits remained flat throughout this period.

A breakdown in pattern-maintenance symbols, beliefs and structures

Perhaps the most important indication that the old cultural order was in decline was a deterioration in labour–management relations, which was given extensive coverage in Japan's mass media and abroad, and which seriously damaged Nissan's public image. Nissan's growth during the 1960s and 1970s had owed a great deal to labour–management co-operation, and in many ways this tacit pact between workers and managers was at the heart of Nissan's culture. The point when labour and management could no longer carry on an effective dialogue was the point at which pattern-maintenance symbols, beliefs and structures were recognised to have broken down.

A new leadership and a new set of assumptions

In 1985 a new President of Nissan, Mr Yakata Kume, was appointed. He put forward the motto that 'management and the labour union should both discharge their duties properly' and appealed to everyone 'to change the traditional currents and create a new corporate culture'. Kume exhorted his workforce to focus on the marketplace without being restricted by the company's hierarchical structure and past customs. The new corporate philosophy emphasised customer satisfaction, the importance of expanding the company's customer base, the need to create attractive products, and the need to develop people.

Conflict between proponents of the old and new leadership

While Dyer's model predicts conflict, and such a prediction seems very plausible, Japanese organisations being what they are there is little direct evidence for it in this case.

Resolving the crisis establishes a new cultural elite

Interestingly, coinciding with Kume's reforms Nissan experienced a further blow: a sharp appreciation of the yen led to an increase in prices, inevitably translating into a decline in competitiveness in overseas markets. The combination of sluggish domestic sales and a drastic reduction in profits on exports to the US meant that Nissan posted an operating loss of Y20bn for the first half of the fiscal year 1986. Gradually, however, the drive for reform began to achieve tangible results. A limited production model called the Be-1 proved a great success at the 1985 Tokyo Motor Show and two years later the Cima was again a smash hit. In recent times the organisation's extensive overseas operations in the US and the UK have also been interpreted as useful assets by once critical commentators.

The culture is sustained through new pattern-maintenance symbols, beliefs and structures

Kume has made a number of attempts to introduce new pattern-maintenance symbols, beliefs and structures. He visited the company's offices, dealers and affiliated firms throughout Japan and also made bold attempts to improve communications with employees and other companies in the Nissan group. More importantly still, he encouraged all employees to address each other as 'mister', regardless of the other person's rank in the company, which represented a fundamental break with the previous practice of addressing other people by their titles. Other significant attempts to remould pattern-maintenance symbols included stopping the wearing of uniforms by female employees and the introduction of flexible working hours. Kume also ordered a review and subsequent improvements of the manner in which visitors were received by receptionists and discontinued visitor badges.

Culture change?

Has real culture change occurred at Nissan? According to Yasuhiro Ishizuna the process of transformation has only just begun: 'A long road lies ahead that is crossed by many hurdles. Whether or not we can meet the challenges before us will be the true test of Nissan's transformation. We are vigorously channelling our energies toward the attainment of the specific goal of constructing a network linking the company's global operations. Once that network has been completed, then we will be able to celebrate the completion of Nissan's transformation.'

Questions

1 Is Nissan experiencing a serious attempt at culture change?

2 Has Nissan undergone culture change?

3 How convincing an illustration of Dyer's model is this account of change management at Nissan?

4 What learning points are there here for other organisations attempting culture change?

5 How useful do you think Dyer's model is for understanding culture change?

Source: adapted from *Long Range Planning*, Vol. 23, No. 3, Ishizuna, Y. 'The Transformation of Nissan: Reform of Corporate Culture', pp. 9–15, © 1990, with permission from Elsevier Science.

As with Lundberg's model Dyer's framework is notable for its generality and simplicity. This means that much of the detail of the processes by which culture change occurs is omitted. Furthermore, culture change is said to be crucially dependent on leadership, specifically the introduction of a new leadership team with a new vision. Those commentators who assert that culture is as much a spontaneous creation of ordinary employees as it is a response to the directives and personality of leaders will find Dyer's model unappealing. In fact, even many of those theorists who consider that leaders are key to understanding the development of culture will not be prepared to endorse Dyer's suggestion that leaders *in situ* are unable to alter fundamentally the cultures that they have helped to create. Despite these misgivings it is apparent that Dyer's model is, like Lundberg's model, an interesting, coherent and intelligible approximation of at least some elements of culture change.

Schein's life-cycle model

Based on his model of culture (see Chapter 1) Schein (1985b) has developed a life-cycle model of organisational culture change. This suggests that organisations pass through distinct phases of development, each associated with a different sort of culture serving different sorts of functions and susceptible to change in different ways. These phases are *birth and early growth, organisational midlife* and *organisational maturity*. An overview of Schein's framework is provided by Fig. 4.3.

Growth stage	Function of culture	Mechanism of change
I. Birth and early growth • Founder domination, possibly family domination	• Culture is a distinctive competence and source of identity • Culture is the 'glue' that holds organisation together • Organisation strives towards more integration and clarity • Heavy emphasis on socialisation as evidence of commitment	1. Natural evolution 2. Self-guided evolution through therapy 3. Managed evolution through hybrids 4. Managed 'revolution' through outsiders
Succession phase:	• Culture becomes battleground between conservatives and liberals • Potential successors are judged on whether they will preserve or change cultural elements	
II. Organisational midlife • New-product development • Vertical integration • Geographic expansion • Acquisitions, mergers	• Cultural integration declines as new subcultures are spawned • Crisis of identity, loss of key goals, values and assumptions • Opportunity to manage direction of cultural change	5. Planned change and organisational development 6. Technological seduction 7. Change through scandal, explosion of myth 8. Incrementalism
III. Organisational maturity • Maturity of markets • Internal stability or stagnation • Lack of motivation to change	• Culture becomes a constraint on innovation • Culture preserves the glories of the past, hence is valued as a source of self-esteem, defence	9. Coercive persuasion 10. Turnaround 11. Reorganisation, destruction and rebirth
Transformation option:	• Culture change necessary and inevitable, but not all elements of culture can or must change • Essential elements of culture must be identified, preserved • Culture change can be managed or simply be allowed to evolve	
Destruction option: • Bankruptcy and reorganisation • Takeover and reorganisation • Merger and assimilation	• Culture changes at basic levels • Culture changes through massive replacement of key people	

Figure 4.3 Growth stages, functions of culture and mechanisms of change

Source: reproduced with permission from Schein (1985a)

Birth and early growth

The first phase of the model, 'birth and early growth', may last varying amounts of time from a few years to a few decades. During this stage culture fosters cohesion while an organisation develops and matures. Schein speculates that culture change will only become an issue if one of two conditions is met: first, the company faces economic difficulties, or second, there is a succession problem, with the founder of the organisation giving way to professional managers. Under these circumstances culture change may occur by means of four mechanisms.

Natural evolution

The culture evolves according to what seems to work best over long periods of time. Two basic processes are involved here. First, *general evolution* towards organisational midlife as a result of diversification and increasing organisational complexity, differentiation and integration. Second, *specific evolution*, which is the adaptation of particular organisational functions (such as research and development, data processing and marketing), to fit the environment. For example, a biotechnology company may well evolve a sophisticated R&D function, while a consumer electronics firm may develop its marketing skills.

Self-guided evolution through organisational therapy

This change mechanism involves outsiders (generally consultants specialising in change management) entering an organisation and facilitating cognitive change. The idea is that the outsiders enable key organisational participants to recognise dysfunctional elements of their culture by providing an analysis of how the culture is operating. If the consultants are successful in unfreezing the organisation and skilled at providing psychological safety mechanisms for individuals (so they do not experience too much distress), while still facilitating cognitive redefinition, then the process can work. This is generally the case only when the client organisation is highly motivated to change.

Managed evolution through hybrids

This change mechanism occurs when an organisation's leaders recognise a need for change, and attempt to implement it by systematically selecting for key jobs those existing members of the old culture who are most sympathetic to the new order the leaders wish to create. These people are hybrids who have credibility in the eyes of other employees by virtue of being 'insiders', and yet whose basic assumptions are sufficiently deviant to accommodate a new culture. A special case of this process are those instances where an outsider is brought in to an organisation as an 'heir apparent', and asked to serve for a number of years on the board in order to become enculturated.

Managed 'revolution' through outsiders

Following Dyer (1984) Schein suggests that (especially young and growing) organisations experience what are perceived to be crises; for example, declining profitability. At the same time the existing culture is challenged by a loss of some powerful supports such as concentrated ownership. At this juncture outsiders may be brought in to fill important positions on the grounds that the organisation needs to be more professionally managed. Conflict with the old culture is almost inevitable, and scepticism, resistance and sabotage are all possible. Eventually a dominant perception emerges that the organisation's performance has improved due to the ideas introduced by the outsiders, or has not. In the former case culture change may crystallise, while in the latter case the outsiders are likely to be forced out. This cycle may be repeated several times with a variety of outsiders before culture change is evident.

While it is tempting to think of these change mechanisms as discrete occurrences, they may often occur simultaneously. For example, an organisation that is diversifying and increasing in complexity may choose to engage consultants, promote hybrids and manage change by bringing in outsiders. The latter three of these culture change mechanisms are evident in Mini Case 4.3 focused on the Garibaldi School.

Mini Case 4.3

Birth and early growth: culture change at the Garibaldi School

Introduction

The Garibaldi School was located in Mansfield next to a large council estate. It was a state secondary school with 800 pupils and 45 teachers, and prior to 1989 was regarded as the sort of school that no one would send their children to unless they had no other choice. Adjectives such as 'ugly' and 'rough' were most usually used to describe the school. Indeed, having suffered two serious fires about 15 years previously, a popular local saying was 'Red sky at night, Garibaldi's alight'. For the 20 years to 1989 the school had been run by a head teacher who emphasised hierarchy and made decisions autocratically. Not unnaturally other teachers had become very defensive about their power, and the organisation's decision-making mechanisms were rigid, ponderous and slow.

Managing culture change

In 1989 a new head teacher, Bob Salisbury, was appointed. He discovered at Garibaldi a demoralised staff, a chronic lack of funds, and a lot of children failing to realise their full potential. His first move was to institute an open-door policy which encouraged staff and pupils to talk to him on an open basis. Within a term, two out of the three deputy heads left, while the remaining deputy head was convinced by Bob of the need to change. Two new deputy heads were immediately appointed, both of whom were sympathetic to Bob's vision.

While the school rule book stated that pupils should be treated with dignity and respect, before 1989 there was little indication that this was the case. One symbol of the school's lack of regard for pupils was the fact that they were banned from being in the school buildings at breaks and lunchtime. This was soon altered by Bob, with the result that not only did staff no longer suffer from the stresses of maintaining a siege within the buildings, but damage to the premises reduced dramatically. As the morale of pupils rose, so too did that of the teaching staff. Their self-confidence was boosted still further by Bob's policy of encouraging innovation by words and extra monetary payments. As he later said: 'mistakes are good, if you try something and it doesn't quite work, you are not hauled on the mat anymore. Instead you get a pat on the back for having a bash, inertia is the greatest sin . . . the money is nice, but it isn't that, that gets people going, it is the trust you are offering them …'.

Bob also attempted to flatten out the hierarchy by recruiting younger members of staff and changing individuals' job titles and responsibilities. The level of resistance to this strategy and his policy of speeding up decision making within the school by means of weekly staff meetings was very low. In part this was a reflection of Bob's personal qualities, but it was also testament to his ability to find individuals niches which satisfied both them and Bob's culture change programme.

It was, nevertheless, recognised that there was still considerable work to be done raising the profile of the school in Mansfield. Following a discussion with staff it was decided that Bob should approach the managing director of the local Mansfield Breweries (who was also a member of the school's governing board). He arranged for a local marketing consultancy called Miles Communication to provide help and advice to Bob concerning how to market the school. As a result, the school developed a fortnightly newsletter for parents, negotiated a series of feature articles in the local paper, and sent out a questionnaire in order to evaluate people's perceptions of the school and how it could be improved. The school also developed a mission statement, wrote a three-year marketing plan, developed roadshows to be put on for primary schools in order to attract students, encouraged local primary schools to come and use their facilities, took steps to improve the school's appearance, and tried to get on to local radio and television.

As the school became a more egalitarian, more person-respecting, and more innovative institution, financial pressures came to the fore. In response to these Bob approached a local theme park called 'The American Adventure'. He suggested that the company should provide the school with promotionally based tickets which it would sell in return for a cut of the profits. A deal was signed, and within three months the school had sold over £17 000 of tickets, the proceeds from which it used to help purchase a mini bus. So successful did this venture prove that a larger theme park (Alton Towers) approached the school with a better deal – which Bob was quick to take.

In addition to a range of smaller excursions into the world of business, Bob also signed a big deal with British Thornton, a scientific and educational equipment manufacturer: the result was a new modern languages centre, a new science laboratory, and a new home economics room, all fully equipped. What is more, because the company were allowed to use the classrooms as showrooms during slack periods, the school also received a 3 per cent commission on any orders generated.

In the mid-1990s the full impact of Bob's policies was not difficult to gauge. The school appeared to be much improved, many of the facilities were impressive, and many new courses had been put on for pupils and adults. It was also the case that numbers attending parents meetings had gone up from 30 to 300, pupil attendance had risen to 95.7 per cent, there had been no recent instances of vandalism, and the number of students staying on into the sixth form increased from 8 to 115. There was also evidence that exam results in some subjects had improved 300 per cent.

While Bob himself spoke of culture change still being in progress rather than accomplished, it was clear that a revolution in culture had already been managed by Bob with the help of consultants and hybrids.

Questions

1 Is the Garibaldi School experiencing a serious attempt at culture change?

2 Has Garibaldi undergone culture change?

3 How convincing an illustration of the 'birth and early growth' phase of Schein's model is this account of change management at Garibaldi?

4 What learning points are there here for other organisations attempting culture change?

5 Are there any special reasons why the culture of schools may be easier to alter than the culture of most other sorts of organisation?

6 How useful do you think Schein's life-cycle model is for understanding culture change?

Source: adapted with permission from Boyett and Finlay (1993)

Organisational midlife

The second phase of the model, organisational midlife, refers to the time when an organisation is well established and faced with complex strategic choices concerning growth, diversification, and acquisitions. The culture of the organisation is now formed and deeply embedded in its routines and structures. Strong subcultures may also have developed, making full understanding of the culture difficult for leaders to appreciate, though this understanding is what they need in order to bring about change. Schein identifies another four mechanisms by which culture change may occur.

Planned change and organisational development

This involves unfreezing the organisation, facilitating change and refreezing the organisation once again. This process generally requires the discovery of the assumptions of the dominant culture and subcultures, the creation of mutual insight, and the development of means of knitting them together in order to pursue superordinate company goals. The mechanism assumes that one of the decisive spurs to change is conflict between the dominant and other cultures within the organisation.

Technological seduction

The introduction of new technology can cause culture change in two basic ways. First, new technologies mean new patterns of social interaction and interpersonal relationships. In other words, when, for example, a new computer system or production line is implemented, people who have been used to working with each other in a particular way often find that their relationship has changed. This alteration in social behaviour can then cause reassessment of the assumptions on which the old patterns were built, and culture change becomes possible. Second, new technology can also mean that the nature and mission of the organisation itself comes to be re-examined. For instance, people may find that their power base is threatened by the availability of information promised by a new networked computer system, while others may find themselves threatened with redundancy.

Change through scandal, explosion of myths

This occurs where an organisation espouses a particular set of cultural values and beliefs and practices another set (see Chapter 1). Where such an incongruity exists there is always the danger that it will be dramatically exposed. For instance, an oil company which claims to be environmentally aware may be prosecuted for pollution or an organisation which claims to be an Equal Opportunities employer could lose a sex discrimination case. Such events expose a part of a culture to thoroughgoing re-examination and change.

Incrementalism

This form of culture change involves leaders making decisions which are designed to achieve a new set of assumptions in the very long term. The point is that each individual decision represents a very small change from the status quo, thus making incremental decisions almost indistinguishable from decisions which preserve the current order. This process was first described by Quinn (1978) to describe how leaders actually seek to implement their strategies.

Organisational maturity

The third phase of the model, organisational maturity, refers to a time when an organisation is highly stable, is exploiting mature markets, and lacks the motivation to change. It is at this time that its culture may become dysfunctional. Environmental change might require an organisation to become more dynamic and flexible, but if one set of assumptions has led to its being successful, then employees may be extremely unwilling to change. A lot of complex processes are probably happening here. For example, the cultural assumptions are likely to be a source of pride and esteem for members, they may also be a source of power, and will almost certainly be acting as perception filters which make it difficult for people to understand potential new strategies or if they are understood, to implement them. An organisation in this state has two choices to regain its competitiveness, first, *turnaround* (rapid large-scale change of elements of the culture), and second *total reorganisation* (such as the destruction of the group or merger with another organisation). Three culture change mechanisms appropriate to this phase in an organisation's life cycle are identified by Schein.

Coercive persuasion

This involves the leadership forcing through cultural change in situations where employees have no alternative but to accept the new reality because they have nowhere else to go. Because people have no other options they are more likely to accept the discomfort of change and accommodate new ideas. Coercive persuasion has a good chance of succeeding when employed by highly skilled change managers who are able to manipulate people's understandings of what is going on, and who are able to deliver results quickly.

Turnaround

This is a very general category for Schein that involves the use of many other change management techniques to encourage unfreezing, change and refreezing. It requires a sense of vision, a variety of leadership skills, the power to implement the new culture, and a host of change management skills to overcome resistance without alienating the workforce. In short, all the other change management mechanisms considered above may come into play here, though it is the leader's ability to coerce that Schein claims is essential for a successful turnaround. An example of cultural change through turnaround at the Swedish company BAHCO is provided by Mini Case 4.4.

Reorganisation, destruction and rebirth

Schein has little to say about this mechanism, except that almost nothing is known about it. The real point here is that total destruction of an organisation (and therefore its culture) is rarely used as a deliberate strategy, perhaps because it is so traumatic a process.

While Schein has attempted to formulate a coherent life-cycle framework for understanding the mechanisms of culture change, he is the first to acknowledge the difficulties and complexities associated with this field of inquiry. He thus exhorts us not to oversimplify our understanding of culture (see Chapters 1 and 2), not to forget how culture is learned through positive feedback and trauma (see Chapter 2), and not to assume that more culture or stronger culture is necessarily better. In contrast with the pessimism of Lundberg, Schein asserts that: 'If we give culture its due, if we take an inquiring attitude towards the deciphering of culture, if we respect what culture is and what functions it serves, we will find that it is a potentially friendly animal that can be tamed and made to work for us' (Schein, 1985a: 42).

Organisational maturity: turnaround at BAHCO

In 1983 BAHCO was a diversified and over-stretched Swedish-based tools and equipment manufacturer. It was also losing considerable amounts of money, Skr 200 million (£20 million) in 1982 and Skr 70 million (£7 million) in 1983. BAHCO had got into difficulties following an ambitious diversification strategy through which it acquired companies in France, the UK, Germany and Argentina. These companies, while theoretically supposed to be working in co-operation did their best to avoid doing so. One reason for the improvement in the 1983 figures was that in May that year Anders Lindstrom had taken over as managing director. At the time Lindstrom was a 42-year-old Swede with a reputation for turning round problem-ridden businesses. This is a brief description of how he did it.

Lindstrom was sensitive both to the history and traditions of BAHCO, a company that had originally invented the adjustable wrench in 1893. He was also keenly aware that the subsidiaries in different countries 'hated each other', and that these conflicts were exacerbated by BAHCO's structures which, imposed the need for them to co-operate, quite unnecessarily in Lindstrom's view. One of his first moves was to simplify reporting relationships, abolish regional co-ordination centres, and reduce HQ staff from 70 to 15. With the company still in a state of despair Lindstrom set about courting the press, shareholders and employees in an attempt to raise morale. He put on a reception for the local and financial press, produced pamphlets and a video for distribution to staff, and announced the doubling of BAHCO's capitalisation – a bold move that was welcomed by the shareholders.

There were, however, some tough decisions still to be made. Twenty-six per cent of the workforce (2000 people) were laid off, all of whom Lindstrom insisted had to be found alternative employment outside the company. By helping those people no longer employed at BAHCO to find jobs he hoped to build trust and confidence in himself and the organisation from the remaining staff. He also had a radical impact on the promotion system. Travelling around the organisation asking questions he quickly noticed who responded quickly and straightforwardly and who were passive and evasive: those who impressed him were rewarded with promotion, those who did not were passed by. Perhaps more than anything else he recognised that he had to lead by example, and when one day he arrived at a West German plant that had laid on a big reception for him, he casually walked by it and into the factory, asserting that there was no time for ceremony and that 'beer and sandwiches' should be sent in. The message was clear: expensive frills were no longer acceptable, and hard work was now required.

1984 was declared by Lindstrom to be 'the year of sales'. As a first step towards improving sales Lindstrom persuaded all his managing directors to spend 10 per cent more of their time either in the field or talking to customers. He then set up a series of internal competitions between companies designed to motivate them to increase sales and open markets. The winners of these competitions were rewarded and their achievements advertised throughout the organisation. In order to facilitate the exchange of good ideas travel between subsidiaries was encouraged, and by the end of 1984 BAHCO was £10 million in profit. 1985 was then declared the 'year of ideas', with the emphasis not just on new products but anything that would save money, improve quality and increase effectiveness. The result was that by May 1985 320 implementable ideas had been examined and their progenitors rewarded. By the end of the financial year the organisation had made a profit of £20 million.

Epilogue

At the end of 1986 Lindstrom left BAHCO following a change in the organisation's share ownership profile that weakened his authority. As he said himself: 'I could have been head of their industrial division, but I didn't want that . . . I'd be maximising short-term profits for the owners and that's not how I operate.'

Questions

1 Has BAHCO experienced a serious attempt at culture change?

2 Has BAHCO undergone culture change?

3 How convincing an illustration of turnaround is this account of change management at BAHCO?

4 What learning points are there here for other organisations attempting turnaround?

Source: derived from Hampden-Turner (1990). Students are recommended to see this original source for a fuller account of Lindstrom's exploits at BAHCO.

Evaluation

Schein's framework presents the important possibility that different mechanisms for culture change operate in different phases in an organisation's development. This is a radical departure from those models which suggest that there is one over-arching framework into which all instances of organisational culture change will fit. It suggests that culture change can occur in a variety of circumstances and is not dependent on the precise conjunction of sets of internal and external variables. In fact, no one factor has to be present (such as a perceived crisis or leadership change), and this flexibility is surely to be welcomed. Moreover Schein provides considerable insight into a wealth of different means for effecting culture change which we can use to further our understanding of these most complex of organisational processes.

While opening up a range of possibilities for understanding culture change, Schein's framework offers relatively little insight into the detail of how such mechanisms operate. Indeed, some mechanisms are so vaguely spelled out, such as 'reorganisation, destruction and rebirth', that it is difficult to know what is being described. We may also question the extent to which it is true that organisations pass through neatly divided developmental phases as the life-cycle model implies. Questions can also be asked of the degree to which each culture change mechanism identified by Schein uniquely applies to a given developmental phase. For example, even very recently created organisations may need to be subject to turnaround if their performance is poor, and may need to be altered through coercive persuasion. Thus despite the apparent plausibility of Schein's framework and the undoubted importance of the culture change mechanisms it embraces, further elaboration and refinement are required in order to render it fully acceptable.

Gagliardi's model

Gagliardi's (1986) framework for understanding culture change is based on an appreciation of the essence of culture as assumptions and values, with symbols, artefacts and technologies being of secondary importance. This conception of culture is essentially similar to those held by Lundberg, Dyer and Schein. His model of culture change differs from those of Lundberg and Dyer in that it is a development of his ideas on how cultures first form. Gagliardi's framework also has a different focus than those devised by Lundberg and Dyer, namely, incremental rather than radical change.

Gagliardi suggests that there are four phases in the genesis of an organisational value. In phase one a leader employs a vision (set of specific beliefs) for evaluating tasks and defining objectives. While not all the members of the organisation may share these beliefs, the leader has the power to orient those under his direct control in the direction that he or she desires. In phase two the belief is confirmed (i.e. found to work) by experience, and comes to be shared by all members of the organisation. In phase three employees turn their attention away from the effects of the belief, coming instead to focus on the belief as the cause of something desirable. The practical consequences of this are that employees will assert their faith in the efficacy of, for example, 'continuous innovation' or being 'production-led' even in the face of (what looks to the outsider like) incontrovertible evidence that such beliefs are damaging. Finally, the value comes to be shared unquestioningly and unconsciously by all concerned. For Gagliardi this is a process of *idealisation* in which a belief is *emotionally transfigured* (i.e. held on emotional rather than rational/logical grounds). In Schein's terms the value has become an assumption.

Gagliardi asserts that organisations do not learn from negative experiences. Thus when a problem emerges which cannot be solved using the potential for action offered by the existing culture, immediate culture change does not occur. Instead, the organisation is more likely to engage in a search for excuses and scapegoats, and in established behaviour patterns associated with the old (and now discredited) culture. These periods are accompanied by an increase in group tensions and a decrease in confidence, cohesion and efficiency. The need for large-scale culture change is, however, discernible by those who are not deeply involved with the dominant culture, because they are either members of deviant subcultures or outsiders. Substantial culture changes therefore require a change of leadership, for only then can problems be correctly diagnosed and the cultural identity of the organisation reconstructed. Cultural revolution in Gagliardi's terms is costly, and requires that many of the old guard leave, that new recruits are brought in from outside, and that the old symbol set is replaced by a new symbology. Gagliardi offers the interesting observation that such cultural revolutions are best described not so much as large-scale changes as the old firm dying and a new one being born.

Gagliardi then presents an incremental model of culture change (see Fig. 4.4), which he suggests is the only form of organisational adaptation that we can meaningfully describe as a change in culture. According to this model, when a problem is recognised by an organisation the survival strategy adopted does not imply that the old culture has to be destroyed, just that its range of options are expanded. This means that new values must be incorporated into an organisation's culture. The process begins with the exercise of a new competence or new way of doing things that is not radically different from past practice and is founded on values which can be fitted in to the organisation's pre-existing hierarchy of values. If the organisation then experiences success the idealisation process may lead to the new values being subscribed to on emotional rather than rational grounds.

This process is likely to be accompanied by an increase in tensions and conflict which must be attenuated by reconciliation myths promulgated by the leadership. These myths convince people that the organisation's success is due to the new prac-

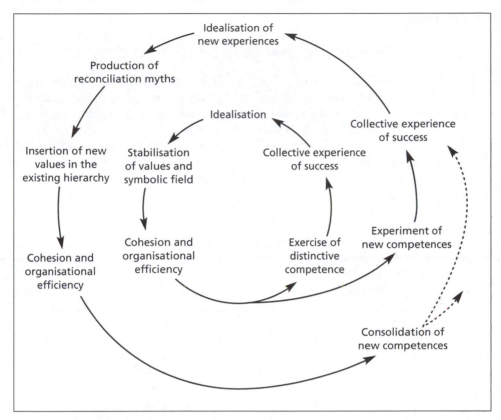

Fig. 4.4 Cultural change as an incremental process
Source: reproduction with permission from Gagliardi (1986)

tices. In reality, of course, success may be due to any number of internal and external factors unrelated to the new ways of doing things. Over time the result will be the insertion of a new value (or values) into the existing cultural hierarchy. Assuming that the idealisation process has been entirely effective, and that the new status quo continues to be linked to successful activity in the minds of employees, then the organisation is likely to become more cohesive and efficient, leading to the consolidation of the new competencies. Cultural change, then, can be an incremental process that requires skilled leadership (see Mini Case 4.5):

> In cultural change, then, the role of the leader is, above all, to create conditions under which success can visibly be achieved, even if only in a limited or partial way, and to rationalize positive events after they have happened, even if accidental. (In the light of this, Napoleon's habit of promoting only 'lucky' men to the rank of general seems rather less a caprice on his part than a selection criterion based on an intuitive grasp of these processes.) A leader does not reinterpret past history to justify retrospectively his own proposals, nor does he go against existing myths; rather, he reinterprets the recent past and the present in such a way that he promotes the insertion of new emergent values into the hierarchy of current operational ones and encourages the birth of new myths which are superimposed on the old ones and reconcile new contradictions. (Gagliardi, 1986: 132)

Incremental culture change at Industrial Products Limited

Exercise of a distinctive competence

Based in the south of England, Industrial Products Limited (IPL) was a medium-sized manufacturer of electronic components. Ever since the company was set up in the mid-1970s Bulstrode (who was one of three partners and IPL's chief executive) had promulgated a consistent vision: IPL was destined to become the UK's leading manufacturer of electronic components. In order to fulfil the vision Bulstrode insisted that the organisation concentrate its efforts on producing high-quality and reliable components for which it could charge a premium. Bulstrode's two partners had originally suggested that they should consider pursuing a volume strategy in which quality would play a less important role than producing in large volumes at least cost. Bulstrode was, however, the senior partner, and it was his vision of what IPL's distinctive competence should be that came to dominate. One notable feature of this vision was that it ascribed only a limited role to exports, which were handled by a small 'export department'. As Bulstrode said, 'if at the end of the day there is anything left over to sell, it will do for the foreigner'.

Collective experience of success

Over the course of the next decade IPL generally returned what the partners considered to be adequate results, and occasionally the firm had some exceptionally good years. As the organisation expanded Bulstrode's formula gained widespread acceptance. Questioning of the senior and middle managers revealed that no strategic possibilities other than that advocated by Bulstrode were seriously entertained. It was arguable that the experience of success that Bulstrode's culture had engineered had come to be valued *per se*, that is, that idealisation had occurred. If there were any signs of dissent they came from the sales/marketing department, which argued that there were sizeable international markets that were not being exploited. Such views were paid scant regard by

Bulstrode, who could see risks as well as opportunities associated with expansion overseas. His opinion was that the company was stable, cohesive and efficient, and that even if his vision was limited it was at least a vision that worked.

Experiment of new competences

Towards the end of the 1980s, however, IPL's profits began to deteriorate. By this time the organisation had grown significantly, and while Bulstrode's quality formula was accepted by everyone, the original three partners now had a lot of additional expertise to draw on in framing their decisions. It was concluded that the downturn in IPL's profits was attributable both to the UK's economic recession, and to increased domestic competition. A lengthy debate then ensued concerning how best to meet the challenges of the 1990s. One of the foremost issues discussed was whether the organisation could and should attempt further penetration of European markets, especially since trade barriers across Europe were soon due to be dismantled. Finally Bulstrode agreed to a limited expansion of IPL's export department, which fundamentally involved taking on new staff experienced in making international sales.

Collective experience of success

In retrospect it was clear that IPL had appointed some particularly talented staff to the export department, because sales to Europe and the rest of the world increased enormously. Pressure then built up to reconstitute the export department as the company's International Division (a separate subsidiary) with its own managing director and considerable autonomy. As the volume of international business expanded, so did Bulstrode's vision for IPL, which he now described as 'seeking to become Europe's leading manufacturer of electronic components'. In fact, as the organisation became increasingly dependent on the International Division (which continued to grow in size) the beginnings of a more radical orientation in IPL's culture could be detected, with some suggesting that it should set up manufacturing operations in other parts of the globe.

Reconciliation myths and the insertion of new values

The evolution of IPL's small export department into a separate International Division did not occur as painlessly as the above description might be seen to imply. Many people, initially including Bulstrode, were uncertain that the costs of doing business in Europe would be outweighed by the benefits. It was only the seriousness of the company's economic problems that made this option seem remotely attractive. Once the decision to expand more vigorously into international markets had been taken there were many doubters to be pacified. Two arguments (which are interpretable as myths) were employed by Bulstrode and his senior team. First, that it was only now that the time was right to expand sales abroad, because now it was easier to export to Europe. Second, that IPL's

products were only now sufficiently good to take on foreign competition. Faced with such arguments few asked why the time had not been right five, ten or even fifteen years earlier. Most were just concerned to enjoy the continued success of what was now going to become Europe's leading electronic components company.

Questions

1 Is IPL experiencing a serious attempt at culture change?

2 Has IPL undergone culture change? If so, how did IPL's culture alter during the period from its inception to the early to mid-1990s? Did IPL's culture undergo radical or incremental change?

3 How important was Bulstrode to the process of culture change?

4 How convincing an illustration of Gagliardi's model is this account of change management at IPL?

5 What learning points are there here for other organisations attempting culture change?

6 How useful do you think Gagliardi's life-cycle model is for understanding culture change?

Evaluation

Gagliardi's work draws an important distinction between radical and incremental change, and offers the interesting suggestion that the only real sort of culture change is incremental, as radical change implies the destruction of one culture and its replacement by another, that is, an act of creation rather than change. The framework also recognises that values often come to be held on emotional rather than rational grounds, through a process of idealisation, thus explaining part of the difficulty of altering organisational cultures: if culture change could be induced through rational argument it would surely be a far simpler and more easily accomplished process. Furthermore Gagliardi's analysis implicates symbols and myths as the mechanisms by which culture change can be enforced, and while their influence is not spelled out in any detail, these are probably important, and certainly worthy of note.

For Gagliardi the phrase 'culture change' properly refers to a single process (in contrast to the eleven identified by Schein) that, as with many other theories, is heavily dependent on the idea of 'leadership': it is the leader who has the vision, creates the new symbology, and spreads the myths. This ignores the very real limits to the power of individual CEOs and leadership elites, and downplays the role that more junior employees have in shaping culture. More important still is the focus of the model on a single value. According to Gagliardi incremental culture change occurs to individual values in discrete phases, whereas other authors have suggested that whole clusters of values may undergo change simultaneously. In addition, and as with Lundberg and Dyer's models, Gagliardi's framework provides little indication of the timescales over which these sorts of changes can be expected to occur. Rather than castigate a fascinating and useful model, however, it is, perhaps, more appropriate to appreciate it for its insight into the value of factors such as 'perceived success' and 'idealisation', which assist us in our understanding of culture change.

Understanding culture change: Lewin, Beyer and Trice, and Isabella

In this section a compilation model of organisational change based on the ideas of Lewin (1952) as modified by Schein (1964), Beyer and Trice (1988) and Isabella (1990) is examined. Instead of a grand theory of culture change the framework points out some of the complex cultural processes likely to be associated with organisational adaptation. It thus provides a more micro and hence more detailed view of what may be going on in organisations experiencing culture change. The framework, shown in Fig. 4.5, follows Lewin in its division of change episodes into three broad phases: unfreezing, change and refreezing. Each of these phases is associated with certain social behaviours or rites[2] and a particular cognitive state. This reflects the view that culture change has both behavioural and cognitive components.

Contextual	Social	Cognitive
Unfreezing mechanisms	Rites of questioning and destruction	Anticipation
	Rites of rationalisation and legitimation	
Experimentation	Rites of degradation and conflict	Confirmation
	Rites of passage and enhancement	Culmination
Refreezing mechanisms	Rites of integration and conflict reduction	Aftermath

Fig. 4.5 Understanding organisational culture change: three related domains
Source: reproduced from Roberts and Brown (1992)

Unfreezing

The process of organisational unfreezing is begun when some (usually senior) managers develop a felt need to change, generally in response to one or more catalytic events such as declining profitability or falling market share. This evidence of organisational failure provides the disconfirmation (feedback that things are going wrong) that in turn induces guilt anxiety (sense of personal failure) that encourages individuals to be more receptive to notions of change. However, while those individuals directly affected by the catalyst events may begin the unfreezing process, in large complex organisations there is no reason to suppose that this will be anything more than a localised phenomenon. If culture change is to occur then this felt need for change must be cascaded down the organisation.

Two basic types of unfreezing rites have been identified, namely, *rites of questioning and destruction* and *rites of rationalisation and legitimation*. Rites of questioning and destruction formally challenge the established order of an organisation, often by presenting the same concrete evidence that individuals or systems are failing to perform adequately that originally induced a felt need to change in the sponsors of the system themselves. These rites commonly take the form of presentations designed not merely to inform but to persuade, generally as part of a calculated 'advertisement' campaign. Other rites of questioning and destruction include bringing in a team of external consultants. Consultants are often less intimidated by an organisation's opinion leaders or informal norms than organisational members themselves, and this intellectual distance allows them to criticise underperforming individuals, systems and practices. Consultants can thus stimulate change-oriented debate and questioning of the basic assumptions of an organisation.

Rites of rationalisation and legitimation sensitise individuals to the significance of the proposed changes by providing explanations of why they are required. The role of the sensitising acts and explanations in organisations is twofold: first, they legitimate the new thinking, making it appear worthwhile, acceptable and necessary. Second, they promote widespread commitment to the proposed change programme. Rites of rationalisation and legitimation mostly involve senior managers and training/education programmes. Many commentators have suggested that top management support for culture change is vital in order to ensure adequate resourcing, to establish and approve new organisational structures, roles and responsibilities, to mediate in conflict situations, and especially to provide the disconfirmation of present behaviour in order to initiate the unfreezing process. Equally important for initiating the unfreezing process are training and education programmes. It is through education that individuals gain awareness of the need to develop formal policies and procedures, distribute responsibilities, alter the way in which decisions are made, and learn to apply different project planning methods. For example, as part of Johnson Matthey plc's attempts at culture change 150 senior and key middle managers were sent on a week-long quality education course run by an internationally renowned consultancy firm.[3] Fifty-five of these individuals were then selected to attend a further two-week course in order to prepare them to teach quality courses for the rest of the workforce. The re-educational process continued on the job with the formation of quality improvement teams (Williams *et al.*, 1993).

At this time individual employees will generally be undergoing intense psychological strain. Isabella describes this as a period of anticipation, in which individuals assemble and exchange rumours and hearsay concerning the nature and extent of the putative changes, collate and integrate the as yet incomplete information they discover into a coherent picture, and thus attempt to arrive at sufficient understanding to decrease anxiety levels.

Change

This is the phase where actual culture change occurs. According to the Lewin–Schein model, if the unfreezing stage has been successfully negotiated, employees will actively seek to change without much further prompting. The framework suggests that this stage is associated with two further sorts of rites, *rites of degradation and conflict* and *rites of passage and enhancement*. It also argues that during this change phase individuals progress through two distinct cognitive phases, which Isabella refers to as *confirmation* and *culmination*.

Rites of degradation and conflict challenge and undermine the existing status quo. A typical rite of degradation is to replace staff who are unable and unwilling to acknowledge the need for change, and to appoint new staff more compatible with the new desired culture state. The deliberate creation of constructive conflictual situations can also be beneficial during this phase of change. The inception of a task force with its own budget, office and resources can ensure that more conservative vested interests are counterbalanced, that rigorous debate occurs and that sweeping action can be taken. A further means of degrading the old order and creating constructive conflict is to develop new goals, milestones and performance indicators which provide the necessary disconfirmatory cues about current procedures and practices. These targets do not just perform co-ordination, control and monitoring functions, they formalise good practice, serve as a motive impelling action, ensure discipline and instil pride.

At the same time that rites of degradation and conflict challenge people's assumptions and work practices, rites of passage and enhancement may also be employed. These rites are designed to overcome resistance to change, broaden the base of support for the new cultural system, and encourage ownership of the process of change. Education and training programmes are obviously important in this respect, as are acts such as promoting individuals who are willing and able to adapt to the new culture, and changing job titles to reflect the new order of things. For example, the establishment of a quality office at Rank Xerox, the manager of which reported to the director of strategic development, seems to have been an important rite of enhancement in their culture change programme.

During this period of change employees' perceptions of what is going on will change substantially as the consequences of new systems, policies and procedures become clearer. Isabella suggests that once individuals have sufficient information they will naturally attempt to understand events using traditional explanations and deductions based on past experiences of substantial change, which she refers to as a period of confirmation. This tendency to rely on old heuristics can help us to explain those instances where individuals and groups are unable to fully understand the cultural implications of the changes that are being sought by those driving the programme. In fact, it is only when the deficiencies of standard explanations become transparent that confirmation can give way to a phase of greater learning and awareness, which Isabella terms culmination. Culmination thus refers to the phase in which the new culture begins to take shape as individuals come to a greater understanding of the changes required of them.

Refreezing

During the refreezing phase individuals seek an end to the uncertainty and instability that characterise their work tasks and relationships with others by meeting their felt need for change. In practical cultural terms this involves the individual employee in redefining his or her understanding of the functions required of him or her, and learning how to implement the new rules and procedures through and with colleagues. This is essentially a consolidation phase which when complete implies that the organisation has settled into a new stable state. The refreezing phase is characterised by a number of features: the new cultural assumptions are deeply embedded, supporting myths and stories are established, all external consultants have left, and employees are enacting the new culture without conscious effort. From now on the continued success of the culture should produce the confirmatory cues required for it to become deeply embedded in the mind-sets of employees. Refreezing is likely to be associated with *rites of integration and conflict reduction*, in order to encourage a general cognitive shift to a state Isabella refers to as *aftermath*.

Rites of integration and conflict reduction bring coherence to an organisation, reduce the level of conflict between individuals, functions and departments, and reconcile vested interests to the new order of things. These are useful and necessary after a period of sustained and far-reaching change. Comments from senior managers praising people for their fortitude and perseverance are one form in which these rites occur, as are refresher training courses. Rites of integration and conflict reduction thus consolidate the change process. Once the changes have occurred and the new culture is in place, individuals enter the final interpretive stage, aftermath. At this time the changes are evaluated, conclusions concerning the organisation's strengths and weaknesses are drawn, and winners and losers are identified. In the aftermath stage, employees are familiar with the new rules, systems and procedures, personal and organisational uncertainties have diminished, and a new status quo has emerged. In this final interpretational phase, individuals are able to put the changes in perspective, and to work out what they mean both for themselves and the organisation as a whole. Aspects of this model are illustrated in Mini Case 4.6.

Evaluation

The framework is valuable because it brings together a wealth of ideas about culture change that are already well known and accepted and presents them in a coherent and comprehensible manner. It realistically implicates elements of culture (rites) as potential culture change mechanisms and specifically addresses both cognitive and behavioural change elements. Furthermore it suggests that culture change involves a complex series of processes, and provides some insight into the nature of them. The framework is also notable in that its extreme generality makes it applicable across a wide variety of organisations, and that while it makes use of notions such as 'leadership' and 'crisis', these are more fully integrated with the micro-behaviour of organisations and individuals than in many other models.

However, it should also be noted that the framework has not been specifically formulated to account for culture change *per se*, does not entail a well-defined notion of culture, and is equally applicable to, say, technological adaptation as it is to culture change. Moreover it is evident that no organisation which undergoes a significant change programme passes smoothly through Lewin's three phases: different individuals are more (or less) open to change, and this means that the time it takes for them to feel guilt-anxiety and learn new procedures will also differ. This implies that, in certain extreme cases, while one individual is entering the refreezing phase his or her colleagues may still be in the process of unfreezing. In the case of large organisations the same variation is also likely to be apparent between functions, departments and subsidiaries. In addition, and perhaps even more damaging, is the suggestion that different sorts of rites may not be uniquely associated with a specific phase in the Lewin–Schein model. For example, it has been argued that rites of rationalisation and legitimation which promote understanding, commitment and legitimacy will occur throughout change programmes, and not just in the unfreezing phase as the framework asserts. To sum up, then, despite its seeming

Culture change at British Airways

When the Thatcher government decided to convert British Airways (BA) from government ownership to private ownership it was evident that a major culture change was first required. In fact, external pressure on BA to change came not only from the government's threat to privatise it but from deregulation of the industry worldwide. The result was a transformation of BA's culture from one which was bureaucratic and militaristic to one that may now be described as service-oriented and market-driven. The success of this cultural transformation is evident in terms of the company's healthy share price and cargo and passenger revenues. So how was this culture change managed?

Unfreezing

The first step in the unfreezing process was a necessary downsizing of BA's workforce from 59 000 to 37 000 people. This reduction in the workforce was accomplished by early retirement and substantial financial settlements which eased what was inevitably a traumatic time for the organisation and its employees. The second dramatic change at BA was the appointment of Lord King as chairman and Colin Marshall as CEO. The appointment of Marshall was particularly significant as he had a marketing background and was not a retired Royal Air Force officer as had been so many of his predecessors. Supporting the unfreezing process was a large-scale training programme called 'Putting People First'. This was designed for all those BA personnel who had direct customer contact, and aimed to educate line workers and managers concerning the service nature of the airline industry. A whole battery of changes to BA's structures and systems were also implemented, such as the use of diagonal task forces (i.e. teams of individuals from different functions and at different levels), a reduction in the number of levels in the organisational hierarchy, and modifications to the budgeting process.

Change

With BA unfrozen, actual change towards the new desired culture state had to be guided and enforced. This was done largely through a series of training programmes for senior and middle managers, such as 'Managing People First' and 'Leading the Service Business'. These involved considerable personal feedback to each individual concerning his or her job-related behaviour. The continued use of diagonal task forces to facilitate change was also significant. The combined result was an elimination of many dysfunctional business practices and a change in climate to one which was more open, placed greater value on teamwork and recognised that quality of service was all important. Critical to the success of the change programme was undoubtedly Marshall's commitment to the new culture, which he visibly demonstrated in question-and-answer sessions at training programmes. Support mechanisms were also much in evidence in order to reduce the psychological burden of change. For example, emotional support systems were developed for workers suffering from burn-out, personnel staff were retrained to become internal change agents, and a new bonus system was introduced to share the financial gains BA was making more widely.

Refreezing

The continued support of the senior leadership team ensured that the culture changes became a permanent feature at BA. This refreezing process was helped by making it clear that those people who openly supported the new values were more likely to be promoted. Refreezing was also aided by a whole new series of training programmes conducted at a newly purchased training centre. The development of a new performance appraisal system and performance-based compensation system, both of which encouraged good customer service, were also important indicators that the changes were not going to be transitory. Finally, the more obvious BA symbols such as uniforms were upgraded and aircraft refurbished, a new corporate coat of arms was devised with the motto 'We fly to serve' and improved systems for using staff were put into effect. British Airways undoubtedly hopes that its continued use of data feedback on its performance will increasingly make it the world's favourite airline.

In conclusion, it is important to remember that BA's culture change efforts have not always run smoothly. In the initial stages chaos and anger were much in evidence, with serious questions being asked concerning the wisdom of the process. While much of the fear and resentment has now subsided a whole gamut of other problems currently face BA. These range from the fact that high levels of customer service are not always consistently maintained to the threats posed by recession and increased competition.

According to Goodstein and Burke (1991) such difficulties illustrate that while BA has achieved significant success in the recent past, in the future 'managing momentum may be more difficult than managing change'.

Questions

1 Is British Airways experiencing a serious attempt at culture change?

2 Has British Airways undergone culture change?

3 How convincing an illustration of this composite model is this account of change management at British Airways?

4 What learning points are there here for other organisations attempting culture change?

5 How useful do you think this composite model is for understanding culture change?

Source: adapted from Goodsteine & Burke (1991). Reprinted, by permission of the publisher, from Organizational Dynamics, spring 1991 © 1991. American Management Association, New York. All rights reserved

sophistication, the processes of culture change are probably still more varied, complex and unpredictable than this essentially static framework allows for.

LESSONS FROM THE MODELS OF CULTURE CHANGE

In this section we will re-examine some of the common themes that the models of culture change share. There are, of course, some obvious points of difference between them in terms of their particular focus, attention to detail and weighting of various factors. For instance, Lundberg's presentation of culture change as the result of fairly specific combinations of internal and external forces is in many ways very different from Schein's attempt to correlate culture change mechanisms with stages in the organisational life cycle. This said, the similarities between the five frameworks are striking. They all (either explicitly or implicitly) make reference to the notion of a crisis, emphasise the importance of leadership, comment on the role of perceived success, and present change as a form of organisational learning. These four factors, then, appear to be key to our understanding of how cultures change.

Crises

The perception of a problem that must be met with organisational change is pivotal to all the models. Lundberg suggests that precipitating pressures lead to the build up of tension which is released by some triggering event, spurring culture change. For

Schein the perception of a problem or crisis (including leadership succession) is what initiates most mechanisms of culture change. In Dyer's model a triggering event precipitates a crisis, which leads to a breakdown in the means of support for the old culture. Gagliardi's theory of incremental culture change depends on an organisation experiencing difficulties. In terms of Lewin's framework, culture change occurs only when a crisis leads to individuals experiencing a felt need for change by providing evidence for organisational and personal failure.

Leadership

For Lundberg culture change requires a relatively stable leadership team with the requisite vision, power and communication skills to formulate a coherent strategy and action plans. Schein's appreciation of culture change mechanisms shows leadership to be central to most of those associated with the early and midlife stages of organisational evolution and all of those associated with organisational maturity. According to Dyer's model a new leader or leadership team is vital if a new culture is to be promulgated within an organisation. In Gagliardi's model substantial changes require a change of leadership while incremental change must be guided by leaders who exercise new distinctive competencies and circulate appropriate reconciliation myths in order to reduce conflict. Leadership also figures prominently in the ideas of Beyer and Trice, where effective leadership is needed to recognise the nature of the problem faced, organise the rites, establish new roles and responsibilities, and mediate in conflict situations.

Success

In order for a new culture to become established it must be identified as the factor responsible for solving the initial crisis. While this view is implicit in the Lundberg model and the ideas of Lewin, it is held explicitly by Schein, Dyer and Gagliardi. The Lundberg learning cycle could not be completed without the organisation experiencing success because employees would be unlikely to accept the leader's new cultural vision. Likewise, in Lewin's framework a lack of success would lead to a rejection of the new culture in the culmination phase. For Schein, success is critical for most change mechanisms, such as natural evolution and managed revolutions. In Dyer's model the new leader's solutions must work (or be thought to work) in order for the internal conflicts and tensions to be dissolved. For Gagliardi success is vital because it is the experience of success that leads to values and beliefs being subscribed to on emotional rather than rational grounds, and thus transformed into assumptions.

Learning

The models agree that culture change is essentially a process of relearning. Lundberg's model is not only formulated as a learning cycle, but he makes it clear that culture change is only made possible by inquiry and discovery. For Schein, change is a learning process, and this view permeates his culture change mechanisms. Dyer's model is another form of learning cycle, again highly dependent on the notion of a search for new cultural possibilities. In Gagliardi's framework people learn from success, and initially subscribe to certain beliefs and values as a result of learning that they have favourable consequences. Learning is also central to Isabella's ideas, where people learn their way from anticipation to aftermath, and Beyer and Trice's notions, in which education and training are important rites of questioning and destruction and rationalisation and legitimation.

RETHINKING CULTURE CHANGE: THE ROLE OF CULTURE

The models for understanding culture change presented in this chapter suggest that all cultures change in essentially the same way. The only slight variation is offered by Schein, who argues that the mechanism of culture change is dependent on the stage of organisational development. The most striking omission from these models is any reference to the characteristics of the culture undergoing change. Wilkins and Dyer (1988) have forcibly argued that a more coherent and believable theory of culture change would allow that different cultures may change through different processes. One important complication is that Wilkins and Dyer prefer to use the terms 'frame' or 'cultural frame' rather than culture *per se*. Their use of the word 'frame' is, however, almost indistinguishable from what Schein has described as an organisation's basic assumptions. As a first step in determining what cultural characteristics are associated with what change mechanisms they have identified three factors that make cultures more or less persistent. These three factors are: (1) the availability of alternative frames; (2) the participants' level of commitment to the current frame; and (3) the fluidity of the current frame. Each of these merits brief consideration.

Availability of alternative frames

The more available alternatives to the current culture are the more susceptible to change the current culture is. A frame is available to a social group if participants are (1) aware of it and (2) have the skill to quickly develop the rules, norms and routines to support it. A number of factors tend to prevent members from developing alternative frames, such as hiring very young employees with little or no prior organisational experience, a policy of promoting from within, employing those who are sympathetic to the current culture, and discouraging interaction with outsiders. In addition, if there are few alternative sources of employment people are more likely to accept cultural demands placed upon them.

Participants' level of commitment to the current frame

The more committed to the current frame members of an organisation are the less likely culture change is. Participants in a culture will tend to be more committed to the current frame if it is thought to have brought stability and success to an organisation, especially if it is supported by stories telling how the frame has been used to survive past challenges. If employees believe in the moral superiority of the frame and/or have made public decisions committing themselves to an organisation (as those in various churches, voluntary organisations and political parties do), then commitment to the current frame is unlikely to waver.

Fluidity of the frame

Wilkins and Dyer identify three factors that influence the fluidity of a frame. First, highly complex frames, especially those associated with a dominant leader, are prone to change (are more fluid) simply because few people really understand them. When the dominant leader leaves the organisation no one is able to mirror precisely that person's characteristics or espouse precisely the same philosophy, paving the way for change. Second, some cultural frames actively encourage change and adaptation, and may have altered substantially many times within recent memory. Finally, some organisations engage in consistent self-monitoring of their performance, while others do not. Those that effectively evaluate their performance and value their performance data are more likely to consider alternative frames when performance indicators show a decline.

Following Lundberg (1985), Wilkins and Dyer suggest that organisations may be classified as *morphogenetic* (change-oriented) or *homeostatic* (stability-oriented). They also argue that of the three factors they have identified as being key to understanding the propensity for culture change, frame fluidity is the controlling variable. Thus the more fluid the current frame is, the less committed participants will be to it and the more available are alternative frames. Conversely, the less fluid a frame is, the more committed to it employees will be and the less likely it is that they will develop alternatives. Wilkins and Dyer then point out that theories of culture change must take account of whether an organisation is morphogenetic or homeostatic as defined by them in terms of frame fluidity, availability and commitment. They theorise that it may take a serious environmental crisis to engender culture change in a homeostatic organisation, but that evolutionary culture change in response to changes in significant personnel may be possible in morphogenetic organisations. More interestingly, Wilkins and Dyer suggest that what counts as a crisis is likely to vary from one organisation to another, indicating that general models of culture change which rely on the notion of a crisis as a spur to action are in need of far more refinement. The same is true of the very general notions of 'leadership' that so many of the models so heavily rely on (see Chapter 7).

FINAL THOUGHTS

The concepts and models presented in this chapter make it clear that understanding culture change is extremely difficult (see for example, the work of Bate, 1994). Furthermore, it has become apparent that none of the models surveyed here is wholly convincing. Indeed, the mini case illustrations which accompanied each model illustrated their weaknesses and omissions as much as their strengths. This should not, however, lead us to the conclusion that reality is too complex to be appropriately modelled or that the models have no utility. It is suggested here that rather than ignore the difficulties concerned with attempting to understand and account for culture change, this complexity should be embraced and studied, for only then will we ever be able to come to a reasonable understanding of organisational behaviour.

That none of the models so far developed is sufficiently complex to embrace the intricacies of various culture change processes is problematic. When we have more comprehensive and coherent models of culture change, then this will surely make the practice of managing culture change far easier. This does not mean that our existing frameworks are either of no interest or no value. On the contrary they provide valuable 'first attempts' to model what are highly complex and often ambiguous social processes. Further, they help us by emphasising some factors (like *crises, leadership,* and *perceived/attributed success*) that can then become the focus of empirical research, which in turn will either confirm or disprove their importance for culture change. The point is that organisational culture change is a very confusing object of study, and simplifying models such as those examined here can be useful guides through the mass of conflicting information that the study of actual culture change throws up.

SUMMARY AND CONCLUSIONS

This chapter has elaborated four main themes.

1 It was suggested that of the large number of models that have been formulated in an attempt to understand culture change none has as yet come to dominate the field. Part of the reason for this are fundamental uncertainties concerning what culture is and thus what constitutes culture change.

2 Five models of culture change were reviewed in detail. Lundberg's learning cycle was notable for its emphasis on external factors as the drivers of cultural change. Schein's model was an interesting attempt to match particular culture change processes to stages in the life cycle of organisations. Dyer's cycle of cultural evolution had similarities with both Lundberg's and Schein's frameworks, but was distinguished by its joint emphasis on the need for both the perception of a crisis and leadership change. Gagliardi's model was valuable for its explicit recognition of the role that perceived success plays in the development of new values and beliefs and its assertion that incremental change is the only real form of culture change. The composite framework consisting of the ideas of Lewin, Beyer and Trice, and Isabella provided a different perspective on change than the first four models, focusing on some of the micro-details of cultural adaptation. Together these five models summarise much of what is known about the processes of culture change as we understand them today.

3 Four common themes that the models of culture change share were examined. It was pointed out that all relied on the notion of a crisis, suggested that leadership was crucial, attributed an important role to perceived success and portrayed change as a form of relearning.

4 It was argued that more plausible models of culture change may be developed in the future by taking three culture-related factors into account. These factors are: the availability of alternative cultures, the participants' level of commitment to the current culture, and the fluidity of the current culture. It was also suggested that culture change models which relied on the notion of a crisis or general conceptions of leadership require further elaboration and refinement.

KEY CONCEPT

Change
Evolution
Adaptation
Relearning
Definitions
Scale of change
Timescales
Lundberg's model
Learning cycle
External enabling
    conditions
Domain forgiveness
Domain congruence
Internal permitting
    conditions
Change resources
System readiness
Co-ordinative/integra-
    tive mechanisms
Leadership

Precipitating pressures
Triggering events
Cultural visioning
Strategy
Action plans
Schein's life-cycle model
Birth and early growth
Natural evolution
Self-guided evolution
Managed evolution
    through hybrids
Managed revolution
    through outsiders
Midlife
Planned change and
    organisational
    development
Technological seduction
Change through
    scandal

Incrementalism
Maturity
Coercive persuasion
Turnaround
Reorganisation
Dyer's cycle of cultural
    evolution
Crisis
Pattern-maintenance
Conflict
Success
Stabilisation
Gagliardi's model
Idealisation
Emotional
    transfiguration
Lewin, Beyer and Trice,
    and Isabella
Unfreezing
Rites of questioning

and destruction
Rites of rationalisation
    and legitimation
Anticipation
Rites of degradation
    and conflict
Rites of passage and
    enhancement
Confirmation
Culmination
Refreezing
Rites of integration
Rites of conflict
    reduction
Cultural frame
Alternative frames
Commitment
Fluidity
Morphogenetic
Homeostatic

QUESTIONS

1 How would you distinguish between the following terms: change, adaptation, learning and evolution?

2 In framing a model of culture change, why is it important to be clear on issues such as how culture is defined, the scale of change being modelled, and the time span over which change is held to occur?

3 Which model for understanding culture change do you find most plausible? Explain your answer.

4 Do you think that it is correct to suggest that organisations pass through three broad life-cycle phases (birth and early growth, midlife, and maturity)?

5 Why is effective leadership thought to be so important a factor in creating successful culture change?

6 According to Gagliardi the only real form of culture change is incremental. Do you agree?

7 Describe how rites were used to manage culture change in an organisation that you know well?

8 What are the most important commonalities between the five models of culture change?

9 Why is it important for models of culture change to take the nature of an organisational culture into account?

10 Using the information in this chapter and your own general knowledge, create your own general model of organisational culture change.

UNDERSTANDING CULTURE CHANGE AT THE ROYAL MAIL, GAMMA DISTRICT

Introduction to the Royal Mail

Founded in 1840 when Rowland Hill introduced the world's first postage stamp the Royal Mail has been a part of the UK civil service for most of the last 150 years. Today, the Royal Mail is one of the Post Office's four main businesses (the other three being Parcel Force, Subscription Services Ltd and Post Office Counters). A few figures provide a feel for the scope and scale of the Royal Mail operation: over 60 million items of mail are handled every day across the UK, its annual turnover is approximately £4 billion, it employs 180 000 staff, and made a pre-tax profit of £252 million in 1993. The Royal Mail is a considerable organisation, with around 2500 properties and a road transport fleet of 30 000 vehicles.

Prior to the reorganisation which came into effect in April 1992, the Royal Mail business was composed of three main elements: a Royal Mail HQ, four Territories (Eastern, Northern, Western and London) and 64 Districts. The HQ, based in London, was functionally organised with approximately 3000 people employed in functions like sales, network operations, planning, finance and personnel. The territories had a relatively small number of staff, and were primarily responsible for co-ordinating national initiatives, helping to implement local network schemes and auditing the District operations. The Districts were responsible for operational issues within their geographically based area.

The Royal Mail is currently in a uniquely privileged situation, having a monopoly in the letter delivery business for items costing under £1. However, while there is a lack of direct competitors, competition is evident in the form of BT, electronic mail and facsimile services. Senior executives were also quick to point out that 16–18 per cent of all mail is 'direct mail', and that advertisers had numerous other media (television, newspapers and magazines among others) to choose from. The parcel business is in a very different situation, and faces considerable direct competition in the marketplace. Three of the most significant influences on the Royal Mail are the Government, the distribution network and the workforce in a predominantly labour-reliant industry. The Government affects the business by setting the framework in which the organisation operates – monopoly, uniform delivery rate and nationwide delivery service. The distribution network (road, rail and air) has a crucial influence on the quality of the service the Royal Mail is able to provide to its customers – late trains, poor roads and cancelled air services pose constant operational problems for the business.

The following information refers to one district (here called 'Gamma') among 64, and attempts to generalise from Gamma to the whole of Royal Mail should be made cautiously.

The Gamma District

In 1990/91 the Gamma District had an annual budget of £33.5 million and employed 2100 staff, of whom 1550 were postmen. In fact, the vast bulk (93 per cent) of the annual budget was spent paying and maintaining the workforce of the organisation. While 600 people worked at the main sorting office, the other 1500 were employed at nine delivery offices spread across the District. Recruitment had been a difficult problem over the past five years with unsocial hours, a six-day working week, and a national wage structure that forced down wages in a high cost of living area resulting in understaffing. When this was pointed out to senior executives they replied that in 1988 an attempt to vary pay scales by region had resulted in a strike. The organisation consisted of five hierarchical levels, with eight senior managers (termed 'direct reports') answering directly to the District Head Postmaster (see Fig. 4.6). Despite a series of recent changes in the structure and functioning of the organisation the District was not targeted for income, and was thus treated as a cost centre rather than a profit centre.

The District was highly formal, with a plethora of written procedures, rules and regulations governing organisational activities. Reporting procedures, spans of control, and mechanisms to secure co-ordination

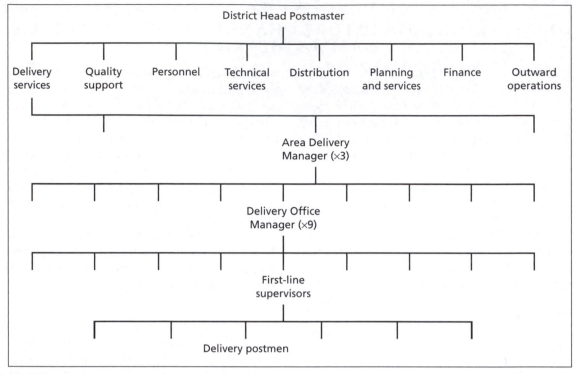

Fig. 4.6 Gamma District: organisation structure

were strictly enforced. This emphasis on formal efficiency and overt rationality was recognised to be causing problems, not least because effective team-building was being undermined by the dictates of a staffing planning process that demanded individuals move between several different supervisors and sets of workmates every day![4] Given the nature of most of the jobs to be performed, specialisation was predictably low, with many employees required to perform a variety of different functions (e.g. sorting, franking, delivery, driving). Furthermore, authority to make decisions was highly centralised, while the degree of collaboration between departments was quite low, with each department tending to perceive its work as self-contained.

Organisational culture
It was the perception of many respondents that the culture of the Post Office in general had been profoundly influenced by its history as part of the UK civil service. In addition, many suggested that it had also been shaped by the large influx of ex-soldiers that were

recruited following the Second World War. These men (and they mostly tended to be men rather than women) were used to strict discipline and could be relied upon to complete a job even when it was routine and repetitive. The fact that employee's duties still commence and end at precise times (for instance 09.22–17.34) is an echo from this past, as are the fond reminiscences of ageing supervisors for the   days when 'you could rely on postmen doing what you told them – you didn't have to watch over them the whole time – not like the youngsters we get   nowadays'. More recent (some thought Government-inspired) changes designed to facilitate greater efficiency and effectiveness, and make concepts such as 'quality' and 'service' more central to the business, have been no less significant. The result is a rich   cultural milieu that deserves to be considered in some detail.

Gamma District sorting office is a large forty-year-old anonymous brick building overlooking a railway station. The entrance is difficult to find, and reception consists of a wooden hut situated next to a driveway. Inside, the building is a maze of narrow corridors and cramped offices. The offices of the eight direct reports were situated along one corridor a considerable distance from any other offices or the sorting office floor. Above each door were three lights used to communicate to intending visitors whether the office was empty, occupied but not to be disturbed, or occupied and available. The functional departments were scattered throughout the building, and it was a rare individual who knew what went on in more than one area. Outside, there was a small car park with spaces reserved for the District Head Postmaster and his direct reports: other employees had to take their chances around the side streets.

Conversations with the staff revealed a rich vein of stories hinting at the extent of the psychological and power-distance between senior managers and junior employees. For example, the story was told about 'the previous Head Postmaster who used to be known on the sorting office floor as "Chalky White", after the character in the *Daily Mirror* newspaper who would appear at resorts and give £5 to the first person to recognise him. On the sorting office floor we ran our own competition where anybody spotting the Head Postmaster would receive a prize. It was rarely won.' Contempt for those in authority was not confined to senior personnel within the District. As one individual said, 'one of the biggest lies uttered by visitors to the Gamma District is "I'm from headquarters and I'm here to help you"'. One casualty of these sorts of attitudes was effective communication: not only did individuals tend only to socialise with others within their department, but there was persuasive evidence that activities and procedures were being unnecessarily duplicated. For instance, both the statistics department and mail department produced traffic forecasts in isolation from each other.

The view was consistently expressed that there were good reasons why activities were conducted the way they were. Anyone questioning the existing status quo was likely to be met with the constant refrain 'have you come from outside the business then?' This phenomenon seemed to be linked to the notion that in order to understand the Royal Mail one had to have joined the organisation soon after leaving school, preferably somewhere at or near the bottom, and worked one's way up over several decades. Indeed, of the ten most senior managers in the District, eight had followed this career track. Another widely held view was that the demands of quality and staying on budget were mutually exclusive, with quality being seen not as an attitude of mind, but a function of expenditure. Furthermore, while senior managers claimed to recognise the need for a quality approach, middle managers suggested that: 'quality is considered important here until we start to run low on our budget – then quality goes out the window. It's not surprising. If a District Head Postmaster fails on his quality service targets he loses his bonus: if he fails on his budget, he loses his job.'

Evidence for change was found, notably in the form of the current Head Postmaster, who unlike his predecessor made a point of walking around the sorting office floor chatting to junior members of staff and making constructive attempts to sort out operational problems. Furthermore, it was generally agreed that since the new Head Postmaster had set the example, all the senior managers were more approachable. The forces for continuity were, however, overwhelming. The development of a Post Office mission statement in 1987 (see Exhibit 4.1) had had little impact: hardly anyone could recall any element of it, despite the fact that it had been placed on notice boards all over the building. Similarly, a recognition scheme designed to facilitate quality was treated with extreme scepticism by most members of the organisation. The overwhelming feeling gained by the researcher was one of a closed community, with its own traditions and language: 'for instance, "buffing" means working overtime (recorded on a buff docket), "steaming" means defaulting on second delivery (the mail then becomes "hot"). We don't talk about work anywhere else, no one would understand us, not even our wives.'

According to the Royal Mail's own literature[5] the cultural values of the organisation include care for the customer, reliability, value for money, accessibility, courtesy, integrity and security. Concerning the Royal Mail's employees, values such as respect, involvement, recognition and reward tended to be frequently mentioned. In practice two different perspectives on employee attitudes were evident. On

Exhibit 4.1
The Post Office mission statement

> As Royal Mail our mission is to be recognised as the best organisation in the world distributing text and packages.
>
> We shall achieve this by:
>
> - Excelling in our collection, processing, distribution and delivery arrangements.
> - Establishing a partnership with our customers to understand, agree and meet their changing requirements.
> - Operating profitably by efficient services which our customers consider value for money.
> - Creating a working environment which recognises and rewards the commitment of all employees to customer satisfaction.
> - Recognising our responsibilities as part of the social, industrial and commercial life of the country.
> - Being forward looking and innovative.

the one hand some claimed that workers had always had a strong customer service orientation, while others suggested that it was clear that the importance of customer service in the Gamma District was minimal except in the most senior managerial cadre. Indeed, belief/value clusters centred on respect for seniority, respect for length of service, and deference to the past, and accepted procedures were far more powerful influences on the day-to-day operations of the organisation than those figuring so prominently in the publicity material and internal reports of Royal Mail suggested. These attitudes had obviously exerted a profound effect on the extent to which IT was employed. Walking into the sorting offices was like stepping back in time: there were almost no hand-held calculators and few desktop computers. Instead, there was a heavy reliance on 'museum-piece' manual calculators of a type that anyone under the age of 35 is unlikely ever to have seen.

In summary, the prevailing view at the District was that the Royal Mail was a 'special' organisation that should be given preferential treatment by the Government, because 'no one else can do the job we do'. Its organisational processes were influenced and constrained by somewhat arcane working practices that had developed over the decades into what many considered to be manifestations of incontrovertible canons of wisdom. Seniority and experience were portrayed as buttresses against political activity and favouritism, and reflected the interests of an older coterie of employees. While the organisation was in many ways a formal bureaucracy its control systems were sometimes extremely loose: there was no clocking-in procedure, work was rarely checked for accuracy, and postmen and sorters were largely left to perform their work on trust.

Individuals at all levels were fatalistic about the future of the organisation, with only the most senior personnel expressing a belief that they could have a meaningful impact on the District. While communication was found to be open between workers of the same level and experience and within the same department, vertical communication upwards and lateral communication between departments was limited. The inevitable result was that problems of integration, co-ordination and control were reflected in problems with quality, efficiency and effectiveness.

Change in the Gamma District:
TQM and business development

In 1975 the Post Office made a loss so large that it made *The Guinness Book of Records*. According to the chief executive Bill Cockburn this 'shocked the system' and began the search for ways out of 'a monopolistic, bureaucratic, operational culture' in which customers were the 'general public'. While a mixture of price rises and economies meant that the organisation was back in profit by 1976, the will to change had crystallised among the senior executive team. The result of taking customers and issues of quality more seriously were striking.

In the late 1980s it was apparent to everyone within the industry that Royal Mail was facing increasing competition for business. There was also much speculation that the Royal Mail could, in the not too distant future, be subject to privatisation. Thus despite the results of customer satisfaction surveys which consistently showed that the Post Office was more highly regarded than some of the most famous retailers (including Boots and Marks &

Spencer), change was considered vital. When quizzed, senior executives argued that this was a positive step, and that unlike almost all other organisations the Royal Mail decided to embrace large-scale change from a position of considerable strength. After all, they argued, the Post Office business had quite recently undergone structural change (which had created the discrete businesses), was considered highly successful by most independent bodies, and had been profitable since 1976. There was, however, a realisation that there was still considerable scope for performance improvement in customer service, product development, operational processes, employee relations and leadership, quality and profitability.

Two important change programmes were being implemented at the District while this research was conducted, one entitled 'Total Quality Management' (TQM) and the other 'Business Development' (BD). Royal Mail first announced that it was to introduce Total Quality Management (TQM) in 1987/8. Since this time a quality support manager (QSM) has been appointed to all 64 Districts, and these people report directly to the District Head Postmaster. An HQ quality department has also been set up. While recruitment to these posts was mainly from within the Royal Mail, at Gamma District an external appointment was made. In the 1990/1 annual report for the District TQM was described as follows: 'Total Quality is the chain of events that a company uses to get the product to the customer. If you get all the steps in the process 100 per cent right first time, you've got total quality.' In practical terms the TQM initiative as interpreted by senior managers in the Gamma District is aiming to:

- improve the performance review procedure by encouraging open discussion of employee strengths and weaknesses;
- encourage more senior staff to be open and accessible to their subordinates, and generally to promote freedom to change and question;
- persuade supervisors to demonstrate more trust in their immediate subordinates;
- enlarge the opportunities for self-improvement through training and facilitate promotion on merit rather than length of service;

- introduce recognition schemes that de-emphasise the traditional adversarial style of management by saying 'thank-you' to high-performing members of staff.

Closely linked with this quality initiative was the implementation of a 'Customer First' programme in January 1989. This involved preliminary training and education, the promotion of an external customer focus, the idea that there were customers and suppliers within Royal Mail, the encouragement of teamwork, and the introduction of a formal process for benchmarking against other organisations. More sophisticated methods for measuring customer satisfaction were also introduced. At the same time the organisation made significant attempts to change employee relations, practices and policies, and raise the profile of employee satisfaction measures which have since become a key part of Royal Mail's success criteria.

Business Development, on the other hand, was an ambitious scheme to reorganise the whole of Royal Mail in order to increase efficiency and improve customer service and quality. According to the operations director (a senior HQ figure, whose thinking had doubtless been influenced by external consultants brought in to help make the senior executive team more effective), BD enshrined certain key values, namely, *involvement, empowerment* and *teamworking*. There were two main thrusts to this programme:

1 Redesign the organisational structure of the business so as to satisfy the requirements of the mission statement. This involved replacing the Districts and territories with nine operating divisions, downsizing by offering early retirement to large numbers of employees, making the divisions profit centres rather than cost centres, and introducing a radically new management process: 'Our new management process will be based on five key strategies – profitability, operational effectiveness, customer satisfaction, quality, and employee satisfaction. We will have a director responsible for each of these strategies. The strategy-based management process will be used to eliminate the negative aspects of functionality.'

2 Assess everybody in the organisation who was not a postman or first-line supervisor, the type of

assessment being based on the seniority of each individual. The aim was to measure the capabilities of each person across a range of skills, both analytical and interpersonal, with the intention of making the allocation of tasks to individuals less of a random process. It was also hoped to identify the training and development needs of individuals with a view to improving the organisation's provision of management development and training courses.

While 15 000 people had been assessed at the Post Office Management Centre at Rugby by the time this research was conducted, the results were difficult to quantify. Some argued that one safe conclusion to draw was that unless and until postmen were subject to the assessment process the results were always likely to be less than wholly satisfactory, but more senior executives suggested that this would be a pointless exercise as the nature of their duties had not (and would not) change.

The change process

Many people at District level considered that while lip service had been paid to senior management's intention to manage change through participation and consultation, it was by a mixture of re-education and coercion that results were really sought. Thus despite the fact that HQ had involved 2000 people in focus groups briefed to help design the content of BD, and although senior executives claimed to have purposefully constructed and implemented that programme as openly as possible, there was nevertheless considerable unease. Furthermore, for frontline employees, Customer First, the training and re-education programme, was, in the first instance, directed only at staff in main sorting offices, though there were plans to extend training and development throughout the organisation in due course. Delivery postmen were effectively ignored. There was considerable disquiet among employees at all levels concerning the proposed changes. For example, the eight direct reports expressed concern that they were likely to lose their jobs if the reorganisation implicit in the Business Development programme was ultimately realised. Lower down the hierarchy of management the firstline supervisors were beginning to interpret the changes required by TQM as a threat to their authority, as well-trained sorting office staff

appeared likely to need less supervision and guidance. Although levels of resistance were hard to gauge with any precision, some questioned whether the TQM and BD programmes could ever be implemented without the support of these key groups.

The HQ view was that BD involved them in an extremely delicate balancing act, in which the principles of involvement, empowerment and team-working had to be balanced by the need to meet very tight deadlines and achieve ambitious business goals. There was considerable confidence that the BD team which had been set up to oversee the programme was effective, that a workable plan was being implemented, and that the new key values had not been compromised: 'Using this project architecture, Royal Mail believes that it succeeded in meeting the competing demands for speed on the one hand and for sensitivity and professionalism on the other' (Williams *et al.*, 1993: 284).

Attitudes towards TQM at Gamma District

There were some positive signs of change. For instance, the researcher was waiting to interview the total quality manager, who was discussing training needs with a first-line supervisor: 'See that?' said a passer-by, 'That's new. A PED would never have come up to talk to a direct report a year ago'.[6] On another occasion an employee suggested that: 'You can ask people to do something now that is not in their 318 – previously they would just quote it at you'.[7] This evidence that the organisation was changing must be set in the context of a larger number of more confused and even critical comments:

Signs and mission statements? People don't even notice them. Especially as there are so many of them now you can't even see the wall.

TQM is for managers. It doesn't affect us on the floor.

I don't know how the recognition scheme works. Something to do with the relative position of the sun and the moon.

My attitude to quality depends on how I feel that day. On a bad day I feel 'never mind about missorts'. On other days I take more care. That's the same for most of us.

Attitudes to BD

From an HQ vantage point, BD could be interpreted as a fair success: it had shattered people's percep-

Exhibit 4.2
Letter from the Personal Assistant to the Chief Executive of the Post Office

An earlier version of this case was read by the Personal Assistant to the Chief Executive of the Post Office, who expressed his views in a letter to the author, as follows:

Chief Executive's Office
148 Old Street
London
EC1V 9HQ

28.2.94

Dear Dr Brown,

Thank you for taking the time to see me last Monday and to listen to my concerns and comments on your proposed chapter.

As I explained to you, my prime concern is one of emphasis. On a first reading I was left strongly with the impression that your chapter described an organisation in crisis and unsuccessfully trying to implement change. I believe that this is far from the truth as The Post Office has been a very successful organisation over the last 17 or 18 years. For instance, we are virtually unique in being the only postal administration to be profitable without Government subsidy; we have a leading edge Quality of Service – value for money provision to our customers; we have increased our productivity by some 30% over the last decade, broadly double other public sector organisations; our prices have reduced by some 10% in real terms over a similar period, and we are recognised world-wide by postal administrations and by other public and private sector companies alike as being a good role model of an organisation striving to achieve excellence focused on meeting researched customer requirements.

That is not to say that everything in the garden is roses – far from it. We believe we are still in the foot hills and have considerable further opportunity to both improve service and product range for our customers; working conditions, morale and satisfaction of our employees; and generally our efficiency standards. But these things do not happen overnight particularly in an organisation with nearly 200,000 direct employees and 20,000 agency sub-postmasters . . . .

I am very happy that we should be involved in these sorts of management textbooks; it is important for us to be used as a benchmark. I don't want to water down the size of the task which is still ahead of us in terms of radically changing our organisation and culture but equally you will understand that I do want to maximise the impact of the success which we have had to date . . . .

I look forward to being in touch again shortly.

Yours sincerely,

Peter R. B. Lewis

Personal Assistant to Chief Executive

tions that Royal Mail was a safe, stable and secure business that offered a job for life, and encouraged a more forward-looking orientation among many middle and senior managers. On the ground in the Gamma District, however, it was difficult to discern much other than fear and anxiety. Most people accepted that the programme would continue to go ahead, but it was a rare individual indeed who could be described as enthusiastic. Employees were obviously keen to put the programme behind them as soon as possible and return to the safe working environment they had grown accustomed to. Two trends of opinion are worth noting here. First, many complained that they should have been better informed: 'There's a lack of communication – people don't know what's coming after the assessment. Will they have to change job? Location? The trouble is that the people who are supposed to tell us what is happening don't themselves know'. Second, there was a widespread suspicion that the whole exercise was designed to cut staff, cut costs and tighten up budgets: 'The Business has been tightening the screw for years. This is just an excuse to get rid of a whole load of people'.

Conclusions

As this piece of research came to an end the change programmes at Royal Mail were still at a relatively early stage in their development. Thus while optimism among senior executives at HQ seemed to be matched by pessimism in the Gamma District, no clear picture of how events were going to develop nationally had emerged. Senior executives at HQ were at pains to emphasise that they realised both the nature and the scale of the problems faced by the districts. Their view was that Business Development was a preliminary attempt to alter the culture of a vast and complex organisation steeped in traditions and subject to the will of Government. They stressed that theirs was a massive task and that it would take years before any proper evaluation of the change process could usefully be made. It was suggested that this research had been conducted midway through the 'unfreezing' process that had been deliberately planned, and that the comments of employees in the Gamma District could be inter-

preted as evidence that the traditional Royal Mail culture was melting (see Exhibit 4.2).

It was quite obvious that the Post Office as an institution had made giant strides in terms of its professionalism, dealings with employees, and developing a business orientation. There was now evidence that senior executives realised that the organisation had a culture that could and should be managed.[8] In addition, senior executives were able to point to some impressive statistics that appeared to indicate that their strategies had been successful. While only 74.5 per cent of First Class mail was delivered the next day in 1989, by 1993 this figure had reached 92 per cent. Profits have also risen, from £116 million in 1988–90, to £247 million in 1993. Further indicators of success are not hard to find: mail volume increased by 50 per cent in the 1980s; prices ran 13 per cent behind inflation; productivity has increased 25 per cent since 1989 and a £750 million cash surplus has been created. Reflecting on these success indicators and the data he had collected, the researcher thought that he could make some fairly accurate long-term predictions based on the history and culture of the Royal Mail.

Questions

1 Summarise the culture of the Gamma District using Schein's model.

2 Given the strategic intentions of PHQ, what are the strengths and weaknesses of the District's culture?

3 How confident are you that (a) TQM and (b) BD will be successfully implemented in the District? Explain your answer.

4 According to one senior executive at Royal Mail HQ one of the main learning points to emerge from BD was that 'the more you communicate with people, the more they need to know'. Discuss.

5 You are a highly paid management consultant brought in to advise and facilitate the desired changes in the District's mode of operation. What advice would you give, and what action would you take?

6 Which, if any, of the models outlined in this chapter usefully enhance our understanding of events at Royal Mail? Explain your answer.

NOTES

1 The 'Brown Corporation' is a pseudonym used to protect the identity of the organisation.

2 Rites may be considered as planned sets of activities that convey important messages within an organisation. They are social vehicles for the communication of information, and can act as symbols of senior managers' intentions and beliefs.

3 Johnson Matthey plc is a firm specialising in advanced materials and precious metals technology. It employs more than 7000 people in 24 countries. The culture change programme was inspired by severe financial problems in the mid-1980s. For a more detailed account of events, see Williams *et al.* (1993: 224–31).

4 At this time the manpower planning process had been recognised as a problem by senior executives at Royal Mail HQ, but was being maintained at the insistence of the Union of Communication Workers (UCW).

5 Royal Mail (1989) 'Customer First', internal report.

6 PED (Postal Employee, level D).

7 P318 (the document title that gives an individual's job description).

8 For example, a unified system of awards for length of service were introduced. This produced an amazing backlog of 78 000 veterans. It is reported that the opportunity this provided was eagerly seized by some districts: in Nottingham, for example, people still talk about the two huge dinner dances that were staged.

CHAPTER 5

Managing organisational culture change

To enable students to:

- understand some central issues is managing culture;
- become familiar with a framework for managing culture;
- assess the importance of human resource management in the management of culture;
- evaluate the significance of symbolic leadership in managing culture;
- appreciate the role of rites in the management of culture;
- consider various strategies for cultural change;
- comprehend the difficulties and complexities in providing general guidelines for culture management.

INTRODUCTION

This chapter is concerned with the practical approaches that have been devised for managing organisational culture. It has seven main sections. First, the debate regarding whether culture can be managed is reviewed. Second, a simple framework for managing culture is elaborated. Third, the role of human resource management in the management of culture is considered, with particular attention paid to the importance of recruitment and selection procedures, induction, socialisation and training, performance appraisal and reward systems. Fourth, the significance of symbolic leadership for issues in culture management is explained and the potential for managing culture through rites is explored. Fifth, Bate's strategies for managing culture change are discussed. Sixth, an integrative model which puts forward a coherent approach to the management of culture change is examined. Finally, an attempt is made to synthesise some of the principal issues touched on in this chapter. The material presented here then provides a basis on which to discuss strategic and performance issues in Chapter 6.

THE FEASIBILITY OF MANAGING ORGANISATIONAL CULTURE

There has been considerable debate concerning whether culture can actively be managed, much of the debate centring on the extent to which a culture can be modified to resemble a pre-stated ideal. The effective management of a culture, however, requires the ability both to introduce change and to maintain the status quo. This is an important point. Many commentators have tended to think of cultures as fundamentally static phenomena which managers can alter through various intervention strategies. As the preceding three chapters have made clear, cultures are in fact highly dynamic entities which are prone to change as a result of a variety of internal and external prompts. Thus for it to be convincingly argued that managers can manage culture it must be shown that they can act to prevent change as well as to induce it. Indeed, it could be argued that the ability to manage culture implies not just a capacity to change and maintain it, but to create, abandon and destroy it as well (Ogbonna, 1992/3). Some authors, for example Berg (1985), have suggested that it is too early to reach a judgement about whether it is possible to develop a culture in a planned way because of the theoretical weakness of the field and the lack of empirical evidence. Others find it ridiculous and possibly even unethical to talk of managing culture, which they see as an expression of people's deepest needs. Yet for the most part there is agreement that culture can be managed, with culture specialists ranging along a continuum, at one end of which are those who emphasise the ease of culture management and at the other those who stress the difficulties.

As Anthony (1994: 4) has pointed out, very wide claims for the success of cultural change have been made, and these have led some to regard this field as 'one of the most significant advances in the history of organisational studies and as the herald of a new renaissance in management'. A word of caution is in order here. Those commentators who emphasise the ease with which cultures may be managed are often motivated by an interest or need to believe their case. It is not, for instance, unknown for proponents of this position to make substantial sums of money as consultants to organisations convinced of the need to manage culture. For these authors, culture is the key to improved productivity and profitability, and a failure to recognise the necessity for its management is evidence of arrogance or ignorance (Martin, 1985). The advice given to managers intent on culture management frequently involves efforts to facilitate organisational learning through the use of symbols, role models, communication and rewards. Such advice also generally involves exhorting senior leaders to engage in symbolic actions in an attempt to manipulate their employees' understandings of what is expected of them. Ouchi's (1981) procedure for creating a 'Theory Z' culture, Peters and Waterman's (1982) advice on how to create 'excellent' companies and Deal and Kennedy's (1982) views on the making of corporate heroes are situated on this end of the opinion spectrum.

While few authors now underestimate the difficulties of culture management many choose to emphasise them. Burack (1991: 88), for example, has admonished the popular press for publishing a rash of articles which 'have often abused or distorted the ease of culture change efforts'. As long ago as 1983 Fortune magazine carried an article which suggested that 'anybody who tries to unearth an organisation's culture, much less change it, is in for a rough time' (Uttal, 1983: 69). More thoughtful accounts of the limitations on the degree to which culture can be managed have been provided by authors such as Nord (1985) and Trice and Beyer (1990). The view of these theorists is that the management of culture is constrained by diverse factors ranging from the multiplicity and complexity of embedded subcultures to conflicting political interests, bad timing and communication failures. Ultimately, however, the differences between those who stress the ease and those who emphasise the difficulties of managing culture are of a relative rather than an absolute nature.

Experience of the realities of culture management has in very recent times brought both sides of the debate even closer together. It is, for example, noteworthy that even those commentators who consider culture to be a critical lever which can and should be pulled to maximise organisational effectiveness also generally concede that it can be an expensive and time-consuming business. This hints at the sort of compromise position recommended here. It is just not meaningful or helpful to state unequivocally that cultures can or cannot be managed or that their management is more or less difficult. Rather there is a better case for pursuing Siehl's (1985) advice that we change the question from 'Can culture be managed?' to 'When and what aspects of culture can be managed?'. This then allows us to explore the possibility of managing culture in general and culture change in particular through an examination of the different variables in play in these complex situations. As a first step in this direction it is worth considering the findings of a literature review on this topic by Hassard and Sharifi (1989), which are summarised in Exhibit 5.1.

Resistance to change

In addition to the whims of senior executives there are a vast range of factors currently operating on organisations to encourage them to change their cultures. These include rapid advances in technology, a tremendous expansion in the rate at which knowledge is being generated, increasingly rapid product obsolescence, demographic changes, a new-found interest in the quality of working life, and new trade legislation. This list is by no means exhaustive. That many organisations are not constantly changing in response to these internal and external pressures is testament to the powerful inertial forces that act within them. These inertial forces may be identified at both the level of the individual and the organisation. Among the most common sources of individual resistance to change are:

- *Selective perception* Every individual has a unique view of how their organisation works and their role within it. Plans for change which seem to threaten some cherished element of this world view or which appear misguided or unfair are likely to be met with resistance.
- *Habit* Everyone has habits which allow them to deal quickly and easily with routine situations, and which therefore provide a degree of comfort and security. Proposed changes to employees' habits, especially where these are ingrained and appear reasonable and rational to people themselves, may well be resisted.
- *Security* Current working practices are often more familiar and thus less threatening to the psychological security of individuals than new methods and procedures. In extreme cases some individuals may even forgo promotions because their need for security is so great and fear of the unknown so intense.

- *Economic* Any change which might threaten an individual's basic pay, bonuses, pension, company car or other element in an employee's reward package may be resisted by that person.
- *Status and esteem* Changes which an employee interprets as likely to lead to a reduction in his or her esteem and status may often be the cause of that individual's resistance to the proposed alterations.

Exhibit 5.1
Principles of cultural change

From their review of the culture management literature Hassard and Sharifi suggest the following general principles and guidelines:

- Organisations possess values and assumptions which define accepted and appropriate patterns of behaviour.
- Successful organisations tend to be those which possess assumptions and values which encourage behaviours consonant with the organisational strategy.
- Successful culture change may be difficult to achieve if the prevailing values and behaviour are incompatible with strategy.
- If an organisation is contemplating change it first needs to check to see whether the strategy demands a shift in values and assumptions or whether change can be achieved using other means.
- Senior management must understand the implications of the new culture for their own behaviour and be involved in all the main change phases.
- Culture change programmes must pay special attention to an organisation's 'opinion leaders'.
- Change programmes must also take an organisation's culture transmission mechanisms (such as management style, work systems and employment policies) into account.
- In order to create a change in culture, channels should be programmed with new messages and old contradictory ones eliminated.
- Every opportunity should be taken to reinforce the key messages of the new values and assumptions.

Qualifications

- The deeper the level of culture change required (artifacts being the most superficial and assumptions being the deepest), then the more difficult and time consuming the culture change programme is likely to be.
- If there are multiple cultures and subcultures then this will make the change programme still more difficult and time consuming.
- Some of the easiest changes to effect are alterations in behavioural norms.
- Managing the deepest layers of an organisational culture requires a participative approach.
- A top-down approach may work when there is only a single culture or when the focus in on changing norms rather than assumptions.
- Top-down approaches yield changes which may be difficult to sustain in the long term, because they produce overt compliance but not acceptance.
- Participative approaches are most likely to be successful and are the only real option if assumptions are to be altered. However, they are difficult to implement and extremely time consuming to enact.

Source: adapted from Hassard and Sharifi (1989)

Organisations and their various subsidiaries and departments are often as resistant to change as individuals. Most large organisations have a well-defined organisational structure and a variety of established rules and procedures which effectively consolidate the existing status quo. Such organisations have usually committed many of their scarce resources to projects (such as new product developments) which cannot easily be given up, and have entered into contracts with purchasers, suppliers and unions which cannot simply be disregarded. In addition, in any organisation there are those groups who perceive that they have power (over decisions, information or other resources), and they are rarely likely to concede their privileged position without a struggle. Perhaps the most pervasive force for resistance in large numbers of organisations, however, is their culture: as was hinted at in Chapter 4, prevailing dominant patterns of beliefs and values cannot generally be altered swiftly, while some have questioned whether basic assumptions can be changed at all. An established organisational culture can, then, be a powerful block on the initiation of new cultural patterns (see the case study at the end of this chapter).

As a general rule it seems plausible to suggest that the more radical a proposed change in the content of a culture, the greater resistance to change will be. For instance, change which involves modifying or eradicating shared assumptions will tend to meet with greater resistance than modifications to artefacts such as the corporate logo. It is also usually true that the level of resistance to change will be greater in strong cultures compared with weak ones. Thus Sathe (1985a, b) has suggested that the degree of cultural resistance may be expressed using the following equation:

$$\text{Resistance to culture change} = \text{Magnitude of the change in culture} \times \text{Strength of the prevailing culture}$$

A FRAMEWORK FOR MANAGING ORGANISATIONAL CULTURE

It is a striking fact that the many 'how to do it' frameworks that have been proposed by consultants and academics all have a similar intellectual core. Wilkins and Patterson (1985) have expressed the kernel of this generally accepted framework in the form of four questions:

1 where do we need to be going strategically as an organisation?
2 where are we now as a culture?
3 what are the gaps between where we are as a culture and where we should be?
4 what is our plan of action to close those gaps?

A more widely known form of the framework has been promulgated by Kilmann (1984). He suggests that there are five steps for managing culture:

1 surfacing actual norms (for Kilmann norms are more or less synonymous with culture);
2 articulating new directions;
3 establishing new norms;
4 identifying culture gaps;
5 closing culture gaps.

On the face of it, according to this framework managing culture is a relatively straightforward managerial task. Having worked out the actual and ideal state cultures for an organisation, senior executives have to take steps to bring the former into alignment with the latter. The key question is, of course, *how*? Disappointingly (but unsurpris-

Exhibit 5.2
Some problems associated with culture analysis

Organisations are highly political entities, and political antagonisms can often cloud rational economic judgements. Individuals' understandings of how their organisation works are often incomplete or defective. Consultants brought in to advise on cultural matters are often under pressure to perform quick and simple analyses in order to save time and money. Thus the potential for error in cultural analyses may often be great. In arriving at an understanding of an organisation's culture care should be taken that the following do not occur:

- *Displacement* Suggesting that culture is the root cause of problems which are the result of, for instance, an inappropriate organisational structure, a failure to invest in new technology, or poor financial control systems.
- *Whitewashing* Declaiming that senior executives are not to blame for problems, but that it is the mass of ordinary employees who require their cultural orientations to be altered.
- *Scapegoating* Identifying a particular group as culturally 'deviant', and blaming them for the organisation's ills.
- *Simplification* Taking the view that an organisation has a single unitary culture when in fact a number of subcultures are discernible.
- *Redefinition* Arguing that strong subcultures are a source of weakness, when they may in fact be contributing in a positive sense to the cultural identity of the organisation as a whole.
- *Missionary zeal* Believing that the employees in a complex and diverse organisation can be made to share a single purpose and vision that overrides subcultural interests.
- *Illusion* Failing to understand an organisation's culture, history and traditions and how they are linked to the organisation's environment.

These potential errors, derived from Anthony (1994), do not constitute an exhaustive list, but they do give a valuable indication of the range of biases and prejudices that afflict culture analyses.

Source: adapted from Anthony (1994)

ingly) there are rather fewer commentators willing and able to provide intelligent advice on this point than on the general framework. Even more alarmingly, some authors have questioned whether this sort of framework really describes what actually occurs when organisations attempt culture change. For example, Anthony (1994) has suggested that even the apparently simple tasks associated with the process of identifying the existing culture of an organisation are prone to a large number of errors and pitfalls (see Exhibit 5.2). In the rest of this chapter we will consider various mechanisms for managing culture. These may be divided into two categories: (1) those relying on various human resource programmes, policies and systems, and (2) those involving leader action and inaction. By far the greatest attention will be paid to the means by which organisations can attempt to manage culture through human resource devices, as it is these that seem to offer the greatest scope for action and which probably have the greatest chances of success in the long term.

MANAGING CULTURE: THE ROLE OF HUMAN RESOURCE MANAGEMENT

The close historical and conceptual relationship between organisational culture and human resource management was noted in Chapter 1. There it was suggested that the two fields of interest had evolved together over roughly similar time spans and jointly reflected a growing concern with people in organisations. It is, however, possible to detect still more intimate links between the two. See, for example, the work of Ulrich (1984), Albert and Silverman (1984a, b) and Guest (1990).

It is popularly argued that human resource professionals are able to play a crucial role in managing key elements of culture, including symbols, rites and rituals, norms of behaviour, beliefs and values, and possibly even assumptions. For instance, the human resource departments of many large organisations are responsible for managing cultural symbols such as office space, office decor and equipment, and car park space. The human resource function is often centrally involved in rituals and ceremonies such as office parties, staff meetings and award ceremonies. It also usually has a role in various organisational rites, especially rites of degradation like demotions and firings, rites of enhancement in the form of promotions and favourable transfers, and such rites of passage as induction programmes. In addition, norms can be influenced through codes of practice and rule books, beliefs and values may be shaped and conditioned by mission statements, and assumptions can be moulded over time by training programmes, the reward system and the performance appraisal process, all of which are (at least in large organisations) generally within the remit of the human resource department.

Human resource systems, policies and practices thus have great leverage over an organisation's culture. The precise nature of this leverage and dynamics of the interactions between a given system or procedure and any element of an organisation's culture is, though, likely to be highly complex. One consequence is that the results of any deliberate attempt to manage culture using the weapons in the human resource department's armoury may well be hard to predict. What is clear is that the human resource function can most effectively manage culture using what might be termed a *consistent cues approach*. The consistent cues approach states that all aspects of every human resource programme must unequivocally promote the desired state culture. The idea is that by consistently promoting certain norms, values and beliefs other cognitive and behavioural dispositions which the organisation has defined as 'deviant' will disappear. In short, if you want to create a culture of, for example, highly competitive entrepreneurs, then make sure that your reward system rewards competitive and entrepreneurial behaviours. If you want people to value quality, then appraise employees according to their concern for quality. While this strategy may sound simple and obvious it is in fact neither. In the first place it is extremely difficult for organisations to correctly analyse the full implications of, for example, a particular reward system or promotions policy. This is partly because the full mechanics of any policy or system are often not worked out in sufficient detail, partly because those operating the systems and policies do not always follow procedures to the letter, introducing unintended consequences, and partly because different employees (and whole subcultures) will tend to interpret the results according to their own often highly personal criteria. It is this variation of interpretation which massively complicates cultural life, especially attempts to manage culture, and it is a theme to which we will return later on in this chapter.

We will first consider the consistent cues approach in more detail with specific regard to recruitment and selection procedures, induction, socialisation and training programmes, performance appraisal systems, and reward systems.

Recruitment and selection procedures

Recruitment procedures are those means used by an organisation to generate an applicant pool for a vacant position. *Selection* refers to the sorting processes by which those applicants who do not meet a set of agreed criteria are eliminated from further proceedings. The process of selection ends when a job offer is made and accepted. Recruitment and selection mechanisms are an extremely powerful means of managing how an organisational culture develops as they directly control what sort of people an organisation employs. This said, their influence is probably greatest during a period of rapid organisational growth when many new recruits are being employed, and least significant when the workforce is static or decreasing. Given their often considerable impact on how a culture evolves over time, it is surprising how few organisations take appropriate steps to ensure that people supportive of (or at least compatible with) their desired state culture are taken.

For those organisations intent on managing their culture the aim of recruitment should be to generate a pool of people who have some degree of prior enculturation – in other words, people who are familiar with the organisation and its culture, and who themselves think that they would fit in. With this objective in mind it is clear that the recruitment of existing employees from other parts of the organisation or ex-employees of the organisation may often be an optimal solution. There are of course many situations in which such strategies cannot be pursued: in the former case, perhaps because actual expansion of the workforce is required, and in the latter instance, because ex-employees are unavailable or have damaged their reputations as loyal organisational members by having left in the first place. In these situations the next most obvious sources of applicants are the relatives and friends of current employees, who can be expected to have a better understanding of the organisation's culture than most people outside it. In the vast majority of instances, however, organisations will have to resort to advertising for external applicants through newspapers, trade journals and recruitment consultancies. While this is sometimes thought of as very much a 'hit and miss' process, attempts can be made to maximise the chances of attracting culturally compatible people through advertisements and follow-up information packs which provide a realistic insight into how the organisation operates and the sorts of people it wants to employ. For example, the UK division of Toshiba produced a video which it used as a Realistic Job Preview to aid the self-selection of those who wanted to work for a 'clockwork' organisation (Williams *et al.*, 1993).

Once the process of recruitment is complete and an applicant pool has been generated, a variety of selection tests and interviews can be employed in order to help choose the most appropriate candidate. While these tests and interviews are often used to discover how competent individuals are at performing particular tasks, they can also be used to assess the extent to which they are likely to support the desired state culture. The suggestion being made here is that organisations should attempt to select individuals who, in addition to possessing the relevant technical skills and experience to perform the job advertised, are also culturally compatible. Selection tests provide one useful tool. A large number of selection tests are employed by organisations, including those for drugs, handwriting and aptitude, though psychometric and personality tests are likely to provide the most valuable insights into an individual's cultural inclinations. These tests can yield impressive insights into how individuals tend to behave in different situations and the beliefs and values which they currently cherish. While smaller organisations may prefer to use standard psychometric tests available from various organisation development consultants, larger organisations have the resources (especially the expertise) to devise their own tests of cultural compatibility.

Interviews are another means by which applicants can be assessed in terms of their ability to work effectively in a given cultural environment. Selection interviews are a very imperfect means of obtaining accurate information about an individual. Research evidence suggests that interviewers tend to make up their minds about an applicant within the first few minutes of the interview, and that a range of cognitive biases (for instance, overconfidence and stereotyping) all affect the final decision about whether or not to offer employment (see, for example, Schuler and Huber, 1993). Nevertheless, interviews are generally used in the process of selection, and can be made more reliable if they are structured and conducted by a panel of trained interviewers. One of the most useful ways of structuring interviews is to work out a standard list of questions focused on individuals' past experiences, on the basis that how individuals have behaved in the past is the best guide to how they are likely to behave in the future.

The argument here is that at least some of these questions should be used to attempt to make a judgement as to applicants' cultural sympathies. For example, applicants could be asked questions about difficult work experiences they have had to deal with and how they reacted. In this way an assessment panel would be able to ascertain applicants' preferences for certain courses of action: whether an applicant was, for instance, more likely to be open and honest or manipulative and political. According to Albert and Silverman (1984a, b) in assessing a potential new recruit questions should be asked about the values and style emphasised by his or her previous organisation, as this will disclose valuable information concerning the individual's expectations about how organisations work in general. Different characteristics will, naturally enough, be valued in different organisational cultures, and the questions asked and the nature of the responses sought from applicants will show great variety between organisations. However, the main point – namely, that selection interviews represent an important means of managing the development of culture by admitting to an organisation some personality types and skill sets at the expense of others – is, in principle at least, a realisable one.

The judicious use of redundancy programmes can also be effective in some instances, especially where it is possible to identify a relatively specific cadre of staff that will not accept the ideals of a new culture: Unisys, the Abbey National Building Society, Jagua and Xerox have all openly embraced this means of managing the development of their organisational cultures. For instance, in the mid-1980s Abbey National discovered pockets of managers uncomfortable with their new management practices and offered them generous early retirement packages, with the result that 150 departed from the organisation (Williams *et al.*, 1993).

Induction, socialisation and training

As was explained in Chapter 2, organisations tend to perpetuate their cultures through a variety of socialisation (enculturation) mechanisms. While many of these means of socialisation are informal and beyond the direct control of senior executives, others are susceptible to control and thus represent a further tool for managing culture. In fact, one of the first opportunities to influence the enculturation process occurs in the selection phase of an employee's active organisational life. For example, the questions asked in the interview stage can be used to create an awareness of what issues are important to an organisation, while follow-up discussions can provide information to the applicant concerning what sorts of answers are considered most appropriate. In those instances where applicants progress through several rounds of interviews with managers of differing seniority and experience, this process of early attitudinal development can be particularly effective. Any organisation intent on managing its culture in this way must, of course, have decided on what sort of culture it wants to develop and thoroughly briefed its selection interviewers on what questions to ask and what responses to look for. While this may seem to be a very simple task, it is likely to require considerable organisational effort. Taking control of the dynamics of socialisation does not, however, end with the selection procedure.

Individuals are at their most susceptible to new ideas and suggestions for new ways of behaving during the early stages of their employment with an organisation. In its weakest form attempts to manage socialisation take the form of chats or lectures about such things as fringe benefits, mission statements, rules and procedures. More progressive organisations such as Procter & Gamble, IBM and 3M are far more opportunistic, and use their induction programmes to inculcate something of their history and philosophy. At organisations such as Intel and Tandem the president conducts the orientation in order to reinforce the significance of the cultural messages the induction programmes attempt to communicate. One of the most extreme examples of an organisation which seeks to mould and develop its culture through its induction courses is Disneyland, as described in Mini Case 2.4. Naturally, the precise means by which cultural messages are transmitted vary between organisations depending on their history, traditions, ethos and, of course, culture. A few of the most obvious transmission vehicles include the following.

1 *Lectures and seminars* focused on an organisation's history, especially its founders and heroes. Such facts are made still more memorable if they are incorporated into a narrative or series of narratives with which people can identify. In fact, such stories are quite easy to construct, for in most organisations there is the latent material for a good narrative. Behind every successful organisation there are stories such as those concerning the brilliant scientist struggling to bring his or her ideas to the marketplace, or the commercially astute entrepreneur who constructed a huge conglomerate.

2 *Role plays* of difficult and ambiguous work situations where it is unclear what course of action an employee should follow. For example, an organisation which values ethical and honest behaviour in its employees may present its new recruits with a theoretical situation where they could make considerable amounts of money for the organisation by acting unethically. In another organisation, which values the maintenance of good long-term relationships with its customers, salespeople may be confronted with a scenario in which they can sell-in large amounts of a product for short-term gain but which action will cause longer-term problems. In each case employees will be taught what course of action they should pursue and why it is valued by the organisation, thus reinforcing the company's culture. Role-playing exercises have, for instance, been used by Hampshire County Council in order to heighten awareness of commercial issues among managers (Williams *et al.*, 1993).

3 *Case studies* describing interesting situations, problems or dilemmas from the organisation's past. These can be used to orient discussions about appropriate and inappropriate beliefs, values, assumptions and actions among new recruits. Again, they are relatively easy to construct and can be a particularly effective means of managing an organisation's culture.

Lectures, seminars, role plays and case studies, among others, are also the lifeblood of management training and development programmes, which again have a key role to play in the management of culture. In fact Albert and Silverman (1984b: 30) have advised business people that:

> Of all human resources programs, management training and development is most important in terms of designing an approach that is consistent with and supportive of your overall management philosophy and values.

This is a helpful recommendation. According to Williams *et al.*, (1993), organisations such as Abbey National and Rank Xerox have made extensive use of training and management development programmes in their attempts to change their cultures. However, many large organisations have extensive and sophisticated training and development programmes which, while technically sound, do not always fulfil a useful culture-management role.

In some instances these programmes are almost culturally neutral in their effects, but in other cases they can be extremely damaging. For example, a training course may be made compulsory by the HRM department in an organisation where the desired culture values individual choice and personal responsibility. Alternatively, it may be insisted that a series of technical training programmes which progress in difficulty must be taken in sequence, with participants attending the easier sessions before they are able to attend those which are more complex. In an organisation which stresses flexibility and adaptability such a rule may appear extremely out of place. Further examples are not difficult to think of: sub-standard courses being run in organisations which emphasise professionalism and quality; external tutors being bought in to organisations which officially state that where possible in-house talent should be employed; and courses whose messages blatantly contradict the desired state values of an organisation – all are possible. The principal point being made here is that such contradictory messages are at best unnecessary and at worst dysfunctional. Conversely, if the training and development programmes scheduled for the employees of an organisation broadcast a consistent set of cultural cues (as dictated by the desired state vision of senior executives), then they represent an important means of strengthening, re-orienting, and possibly in the long run even changing the culture.

Performance appraisal system

Performance appraisal is a formal, structured system of measuring, evaluating and influencing employees in the conduct of their work. The usefulness of a good appraisal system is generally acknowledged to be in terms of, *inter alia*, its ability to reinforce and sustain excellent employee performance, as a vehicle for assessing training needs, and a mechanism for ensuring the fair distribution of rewards and punishments. The performance appraisal system can also be employed in the management of an organisation's culture, as culture change programmes at Unisys (a US-based information systems company) and Marley plc (a UK-based producer of building products) illustrate (see Williams *et al.*, 1993). Indeed, the most fundamental decision of all, whether or not to implement an appraisal system, must be taken in the light of its likely implications for culture. The introduction of a performance appraisal system into an organisation can generally be expected to have a profound effect on superior–subordinate relations, on interpersonal communication, on organisational politics, and on levels of morale and motivation. The precise nature of its impact will largely depend on the nature of the organisation's culture, and the sort of system introduced must often be sensitive to the existing cultural proclivities as well as being geared to create the desired state culture of senior executives. Most importantly of all, any performance appraisal system has a number of different components which can be configured in a multiplicity of ways to reflect different cultural orientations or to promote the development of particular cultural characteristics. In this section we will examine four main elements of an appraisal system and the different sorts of cultural messages associated with them. These can aptly be expressed in terms of the following four questions: What is appraised? What time orientation does the appraisal system take? What appraisal methods are used? Who conducts the appraisal?

What is appraised?

In reaching a decision as to what an appraisal system should appraise, three basic options should be reviewed: the assessment of personal qualities or *traits* (such as intelligence, the ability to communicate effectively and the capacity to cope with change), the assessment of *behaviours* (what people have done) and the assessment of *results* (what people have achieved). An organisation that wants to develop a culture which values people for what they are might choose a trait-based appraisal system. Alternatively, an organisation that wishes to evolve a culture where people generally act in line with its rules for good behaviour may find a behaviour-based performance appraisal system more appropriate. Finally, an organisation desirous of creating a culture where achievement is all important will probably favour a results-based system. The fact that most appraisal systems focus on results is a good indication of the importance of achievement in work organisations.

What time orientation?

In designing a performance appraisal system a fundamental choice has to be made about whether to focus on the past behaviours and achievements of employees, their future potential, or both. While few organisations would deliberately set out to create a system that did not take account of the future potential of employees at all, as a matter of fact many existing systems make this omission. Moreover, although almost all organisations would probably wish to include an element of future orientation, there is still scope for considerable difference. Those organisations which wish to use the appraisal system in order to allocate performance-related rewards will usually develop historically focused systems. On the other hand, those organisations that wish to develop a culture that is highly oriented towards the future and which value the personal development of their staff will be more likely to have a greater future orientation.

What appraisal methods?

A large number of methods for performance appraisal have been developed, many of which are American in origin. These may be divided into two basic categories, *objective* and *subjective*. The objective techniques generally attempt to measure the outputs of employees, while subjective methods rely on evaluations of employee performance. Although in some situations both objective and subjective measures may be used, and there will therefore be scope for a culturally based choice to be made, it is evident that in most organisations there will be no real alternative but to use subjective measures because no objective criteria are available. For example, while production line operatives employed to handmake sweets may be evaluated in terms of how many individual items they make per hour, the objective criteria available for assessing managers (such as profitability, turnover and market share) are all prone to contamination by external variables. Nevertheless some choices can be made with culture in mind. For example, the subjective methods of assessment vary greatly in terms of their sophistication and complexity, and an organisation keen to illustrate its commitment to staff and to the appraisal process may choose a more rather than less thorough method of appraisal. A further good example of the potential for cultural choice is the decision about whether to employ a method which involves numerical data (such as the use of rating scales) or prose: organisations with a numerical bias or which have a preference for complete accuracy may favour a method which allows the compilation of quantitative results, while an organisation which prides itself on its ability to use its interpretive abilities might choose a method which provides qualitative data (i.e. the written word).

Who should appraise?

While performance appraisals are usually conducted by an employee's immediate superior, self-appraisal, peer appraisal, subordinate appraisal of superiors, assessment centre appraisal, customer appraisal and appraisal by members of the human resources department are all possible. The choice of who should appraise, perhaps more than any other, should be made with reference to the desired state culture. For instance, appraisal by one's immediate superior may be used where the intention is to reinforce the organisational hierarchy, while self-appraisal can be used to produce a culture of self-critical, highly individuated employees. For organisations that wish to encourage a culture of openness, trust and mutual respect peer appraisal could play a role, and in organisations that seek to promote responsiveness to the environment customer appraisal might be the favoured option.

It should be noted here that this is a book on organisational culture rather than human resource management and that the intention here is to illustrate the general point that there is the potential for cultures to be manipulated and managed through the process of performance appraisal. There is far more to performance appraisal than can possibly be dealt with here and almost certainly far more opportunities for influencing culture by means of appraisal than the four areas listed above. For example, in addition to the design features of an appraisal system, *how* the procedures work in practice, the openness with which feedback is given to employees, and the ways in which the information gained in the appraisal interview is used all reflect on an existing culture and impact on an organisation's developing culture.

Reward systems

An organisation's reward system represents another powerful means for influencing its culture, as has been illustrated by Kerr and Slocum (1987). Organisational culture is frequently viewed as a mechanism for controlling the cognitions and behaviours of employees. The reward system plays a similar function in that it specifies guidelines for what employees have to do in order to receive pay rises, bonuses, promotions and praise. An organisation's reward system, then, can be thought of as an unequivocal statement of its values, beliefs and assumptions. This has led some authors to assert that the reward system is the key to understanding culture. From the perspective of this chapter, however, it is clear that organisations can tailor their reward systems to influence the evolution of their cultures. One important complication that should be noted at the outset is that large diversified corporations often have multiple reward systems reflecting the demands of different business settings, product life cycles and competitive environments. Moreover multiple reward systems can serve to perpetuate multiple cultures, some of which may even be countercultures (see Chapter 1), by reinforcing natural divisions within an organisation. Managing culture through reward systems in large organisations is thus likely to be a highly complex matter.

As with performance appraisal, reward systems can involve many interrelated processes, and provide plenty of opportunities for moulding culture development. Some of the most obvious and exciting issues that require examination include: whether to reward teams or individuals, how large a percentage of basic salary bonuses should be, how salary increases are determined, how perquisites are distributed, and how promotion decisions are made.

Rewarding individuals and teams

While in most organisations employees draw individual salaries, a choice often has to be made about whether to give bonuses on the basis of individual or team contribution. If the system rewards the individual, then employees may tend to act in their own best interests rather than those of the group, whereas rewarding the team provides a rationale for co-operative behaviour. In sales-led organisations such as Mary Kay Cosmetics, where what is good for the individual saleswoman and what is good for the organisation are directly related, rewarding individuals is a sensible policy. In organisations or parts of organisations where it is important that people work together on a collaborative basis – for example, teams responsible for new product development – it is generally good practice to encourage a culture of co-operation by rewarding the whole team.

Bonuses

Issues such as how large a proportion of total compensation bonuses should be, who decides who should receive a bonus, and whether the size of the bonus awarded should vary with length of service or seniority are important from the point of view of culture management. If bonuses represent only a small percentage of total compensation for individuals, then this is likely to dissuade people from engaging in behaviours which help their career at the expense of the organisation, though it may also lead to the development of a more cautious culture. If an employee's immediate superior decides whether or not he or she should receive a bonus, then this will reinforce the dependence of individuals on their line managers, perhaps resulting in a culture of conformity. If potential bonuses increase by level in the hierarchy, then this tends to emphasise the importance of long-term commitment to the organisation, leading to a culture in which loyalty is seen to be a central value. Considerable thought should therefore be devoted to how bonuses are used in organisations, because their impact (intended or not) on culture can be highly significant.

Salary increases

The criteria used to decide who should get a pay rise and when are also important tools for culture management. Two of the most well-used criteria are length of service and performance as evaluated by senior managers. Where length of service is of overriding importance, then an organisation is likely to end up with large numbers of long-serving middle and senior managers, highly deferential to organisational norms, and possibly conservative and unadventurous. In those organisations where subjective perceptions of employee performance constitute the vital information on which salary decisions are made, then conflict in the form of personal and political antagonisms is often much in evidence. Where salary increases are determined by a rigid pay system, then order and predictability may tend to become ingrained within an organisation. Alternatively, where pay increases are a matter of discretion on the part of senior managers, then the building of close personal relationships, the formation of cliques and an upsurge in self-serving activity might develop.

Perquisites

The distribution of perquisites within an organisation should be carefully thought out by executives keen to manage their culture. As we have seen in Chapter 1 the location of offices, club memberships, the quality of office furniture and first-class travel, among others, are usually important symbols of status and authority. While no organisation can completely eliminate status symbols some companies have attempted to minimise differences in status by not having reserved car parking spaces, replacing closed offices with open plan layouts, insisting that everyone travel standard class and closing executive dining rooms. Other organisations with long histories and rich traditions seem to have decided that such distinctions in rank are integral to their cultures and play an important role in motivating those in more junior positions. The point being made here is not that one approach is right and the other wrong, merely that a conscious strategy for perquisite distribution should be formulated.

Promotions

There are a variety of ways of influencing culture using promotions. One basic choice to be made is whether to favour internal or external candidates for vacant positions. By adopting a policy of internal promotions values such as loyalty and consistency can be strengthened and basic assumptions are likely to remain unchallenged. Conversely, a policy of looking for external appointees is more likely to result in cultural diversity and can more easily lead to cultural change. Some organisations choose to use promotions to expose individuals to different functional areas and thus play a key role in their personal development. Such a policy can contribute to a tight, homogeneous organisation with a common language, experience and values, while also being a palpable indication of the organisation's commitment to its staff. In other organisations promotions are used in a political game to ensure that supporters of particular causes find positions of influence. While highly internally competitive organisations may find this acceptable others often try to eliminate such practices. Again, the argument being put forward here is that these sorts of issues should be actively considered and a coherent strategy formulated by any organisation attempting to mould and direct its culture.

An alternative view

In the preceding sections a very positive view of attempts to manage culture through HRM mechanisms has been given. However, some authors have suggested that the good intentions explicit in the HRM literature to make intelligent use of reward systems and encourage teamwork and participation have not been realised (Purcell, 1989). Rather than as means for managing culture it has been argued that HRM has been employed as a smokescreen for the pursuit of anti-unionism and a reduction in the workforce (Guest, 1990; Keenoy and Anthony, 1992). These authors argue that HRM provides a rationale for increased management control and downsizing, which it asserts are the keys to higher performance. Employees have been encouraged to accept this view as valid and legitimate because they have been conditioned (enculturated) to think of HRM as a positive trend and discouraged from regarding it as a kitbag of tools for manipulating organisations as an elite sees fit (Ogbonna, 1992). The coercive control of organisations is being replaced by control based on commitment, and this employee loyalty and identification with their organisations is being structured and conditioned by executives whose ethical principles are open to question.

Discussion

This discussion of some of the human resource means of managing culture has not been exhaustive. Some of the more obvious omissions include:

- *Transfers and secondments* By moving key people around an organisation many different departments can be exposed to the good influence of suitable role models.
- *Opportunities for participation* Task forces and quality circles are just two of the many methods that can be used to mould people's beliefs and values, as evidenced at the Royal Bank of Scotland and Jaguar.
- *Formal communication* Most cultural change programmes in large organisations are accompanied by, for instance, poster displays, newsletters, internal computer communications, the use of videos, and so forth.
- *Counselling* Where a reasonable number of people need to be quickly persuaded of the advantages of a change programme, then individual counselling can be effective, especially when these interviews are conducted by senior executives rather than members of the HRM department.
- *Employee relations* The relationship between the managerial elite and other employees (whether confrontational, co-operative, relaxed or disinterested) often has a profound impact on the nature of an organisation's culture.

175

One point that needs to be emphasised here is that no single programme, policy or system is likely to have much impact on an organisation. For the human resource approach to the management of culture to have any realistic chance of success an integrated package of initiatives will be required. As Williams *et al.* (1993: 28) have argued:

> It should not be assumed that culture can be changed simply by the introduction of, say, a new appraisal system, new reward practices or new methods of training. All of these are likely to have an effect on culture and each of them could be a crucial element in a culture change programme. In isolation, though, these personnel mechanisms are likely to be subordinated to the existing culture. At best employees will pay lip service to them. At worst, they will be disregarded entirely.

Mini Case 5.1 illustrates some of the HRM culture change mechanisms considered above with reference to First Direct. It is clear that human resource policies, systems and procedures have a highly significant role to play in the management of organisational culture. This should not surprise us. Human resource management is centrally concerned with people, and how people are treated can be expected to have an effect on how they think and act. This represents a marvellous opportunity for executives keen to exert control over their organisations. Certainly there are dangers: systems designed to encourage certain behaviours may have unexpected consequences, and unscrupulous executives may attempt to manipulate their employees into acting unethically or illegally. Nevertheless, in general, it seems reasonable to suggest that these human resource programmes can and should play a crucial part in any serious attempt to manage culture in the long term. The fact that managing culture in these ways is always going to be a long-term strategy has led other commentators to suggest other ways of influencing culture development, notably through leadership.

MANAGING CULTURE

The role of leadership

Few would dispute the assertion that effective leadership is vital to the success of all large-scale change programmes. Research studies have repeatedly demonstrated that the absence of top leadership support for a project is often a key factor in that project's ultimate failure. The successful management of culture also requires the backing of top managers, especially the most senior executive in any organisation. Indeed, Allen and Kraft (1987: 87) have claimed that 'the very definition of successful leadership is the ability to bring about sustained culture change'. The leader of an organisation obviously has a crucial role to play in setting the vision (ideal state culture) that the organisation is going to move towards. The leader also has responsibility for allocating tasks and duties, structuring the organisation, and distributing material and financial resources. If human resource policies, programmes and systems are to be used as cultural levers, then organisational leaders must be centrally involved in their redesign, for it is only they who have the authority to sanction such a strategy. Senior leaders also have more direct and immediate means for managing culture. Peters (1978) has cogently and persuasively argued that the CEO can manipulate culture through symbols, while Beyer and Trice have eloquently elaborated the potential power of managing through rites.

Managing culture at First Direct

Launched in October 1989 First Direct was the UK's first retail telephone bank. As part of the Midland group the organisation provides a full person-to-person telephone banking service 24 hours a day, 365 days a year. This innovative approach to personal banking was inspired by research conducted by MORI which suggested that 51 per cent of bank customers preferred to visit their branches as little as possible while 27 per cent wished that they could perform more transactions by telephone. In order to make the idea work, however, it was recognised that a particular culture would have to be developed which was customer-focused and fixated on quality.

As First Direct is a very new organisation it has not had to bolt on notions of quality and service to existing cultures as other UK banks have attempted. Instead, impressive steps were taken to construct First Direct with quality, service and value for money very much in mind. The result is a flat organisational structure, an ambitious mission statement (to become the best in the world at personal banking), and effective operational systems. The style is very open and democratic, with employees (including 'Kevin' – the chief executive) on first name terms. Most importantly of all, its staff are subject to some sophisticated HRM procedures which help the company maintain its desired state culture.

Recruitment and selection

First Direct explicitly recognises that the quality of service it offers is only as good as the staff it employs. Recruitment and selection are therefore taken extremely seriously, with applicants undergoing various psychometric tests and interviews to discover not just if they have the required analytical abilities but are enthusiastic, motivated, dedicated, extrovert and hardworking. Unsurprisingly, the overriding factor assessed is, of course, their commitment to customer service. Few will find it surprising to learn that 90 per cent of First Direct's frontline staff ('banking representatives') do not have a banking background!

Training

All banking representative recruits receive a minimum of seven weeks' intensive training. This includes four weeks' training in product and systems knowledge, sales, communication and telephone techniques, voice projection, and how to listen to the customer. This is followed by a further three weeks of role playing and tests. While some might consider the amount of training excessive it is vital to First Direct that their frontline staff project a positive and professional image of the organisation. It is also important that raw recruits are socialised into the dominant culture, with its heavy emphasis on quality, service and customers. One important point to note is that training does not finish once basic training is complete: all phone calls are taped and regular feedback is provided to banking representatives concerning the appropriateness and effectiveness of the conversation, including its style and tone.

Rewards

First Direct is very much aware of the importance of positive motivators, and considerable thought has gone in to the creation of its performance-related pay system and rationale for the distribution of bonuses. All the banking representatives are given multiple objectives which go well beyond answering each call politely and effectively. Employees are tapped for good ideas regarding job improvement, and monitored to assess how many calls they take per hour, the amount of time spent per customer and their ability to spot cross-selling opportunities. Rewards are then distributed on an individual basis, to high-performing teams, and according to how the business as a whole performs. Non-financial rewards also figure in First Direct's management systems. For example, a prominently placed 'customer board' contains words of praise from satisfied customers on one side and customer

▶

criticisms on the other: both sides of the board are frequently updated.

First Direct's success as a quality service provider is not in doubt. Four years after being launched the bank had 400 000 account holders, which seemed set to grow to 500 000 within 12 months. In fact, with demand threatening to outstrip its ability to provide a good service the organisation postponed its 1993 television advertising campaign until its operational facilities could be expanded. Moreover recent consumer research revealed that 82 per cent of main account customers were very or extremely satisfied with the service they received, 89 per cent had recommended First Direct to someone else at least once, and 92 per cent thought that First Direct provided a better quality service than other banks.

Questions

1 Are there any dangers or drawbacks associated with attempts to manage culture at First Direct?

2 Why would the same policies for managing culture at First Direct not work in all other organisations?

The role of symbols

According to Peters symbols are the means by which managers achieve their work goals. His argument is that executives:

> do not synthesize chemicals or operate lift trucks; they deal in symbols. And their overt verbal communications are only part of the story. Consciously or unconsciously, the senior executive is constantly acting out the vision and goals he is trying to realize in an organization that is typically far too vast and complex for him to control directly. (Peters, 1978: 10)

Peters identifies a number of different symbolic means by which executives may impose on the culture of their organisation. Among the most interesting of these are: how top executives spend their time, their use of language, their use of meetings, agendas and minutes, and their use of settings.

Use of time

A chief executive can communicate important messages to employees through his or her actions. Most senior and middle managers in organisations are acutely sensitive to what the leader is doing, and spend considerable time working out the implications of what they see and hear for their careers. Roy Ash at the American corporation Addressograph-Multigraph is reported to have understood the power of symbolic actions in managing culture. Having taken over the leadership of the organisation, Ash made a number of breaks with past tradition. He visited some of the widely scattered operations himself rather than summoning subordinates to headquarters, left his office door open, placed his own calls to arrange meetings, and always questioned people in person rather than in writing. He also took measures to reduce paperwork by removing copying machines, and having seen a complaint from an important customer, flew off to visit him saying 'I wanted the word to get around our organisation that I'm aware of what's going on'. All these moves can be interpreted as symbolic acts designed not just to have a substantive impact themselves, but to illustrate what Ash thought was important, his vision of the new direction in which he wanted to take AM's culture.

Use of language

In attempting to manage organisational culture a leader is seeking to manage meaning, that is, how employees think and feel about their colleagues, work activities, the marketplace, and all other elements of organisational life. If a chief executive makes a public announcement that R&D is important, or that quality is the organisation's most pressing concern, then employees will listen. If the chief executive makes the point on a continual basis, and especially if the argument is made forcibly and memorably, perhaps by using anecdotes and stories, then over time people may begin to adjust the way they think about the organisation. Leaders occupy privileged positions which allow them to communicate with all their employees. If an organisation acquires a competitor and the press question the commercial wisdom of the venture, then a leader can help to define the employees' perceptions of the acquisition in a positive light by pointing out all the advantages of the move. In fact, few commercial decisions are obviously completely justified or wholly inappropriate: in most instances there is considerable ambiguity or room for doubt. The role of the leader is to shape people's understandings of what is going on by giving information and explanations packaged in ways which encourage the development of the desired state culture (Pfeffer, 1981a).

Use of meetings, agendas and minutes

Organisational leaders have the power to call and postpone meetings, shape agendas and determine the way in which minutes are written up. They thus possess considerable influence to define those issues which are important to an organisation, and the organisation's official view on key matters. These subtle tools also have a role to play in shaping employees' understandings of what is expected of them, what views are considered *appropriate* for them to hold, and how they are expected to conduct their work activities. When these means are used skilfully and backed up by the use of questions which indicate the direction in which the chief executive wants to push the organisation ('What about quality?', 'What's happening with customers?', 'What's new in R&D?'), then they can be particularly effective. For example, if the chief executive puts discussion of the latest customer satisfaction report top of the agenda and insists on questioning his senior executives on its implications for some hours at every board meeting for the next six months, then this is likely to have a marked impact on how the organisation operates, at least in the short term. If the same customer satisfaction survey is repeated on an annual basis and the chief executive pursues its findings with consistent enthusiasm, then over time this may well have an impact on the underlying beliefs, values and behaviours of employees throughout the organisation.

Use of settings

Leaders exercise their power in various physical settings, some of which reinforce and some of which may attenuate the impact of their messages. Merely by turning up to a meeting or turning down an invitation to attend a meeting a leader can communicate much about the relative importance of teams, functions and issues. If the chief executive always attends top level R&D meetings but rarely bothers with meetings of senior marketing executives, then the importance of R&D over marketing to the organisation will be widely noted. The location in which meetings are held can also be symbolically significant. For example, moving a senior management board meeting from an isolated headquarters to the centre of operations might be employed to signal a genuine attempt by executives to really understand field problems. How leaders choose to use their personal office space and the nature of the buildings in which they choose to house their organisations can also be of symbolic importance. For instance, Lawrence Rawl, CEO of Exxon, has attempted to trim down his organisation, and as such his office mirrors this philosophy, being conspicuous for its lack of symbols. Sir Ralph Halpern of the UK clothing retailer Burtons has also illustrated his sensitivity to symbolic settings in his description of Hudson Mills, the enormous manufacturing site of Burtons in the 1960s and 1970s:

> It was a feudal castle. They had their lunch in the feudal canteen, the feudal barons called Burton turning up and administering the rites, and allowing employment to be granted: and there would be a medical man on the premises and a bit of billiards and a bowling green. So the whole of the village set up was really to show that we could protect you there ...' Hudson Mills was closed as a manufacturing plant shortly after Halpern took over responsibility for the operation: a move which signified that the company was irreversibly a retailer rather than a vertically integrated menswear clothing company. (Johnson, 1990: 192)

Many of the issues discussed here in the abstract are illustrated with reference to two actual leaders at TI in Mini Case 5.2, though for obvious reasons the real names of the company and the individuals concerned have been disguised.

Summary

These, then, are the sorts of means that senior executives can employ in their attempts to manage culture. The central theme that runs through them all is that of *personal enactment*. That is, if chief executives wish to mould their organisations' culture, then they should personally enact the beliefs, values and assumptions that they want to inculcate in others. The same is true for all managers seeking to influence employees in their departments, whatever their size. Most people learn a lot from modelling the behaviour of those they respect, especially when there are other benefits to be derived from so doing. Roger Paine, the chief executive of Wrekin District Council, had an intuitive understanding of this when he attempted to develop a service ethos among his staff by answering questions at the Council's main reception desk every Monday morning. So too did the chief executive of a multinational hotel chain who issued his home phone number to a convention of travel agent directors, asking for a personal report of any problems (Johnson, 1990). To have maximum impact leaders should resort to such symbolic actions *frequently* and *consistently*. They should also back these actions up with the use of *positive reinforcement* in the form of praise and other motivators (money, status, awards) that encourage behaviours consonant with the desired state culture.

The role of rites

As we saw in Chapter 4 rites refer to organised and planned sets of activities that are usually relatively elaborate and dramatic, and which communicate cultural messages. While it was suggested in Chapter 4 that particular rites are naturally associated with different phases in the culture change process Trice and Beyer (1990) have argued that it is possible to use them to manage culture. They assert that rites of passage, degrada-

Mini Case 5.2

Symbolic leadership at Telecommunications Inc. (TI)

Telecommunications Inc. (TI) was a wholly owned subsidiary of a large electronics organisation, and in the early 1980s employed approximately 600 people. The parent company manufactured products which TI (and other external organisations, notably British Telecom) then marketed and distributed. In January 1980 Gordon joined TI as its managing director, having previously been employed by another big telecommunications/computer company and before that the Royal Navy. Surveying his new organisation, Gordon recognised an immediate need for his company to become a more customer-focused organisation in order to differentiate it from similar sales/service firms marketing similar (in some cases identical) products. On the face of it this seemed an enormous task, which implied a need to radically alter the nature of TI's organisational culture.

Use of time

In contrast with some of his predecessors and those who were to come after him Gordon spent large amounts of time out of his office and in the field talking business to all levels of employees. In all such activities he was noted as being extremely open, honest and trusting, while at the same time demanding a high degree of commitment and on-the-job competence. As he talked to people he rarely failed to ask for their opinions on difficult and complex issues and was generally encouraging of good work. Backing up his informed questioning was an extensive knowledge of the business which amply demonstrated to others that he 'lived the company'. Moreover, everyone knew that he pushed himself hard, worked long hours, did not claim all the business expenses for which he was entitled, and purchased expensive bottles of whisky for his direct reports out of his own pocket each Christmas.

Use of language

As befitted an ex-Navy officer Gordon's style was precise and direct. When dealing with peers and subordinates this was a significant asset. Not only did his employees know where they stood with him, but he had the ability to express ambiguous situations and problems in language which everyone understood. A man of vision, Gordon knew where he wanted to take TI in terms of its culture, namely, in the direction of IBM. Time and again his employees heard him say 'that's how IBM do it' when pointing out some good business practice, or 'IBM would never do that' when discussing behaviours he considered ill-advised. Perhaps his favourite aphorism was that TI should be more like IBM in that long-term relationships with customers should be valued above short-term costs and gains. These sayings were central to his overriding objective, namely, the achievement of a change in TI's culture from a preoccupation with technical engineering and a spirit of commercial amateurism, to a highly professional marketing-led ethos. This drive for marketing excellence required Gordon to introduce a whole new vocabulary into the common language of people in TI ('product life-cycle management', 'product range' and 'product differentiation', 'mean time between failure', etc.), which vied with the language of mere technical competence. As a colleague of Gordon's commented, he brought to the conservative and inward-looking world of telecommunications some of the flair and openness to change which characterises the computer industry.

Use of meetings, agendas and minutes

Scrupulously fair and honest, the idea of deliberately manipulating agendas and minutes to reflect his own prejudices probably never occurred to Gordon. Nevertheless, his obsession with customer focus and forceful personality meant that his concerns always dominated discussions, whatever the topic on the formal agenda. His insistence that subordinates should always be punctual to meetings, and that when visitors were present everyone should strive to make things go smoothly, was mirrored by his own behaviour. It was in meetings (especially informal meetings) that his self-understanding and comprehension of others was most impressively demonstrated. No matter the setting or the type of people he was dealing with Gordon was always able to choose appropriate words and phrases which others found meaningful and relevant. In the best possible sense of the phrase he was a natural conversational chameleon who could alter the register of his language to fit the context, always with the result of reducing the power distance between himself and subordinates.

Use of settings

While relatively insensitive to the niceties of organisational settings and careless of the trappings of office, Gordon's own physical appearance and dress sense spoke volumes. A big and powerful man, he was always immaculately dressed, making him a dominating presence wherever he went. A couple of his most obvious idiosyncrasies further underlined his personal code and cultural expectations. First, it soon became known that the trouser pockets of his expensive and stylish suit were sewn up, a potent symbol to employees that idle hands were not to be tolerated. Second, he did not wear his watch on his wrist but in the breast pocket of his suit (the only one not sewn up). When quizzed he replied that the strap had broken and that his wife had promised to purchase a new one for him. As the months passed it became obvious that his wife had forgotten her promise, but it was such a point of honour for Gordon ('a promise is a promise') that he refused to buy a replacement himself or allow anyone else to do so.

Using these symbolic means (largely unconsciously, it seemed) Gordon sought to create a culture which would increase the profit potential of TI in the long run. His vision was of an organisation which was tightly knit and cohesive, hard-working, supportive, open and flexible, and, most of all, focused on the needs and aspirations of customers. Unfortunately for Gordon his attempts to change TI rapidly into a modern sales organisation were interpreted as efforts to create a counterculture by those in the parent company. To some extent it appeared that his bosses just did not understand the need to be marketing-led. The result was a rapid decline in relations between TI and the parent organisation (which Gordon dubbed 'the sales prevention organisation'), and within four years he left the company.

Gordon was soon replaced by Paul. Paul had been the marketing director of the parent division, where he had a relatively small staff, and relished the opportunity of taking on the high profile and demanding job of MD of TI. Before joining this group Paul had worked for a number of leading consumer companies, and thus had significant experience of this market sector. Like Gordon, he was a highly competent leader, though with a very different management style.

Use of time

Paul had a dynamic and immediate style, which meant that he accomplished what he considered to be 'his work' very quickly. On a typical day, while most of his senior and middle managers would arrive at 8.00 a.m. and leave at 7.00 p.m., Paul would arrive around 9.00 a.m. and depart at 5.00 p.m. In addition, he took lengthy exotic holidays in Africa and the Far East and frequently took his wife on long-weekend mini-breaks, during which times he left his senior managers to their own devices. While he was at work, however, he did little other than perform the tasks at hand. In a culture where it was the norm for subordinates to dial their bosses' telephone calls for them Paul always insisted on placing his own. This was part of his philosophy of going direct to the individual most immediately concerned with any problem, opportunity, or other issue. Thus if there was some difficulty with the invoicing procedure he would phone the invoice clerk responsible, discuss the matter, and then advise him or her how to act. This tendency to go direct to the focal person concerned infuriated large numbers of middle and senior managers, who felt that their authority was being undermined. It also meant that things happened fast.

Use of language

Unlike Gordon, Paul was an intensely private man who kept his personal opinions on all non-business matters strictly to himself. Furthermore he never talked about himself, and many employees interpreted this as secretiveness on his part. In conversation he was extremely direct and focused. More than one employee could recall that before they had finished explaining an issue to him Paul was already making his views known. Paul was never known to have told a joke or to have engaged in much casual conversation, and one consequence of this was that none of his work colleagues considered themselves friends of his. Moreover, Paul was, in essence, a pragmatist. He had little concern for ideology or set ways of doing things. If a problem arose or an opportunity presented itself he would not ask 'How has TI historically dealt with this?' but would act as he saw fit. His sole criterion in arriving at commercial decisions was: 'Will this work?' Paul was fanatically results-driven, so much so that he was often careless of the sensitivities of individuals. This led some of his subordinates to think of him as a cold and calculating business machine. To some large extent Paul was immune to their feelings, being far more concerned to find practical solutions to operational difficulties and implement them as speedily as possible.

Use of meetings, agendas and minutes

Paul was extremely effective in meetings. His excellent knowledge of the business and phenomenal memory gave him enormous leverage when dealing with his boss and his boss's boss. His subordinates told stories of him being completely unphased by unanticipated phone calls from the chief executive of the group, which he handled with supreme nonchalance and acumen. An indication of his strength of personality and ability to exert control upwards was Paul's ability to ignore the orders of his bosses while still retaining their good opinion. An example of this was Paul's refusal to merge the two separate companies he had been given, apparently realising that in so doing he would reduce the combined operating profits. (It is worth noting that his successor was not so astute, and having merged the two separate entities, profits then declined and he was sacked!) Likewise, in meetings with his own staff he was always in control. In contrast with many of his predecessors Paul always ensured that meetings were kept short. A typical operational meeting would involve a rapid exchange of information, Paul's decision, the delegation of responsibilities and the setting of deadlines – all with great speed. This seemed to reflect both Paul's impatience with time-wasting and his great intellectual abilities, which enabled him to come to swift (and generally good) judgements.

One significant problem for Paul was that he often trusted people who let him down. Some of his colleagues thought that this was symptomatic of his inability to understand people. Paul's tendency to judge people purely on results further buttressed this view. One particular character trait that merits attention was his habit of apparently agreeing that something was a good idea and giving the go-ahead for it to be actioned, only to later change his mind. So much confusion did this cause that the personnel director took it upon himself to warn those unfamiliar with Paul's idiosyncrasies not to act on what they thought had been agreed immediately, but to wait a few days, just in case the decision was reversed.

Use of settings

Paul was no less physically imposing than Gordon, although of very different build, being both tall and slim. He too took great pride in his personal appearance, dressing in high-quality and fashionable jackets with matching Gucci shoes. Most noticeable of all was his hair, which was always immaculately sculptured: during his time in office no one could every recall a time when a single hair appeared out of place.

▶

Paul evidently had a high need for control, and could be ruthless when he judged that the situation demanded tough action. Two examples illustrate this well. First, on one occasion he had delegated the difficult task of setting next year's sales targets to the personnel director and sales director, who worked long hours attempting to ensure that fair and equitable targets for all the salesmen were drawn up. They then called the sales managers (who were responsible for the salesmen) together and agreed the targets with them. Near the end of the meeting Paul walked in, looked over the figures, and declaimed that they were inappropriate. He then took out his pen and adjusted all the sales targets downwards by 20 per cent. In the second example, the key accounts manager, who was extremely good at his job of securing contracts with big organisations like high street banks, was headhunted by a competitor. When Paul heard this he phoned up the personnel director and ordered him to escort the man off the company's premises immediately. The key accounts manager, who had given many years loyal service to TI, and who very much wanted to work out his three months' notice, was devastated. Paul was not in the least perturbed, and refused to see the man, arguing that 'If you're not for us, you're against us'.

After two years with TI Paul decided to leave in order to join a smaller company where he thought he would have more control.

Questions

1 Compare and contrast the leadership styles of Gordon and Paul.

2 Who do you think was the most effective symbolic leader? Why?

3 What advice would you give (a) to Gordon and (b) to Paul?

4 Who would you most like to work for? Explain your answer.

tion, renewal, conflict and integration may actively be employed to either maintain the existing status quo or accomplish cultural change, depending on how they are configured and the perceived needs of the organisation at the time. While no one individual or department fully control rites in most organisations, it is usually the case that the human resource function and most senior executives play crucial roles.

Rites of passage

These rites facilitate the transition of new recruits from 'outsiders' to 'insiders', so that they become members of the group. Basic training in the military and the police, Zen meditation exercises in some Japanese companies, and extensive testing, screening and assessment exercises in many Western organisations are all examples of rites of passage. Such rites are generally used to maintain the continuity of organisational and occupational cultures. There are, however, no reasons why the messages they communicate cannot be altered in an attempt to modify a culture. For most organisations, what Trice and Beyer (1990) refer to as rites of passage are in fact a mixture of recruitment, selection and induction procedures, and as such have been dealt with above and in Chapter 2.

Rites of enhancement

These are rites which celebrate the accomplishments of one or more members of the organisation, usually by bestowing a selection of rewards including praise, recognition, bonuses, promotions and plaques. Rites of enhancement are a means of reinforcing those behaviours consonant with the desired state culture, and their skilful use can, Trice and Beyer (1990) argue, lead to cultural change. While they can only act as a reinforcement mechanism for those who receive some benefit, rites of enhancement also serve to motivate and inspire others by creating organisationally desirable role models. In addition, an individual who receives a reward as part of a rite of enhancement will usually benefit from increased visibility, authority and control over resources, and can thus exert more influence over others to act as they do, that is, to conform to cultural norms.

Rites of degradation

These involve certain individuals being publicly identified with problems and failures and then stripped of their positions and statuses. One obvious way in which rites of degradation may encourage culture change is by removing members resistant to change or who have come to symbolise significant features of the old regime. These rites are generally infrequently used in organisations, though are quite common following a merger where those in the dominant culture seek to extend its influence by ousting those members of the losing culture. Rites of degradation, then, dramatically inform an audience of who has won and who has lost in any given situation, and which behaviours are acceptable and which are not, and thus teach how to avoid public humiliation and expulsion from the group.

Rites of conflict reduction

During periods of culture change, conflicts inevitably develop. Rites of conflict reduction can help organisations to restore equilibrium in disturbed social relations by acknowledging differences in opinion and providing a means by which both sides can discuss the issues at stake. Some of the more usual conflict reduction mechanisms include union–management committees, grievance procedures and appeal systems. It has been suggested that sports contests between warring factions can play a role in reducing organisational conflicts by involving everyone concerned in shared activities with common goals. Trice and Beyer (1990) have argued that the spoof skits of difficult people which occur at some organisations' annual dinners are also potential means of reducing conflict. Thus while all these forms of the conflict reduction rite provide opportunities for tension reduction and social integration through participation, the precise form they take – formal procedure, sports or humour – is likely to differ radically between organisations.

Rites of integration

These rites help to foster closer social cohesion by reviving common feelings and maintaining individuals' commitment to the continuity of the group. Such rites often involve eating, drinking, dancing and other recreational activities in formalised events such as parties, picnics and festivals. It should be clear that rites of conflict reduction such as sports contests can also serve as rites of integration. Trice and Beyer (1990) suggest that these sorts of events should be deliberately staged by managers during periods of culture change in order to maintain social cohesion and facilitate the change process. They argue that rites of integration, to be effective, must be inclusive rather than exclusive, enjoyable to the vast majority of people, and allow adequate mixing between those of different gender, race and hierarchical position. This is an important point, since many activities which managers conceive as rites of integration do not fulfil this function because, for example, they are reserved for managers above a certain level or do not encourage integration between those of distinct subgroups.

Rites of renewal

These rites help to maintain the organisation in more or less its current form by revitalising social structures so that they can perform effectively again. Rites of renewal are thus essentially system-supportive, and can disguise the nature of problems or convince people that something is being done about them while reinforcing the status quo. Rites of renewal include those change programmes which have little impact and protect the interests of powerful groups, organisation development activities such as team-building exercises which fine tune what already exists rather than create anything new, and employee counselling programmes which help individuals overcome personal and job-related problems for the benefit of the organisation. Rites of renewal, then, can eat up a lot of resources for little apparent gain, are highly conservative, and likely to militate against change. In the process of managing culture change, therefore, these are to be avoided or highjacked and transformed into other sorts of rites as appropriate.

Summary

Rites, then, have a vital role to play in the management of culture. For the most part they are concerned with preserving and promoting what already exists, and this conservation function can be especially important to executives keen to perpetuate a culture under threat. Rites can, though, also help in the management of culture change, especially when old established rites are subtly modified to incorporate new values. The elimination of any rites which express values that are no longer considered desirable and the creation of totally new rites are also possible, but more risky strategies. If an established rite is to be discontinued executives must be certain that this will not create overwhelming resistance to the change programme from its most ardent adherents, and this may call for the creation of a near-substitute for the rite. If a completely new rite is to be created then its consequences for the culture should be thoroughly assessed, for there are dangers in provoking staff more familiar and comfortable with traditional procedures. In the words of Beyer and Trice (1988: 393–4):

> Rites thus clearly can be used to facilitate cultural change. To use them effectively, however, managers and others must recognise the rites and ceremonies already occurring around them and become aware of both their intended and latent consequences. With such an awareness, combined with a healthy respect for the power of rites to help people maintain some sense of stability in the midst of change, managers can begin to use rites creatively and effectively to achieve desired cultural change.

Managers as actors

Some commentators have suggested that the dramatic roles that managers have to play when using symbols and organising rites mean that we should think of them as actors or performers (Jackall, 1988; MacIntyre, 1981). Mangham (1990), has identified a variety of 'star' performers in the business world, notably Iacocca at Chrysler, Sir John Harvey-Jones at ICI, and Michael Edwardes in a variety of roles, for instance at Chloride, British Leyland, Mercury Communications, ICL and Dunlop. The notion that leaders of culture change need to be expert in their use of rhetoric and histrionics, and skilled in role modelling those behaviours they wish others to adapt, is apposite here. It draws our attention to the important idea that in order to be effective a manager's performance must be considered 'authentic' by his or her audience, for only then will people believe in it and be influenced by it (Anthony, 1994). This view also points out the potential dangers of acting contrary to one's real concerns and principles: such actors (managers) must 'suffer the attenuation of selfhood that results from impersonation' (Trilling, 1974: 64), and this could potentially be both morally and psychologically damaging.

Leaders as barriers to culture change

While the primary focus of this chapter is how to manage culture change, it should be borne in mind that it is an organisation's leader (especially if the leader is also the founder) that is often most resistant to change. The reasons for this are evident. Founders have generally made a success of themselves and their organisation for a number of years, and believe that they have a winning formula. Indeed, a belief that their vision is best may have carried them through difficult periods in the past. It is also worth noting here the results of studies into the characteristics of founders (Trice and Beyer, 1990), which suggest that founders are often charismatic individuals who claim supernatural (almost magical) powers. They are generally self-confident, dominant, articulate, good motivators and convinced of the moral righteousness of their beliefs. Despite obvious advantages of such a personality profile, there are also dangers. The problems are often most obvious when there is a really significant shift in technology, markets or competitive structures that necessitates a radical departure from traditional methods. According to Dyer (1986: 59): 'most founders have blinkers on. They are unwilling to listen to advice, collaborate with others, or recognise their own weaknesses. Thus they unknowingly get themselves, their families, and their businesses in deep trouble by fostering cultural patterns that are not amenable to change'.

The point is that even extremely competent symbolic leaders may not always be good transformational leaders, that is, able and willing to create a culture that can cope with change. This is well illustrated by William Millard at Computerland, who although the largest stockholder was forced to resign by investors and franchisees disgruntled by his inability to work with others to make desperately needed changes in the organisation's culture and strategy. Natural leaders, we should recall, can also be unethical people (as recent enquiries into Guinness, BICC, Barlow Clowes and the Maxwell companies have illustrated), and sometimes extremely dangerous, as Adolf Hitler proved.

STRATEGIES FOR CULTURAL CHANGE

Paul Bate (1994) has identified four basic strategies for dealing with organisational culture. These are: (1) *conforming strategies*, designed to adapt, improve and perpetuate existing constructs; (2) *deforming strategies*, which aim to pervert or subvert existing constructs; (3) *reforming strategies*, which mean abandoning or removing existing constructs; and (4) *transforming strategies*, which imply a 'frame-breaking' transition from one set of constructs to another. While conforming, deforming and reforming strategies may be appropriate for managing culture over long periods of time, ultimately all cultures begin to stagnate. When a culture loses its vitality and malaise sets in, transforming strategies are required if the organisation is to rejuvenate itself. Transformation implies a radical second order change in cultural identity, and is often associated with a perceived need to regain creative and/or reproductive capacity.

Some of the dominant symptoms of cultural stagnation include:

1 an organisation's sense that its normal recipes for success no longer work. This seems to have occurred at SAS before Carlzon arrived, and at Disney, which was doing little other than recycling old material, before Michael Eisner;

2 an organisation appears unable to discern better alternatives, a sort of cultural myopia. A case in point is IBM's now well-known initial failure to recognise the coming dominance of PCs;

3 an organisation becomes engaged in compulsive, repetitive behaviour, that in the extreme case becomes a vicious circle of deteriorating performance. The old British Rail fits this picture of decline rather well;

4 an organization is prone to spend increasing amounts of time, resources and effort in structural reorganisation. The UK National Health Service has, since its inception, suffered from this indicator of cultural stagnation, (though it is worth noting that successive governments must take at least some of the blame in this respect).

For organizations experiencing some or all of these problems, Bate outlines four generic strategies for implementing cultural change: *aggressive, conciliative, corrosive* and *indoctrinative*.

1 The aggressive approach consists of a deliberate attack on the culture of an organisation, and is extremely forceful and overtly insensitive. Usually conducted quickly and in the context of organisational crisis, aggressive culture change is most often associated with one dominant leader. The intent of such a strategy is to deauthenticate the existing culture, to undermine its coherency and dissolve old habits. For ordinary organisational members this can be a difficult and fear-provoking experience that leads to the questioning of cherished identity, values and assumptions. As the old culture is undermined so new, usually simple and detailed, learning cues are set up for people to absorb.

2 The conciliative approach seeks change through non-dramatic, gradual and routine means. The emphasis is on reason rather than emotion, and a new culture is grafted on to the old without confrontation. The prevailing spirit is one of accommodation and egalitarianism rather than conflict, on pragmatism not ideology. Coercion is not required, because there is an assumption that organisational members are reasonable people who can be persuaded by argument. Change in this manner tends to be gradual and continuous, commands wide consensus, and is characterised by incrementalism and sensitivity to language and interests.

3 The corrosive approach is, essentially, a political strategy in which individuals attempt to shape change by exercising influence through networks. Power is a resource to be exploited for the selfish advantage of people (individuals and groups), and culture is the result of the influence strategies of different networks and coalitions. In such organisations work colleagues are not so much friends but useful contacts with whom alliances may be concocted for sectional advantage. Culture is changed by the skilful manipulation of ideas and resources by those astute enough to play the complex political games that characterise organisations.

4 The indoctrinative approach emphasises the possibility of inducing culture change through various learning or training programmes. Most usually accomplished through a professionally planned and managed process, this strategy assumes a quite high degree of involvement and willing participation on the part of those whose culture is to be altered. This said, we should not underestimate the extent to which such learning programmes are concerned with control, albeit in a co-operative and good-natured atmosphere. Nor should we overlook the ethical implications of teaching (some might say indoctrinating or culturally conditioning) people to accept certain beliefs and values designed to benefit the organisation rather than individuals or the wider environment (see, for example, Mini Case 2.4).

A MODEL FOR THE MANAGEMENT OF CULTURE CHANGE

Given the importance of organisational culture it is only to be expected that attempts to formulate culture management models would be made. However, the vast number of variables that need to be taken into account by any general, inclusive and coherent model are so numerous that this is a very difficult task. Perhaps the most useful and best known of the models available is that formulated by Stan Silverzweig and Robert Allen as long ago as 1976. Based on a form of the culture change framework considered earlier in this chapter their model provides us with an effective summary of much of the material considered above, while also yielding some new insights into the possibilities for culture change management. While only this model will be considered in detail here, it has much in common with other models of culture change formulated by Allen and Kraft (1987), Kilmann (1984) and Sathe (1985a, b). As with all such models its use is restricted by the notion of culture which it employs. According to Silverzweig and Allen, culture is a set of expected behaviours (or norms) which are generally supported by people in the organisation. Hence the name of their approach, *the normative systems model*. Critics of the model are likely to point out that the model is unconcerned with the 'deeper' layers of culture, namely, beliefs, values and assumptions, and is thus unable to offer a comprehensive guide for managers, though as we shall see some aspects of the model may well have relevance to the management of these elements of culture in addition to norms.

The normative systems model may be illustrated diagrammatically as four inter-locking circles, each representing a separate phase in the change management process (see Fig. 5.1). It is important to realise that this is a generic model which sacrifices specificity for generalisability and that the guidance which it offers needs to be tai-lored to meet the organisation needs in any particular context. This said, the four phases may be characterised as described below.

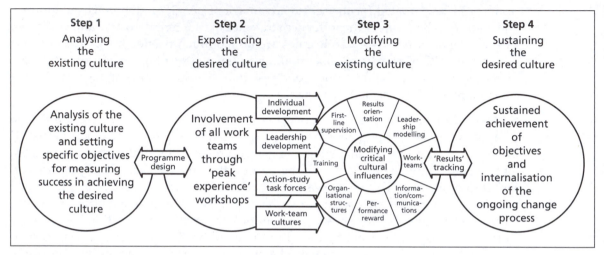

Fig. 5.1 Normative systems model for organisational change
Source: Silverweig and Allen (1976)

Step 1 Analysing the existing culture: establishing a norm gap

During this phase the existing culture must be analysed and the desired culture agreed on and expressed in the form of a set of specific objectives which can be mea-sured on a regular basis. The existing and desired cultures should be established by such means as discussions with workers, leaders and key opinion-makers, the use of survey questionnaires, observation, interviews and the analysis of performance and results. The result is the identification of a 'norm gap' between the actual and desired cultures, which needs to be closed. There are eight critical influence areas.

1 *Leadership modelling behaviour* Leaders exercise power and influence over a culture through their words and actions (symbolic leadership).

2 *Work-team culture* All work-teams have their own subculture which usually devel-ops *ad hoc* without any formal input from managers. Taking control of the development of work-team cultures and moulding them so that they are both posi-tive and contributing (as defined by the desired culture) is important for achieving sustained change in the workplace.

3 *Information and communication systems* Cultures are supported by the communica-tion of information concerning what norms to support.

4 *Performance and reward system* What is appraised and rewarded in an organisation will have an influence on the sort of culture that develops.

5 *Organisational policies, structures, budgets and procedures* These convey important messages from the power structure to employees concerning the organisation's cultural priorities.

6 *Training and orientation* These provide an opportunity for influencing culture, especially during the early phase of an individual's employment with the organisation.

7 *First-line supervisory performance* Silverzweig and Allen suggest that most organisations contain two distinct cultures (managers and workers) which first-line supervisors are expected to bridge, and who if given the tools and support can impact on culture.

8 *Results-orientation* There is considerable scepticism in many organisations concerning whether cultures can be changed. In order to overcome this it is necessary to agree on specific and measurable objectives at the outset. There must also be regular data feedback and monitoring of progress.

Step 2 Experiencing the desired culture: systems, introduction and involvement

The second phase of the model suggests that all members of an organisation should be provided with opportunities to:

1 participate in discussions which determine the preferred organisational culture;

2 share their frustrations about the problems which exist with the current culture;

3 examine existing norms and experiment with new ones together with work colleagues;

4 experience the feelings (hopefully positive) they will have regarding the new culture;

5 commit to objectives that they and their organisation will from then on be striving toward.

In order to facilitate these experiences the authors suggest a series of normative systems workshops which provide 'peak' experiences not easily forgotten by participants, and which serve as a benchmark from which they can begin to measure change.

Step 3 Modifying the existing culture: systems installation

With the involvement workshops complete, the implementation process begins, focusing specifically on the culture influence areas identified in Step 1. There are three principal strands here. First, a programme designed to re-orientate leadership at all junior levels in the hierarchy of management is implemented. This involves the training of line managers and supervisors by those who have demonstrated on-the-job success and thus embody and enact the desired leader behaviours. Second, the participants in the workshops are organised into action-study teams (incorporating all levels of employees) which are briefed to identify problems and recommend solutions in each of the critical culture influence areas. Third, all organisational work-teams meet regularly to modify their culture through a discussion of critical issues and problems. To facilitate this, all team leaders should be provided with relevant training which allows them to develop their work groups as required.

Step 4 Sustaining the desired culture: ongoing evaluation and renewal

If or when positive results are achieved there must be a shift in focus to sustaining the emerging culture. Clearly continuing measurement and evaluation of what is going on using tools such as questionnaire surveys are an ongoing requirement. Only through continual self-critical analysis can the desired culture be brought into being and sustained. According to the authors, if the programme is ultimately to be successful, then it must possess the following characteristics: the involvement of people, an emphasis on results, a total systems approach, build win–win solutions in which all sides benefit, enjoy continuing commitment and focus specifically on culture.

While the normative systems model has tremendous face validity and is, for many practitioners, intuitively appealing, serious questions can be asked of its practical value (Ogbonna, 1992/3). For example, to the extent that the model is dependent on questionnaire surveys to discover actual and desired cultures it can be misleading because the questions asked may reflect only the manager/ consultant's values or preconceived notions of the culture of the organisation as it is or should be. Furthermore the workshops that Silverzweig and Allen have so much confidence in may not be reliable mechanisms for inducing culture change in all situations. It is not, for instance, unknown for people to exhibit behaviours in a workshop setting (out of fear, as a result of careful calculation or just because they are being watched) which they do not repeat when performing their normal duties. It might also be argued that senior leaders do not have a monopoly control of communication channels in organisations and that deviant messages are likely to be transmitted by those resistant to the culture change. More damagingly still, it is evident that even highly consistent messages are subject to different interpretations by different people depending on their knowledge, experience and interests. Other points of weakness with the normative systems model are not hard to identify: is normative or behavioural change really what we want to understand by the phrase 'culture change'? Is leadership change, if not a sufficient condition, then at least a necessary condition for culture change?

It is important to realise that Silverzweig and Allen's model has not been elaborated only to suggest that it is flawed, although it does have serious deficiencies. The normative systems model was described in detail because it is one of the most interesting and coherent of the 'how to do it' frameworks available. In other words, many of the criticisms levelled at the model here are equally applicable to the other frameworks that have been developed. At the very least, the ideas of Silverzweig and Allen provide a good starting point for managers and consultants interested in the possibility of managing culture change in their organisations. Many of the principles outlined in the Silverzweig and Allen framework are illustrated with reference to culture change at Hambro in Mini Case 5.3.

FINAL THOUGHTS

It is clear that organisational cultures are neither static nor permanent. Rather, they evolve over time in response to changes in the external environment, new technologies and products, and various macro-social and political trends. Indeed, small-scale incremental changes occur on a daily basis as some individuals leave and others join, new systems and procedures are introduced and some are modified to reflect changing personalities, the latest fads and fashions, and the recommendations of the most recent training courses. Thus culture change (where 'culture' is understood in its broadest sense) is a feature of organisational life. The real point at issue is how much control managers can exert over the dynamics of culture change processes. While most of this chapter has been taken up with reviewing the sorts of measures that might be employed to engineer change towards a desired state culture, their effectiveness is largely yet to be proven. Many scholars have sought to temper the optimism of enthusiastic executives keen to mould their organisation's culture to match their ideal, and we would do well to recall their arguments.

Culture change is difficult to realise because most employees in an organisation have a high emotional stake in the current culture. People who have been steeped in the traditions and values of an organisation and whose philosophy of life may well be caught up in the organisation's cultural assumptions will experience considerable uncertainty, anxiety and pain in the process of change. For many middle and senior managers change may also seem to threaten a loss in status, loss of power over resources and less security. Even if there are personal gains to be made from altering the habits of a lifetime these are likely to be seen as potential or theoretical only, as against the certainty of the losses. These multiple sources of perceived risk will usually result in resistance to change, resistance which is often culturally based. Depending on the organisation this resistance may be more or less organised and more or less overt, the form it takes being of far less significance than the possible consequence, namely, the gradual failure of the culture change strategy. While most case studies of change tend to focus on the successes as defined by senior executives, it is apparent that in many organisations individuals threatened with change successfully invoke *rites of continuity and renewal* which preserve and protect the old order.

More subtle attempts to modify a culture rather than direct and overt attacks on it may have more chances of success, but our limited knowledge of how organisations work precludes a final judgement. Furthermore, all possible levers on culture are very restricted in their scope and highly dependent on large numbers of variables that are difficult to assess and predict. Using human resource programmes, policies and procedures to manage a culture seems an intuitively plausible plan, but is only likely to have much impact in the long term. This may mean that a given culture management strategy has to be pursued with persistence and enthusiasm for years to have any noticeable effect. The problem is that the turnover of senior executives in some organisations is very rapid, that desired state cultures are likely to be constantly redefined in the light of changing circumstances and personalities, and that even in stable environments and with a stable leadership team organisational strategies are prone to alter in response to the demands of shareholders and the outcomes of internal political machi-

Mini Case 5.3

Managing culture change at Hambro

From its inception in 1971 Hambro Life grew to be the UK's largest unit-linked life insurance company. At the beginning of the 1980s, however, new legislation meant that banks, building societies and even some high street retailers started to compete with Hambro for business. If Hambro was to remain a high-growth organisation, then it was obvious to senior executives that the enterprise would need to transform itself in line with reform of the industry as a whole. The result was a large-scale programme of radical change that aimed to change not just the structure but the culture of the company. One of the first moves made was to change the name of the corporation to Allied Dunbar, itself a powerful symbol of the need for adaptation and relearning. Here we will consider briefly how culture change was sought within two parts of the organisation from the early 1980s onwards, the administration function, and sales and marketing.

Administration

Having decided to take action the first step was to commission an attitude survey (handled by external consultants) for all 2000 employees. The results of the survey were then fed back and discussed by all staff in a lengthy and reiterative process under the guidance of consultants. Following this exercise the whole of the management team was co-opted into discussions concerning the business objectives of the administration function: requirements, expectations, responsibilities and standards, among others, were considered in an attempt to formulate a comprehensive statement of aims and goals. This was a difficult and time-consuming affair that was only sustained because of the extent of the management involvement and commitment from the top. Ultimately a written statement called the 'Allied Dunbar Approach' was drawn up, which was to guide the development of a new culture. Part of the document included a mission statement in which key values and beliefs were

explicitly stated. These included: a commitment to provide a cost-effective service to customers, a declaration that the administration was a paternalistic, caring but demanding employer that looks after the interests of employees in return for high performance, and a belief that a strong and talented leadership team was crucial to the success of the organisation. In addition, eight policy statements were formulated, constituting an inclusive and integrated guide to managing within the Allied Dunbar administration.

With the desired state culture agreed, the next step was to find means for translating the blueprint for a new culture into organisational reality. Four of the principal methods employed were communication, management training, annual action plans and monitoring:

1 *Communication* of the Allied Dunbar approach to all 2000 employees seems to have been effective, with each individual receiving a written statement of it. In addition, it features in the employee handbook and figures prominently in the organisation's recruitment literature and induction programmes.

2 *Management training* programmes are based on the new Allied Dunbar approach, and every line manager in the administration has attended a course run by his or her divisional management during which it has been explained and discussed. Furthermore, all the off-the-job training programmes run by the organisation have been revised to include the approach and policies.

3 *Annual action plans* are now formulated by all areas of line management in which areas for improvement are highlighted against the standards set by the approach.

4 *Monitoring* of the effectiveness of staff against the standards of the approach and policies is accomplished using a specially designed questionnaire which is completed anonymously by

three broad categories of managers. The results are then used to facilitate appraisals, individual development and team-building programmes.

Sales and marketing

While there are over 3000 people working for Allied Dunbar in this area, only 240 managers are employees, the others being self-employed financial management consultants and sales associates. These 240 managers have the task of creating an environment in which consultants and associates can maximise their individual success. Research suggested that significant changes in organisational structure, the managers' contracts and a new management development programme would all be advantageous to the organisation. Perhaps the most significant of these changes was the restructuring, as this had direct cultural implications.

Up until the end of 1984 the sales force was organised around six geographical areas, each with its own management team led by a director in the field. The problems with this arrangement was that the size of the areas was so great that employees had become too far removed from the point of sale. With the coming diversification of product lines this problem seemed set to worsen. Allied Dunbar was faced with the classic difficulty of not wanting to constrain entrepreneurial energy, drive and creativity in the field while ensuring that the centre did not lose control. The solution chosen was to create smaller teams ultimately headed by a regional manager reporting to head office. The new organisation not only improved lines of communication and operational efficiency, it also served as a vehicle for changing the sales managers' values and behaviours.

Before the changes branch managers tended to work in isolation from each other with little overt collaboration. While this sort of stand-alone entreprenuerialism had its advantages, the downside was that pressures on the branch managers were enormous. Regionalisation is the compromise structure that is designed to encourage and foster co-operation through the formation of regional management teams from which branch managers can obtain support and ideas from colleagues. The fifteen heads of region are key to the process of cultural change, and attend a variety of meetings at head office on a regular basis in order to ensure that every one of them is pulling in the same direction. The enthusiasm with which culture change is pursued at Allied Dunbar should come as a surprise for no one, because it is fired by one overriding motivation, profit: 'Our interest in culture is only as a means to an end – sustained, high growth and increased profitability through people who have rewarding and enjoyable working lives.'

Questions

1 Is Hambro experiencing a serious attempt at culture change?

2 Has Hambro undergone culture change?

3 What learning points are there here for other organisations attempting culture change?

nations. Moreover, it is a fact that in many organisations the human resource function is viewed as marginal to the process of strategic management, and peripheral to attempts to manage culture. In short, pursuing a consistent culture management strategy using human resource systems may not be as simple as it at first seems. Indeed, for some complex, quick-acting organisations in unstable environments and with high staff turnover, it may not be a realistic option at all.

Symbolic leadership can certainly be an effective means of managing culture, but is not an easy option for the overwhelming majority of organisational leaders. The appropriate use of symbolic action requires considerable self-understanding and sensitivity to others, supported by a relatively clear sense of direction and knowledge of how organisations work. Whether there are large numbers of talented individuals able and willing to play out the dramatic roles managing through symbols necessitates is an as yet unanswered question. There are similar difficulties associated with the use of rites. Rites are relatively elaborate and dramatic planned sets of activities that need to be well thought out and convincingly executed in order to have the desired effect: not all leaders have the charisma, determination and vision to handle these situations effectively. In addition, the extent to which rites can be deliberately moulded to pursue a desired state culture and the extent to which their form and content is decided by the history, traditions and inclinations of employees is unclear. In the final analysis it may well be the case that the scope leaders have for managing culture through rites is restricted by these contextual factors, making them a rather blunt instrument of control.

It is apparent that if culture change is to be induced, then it can be most effectively accomplished by means which rely on *intrinsic motivation* (i.e. the internalised commitment of employees) rather than by means which involve *extrinsic motivation* (that is, rules, incentives and the threat of sanctions). This is because extrinsic motivators allow employees to overtly comply with the new culture (actions which they are able to justify as being 'required' or 'worth their while'), but does little to adjust their belief/value preferences or assumptions. In contrast, intrinsic motivators attempt to persuade people of the inherent worth of the new culture without resort to either incentives or sanctions, generally by pointing out the negative consequences of not changing (disconfirmation) and the advantages of adopting the new beliefs, values and assumptions (confirmation). To work effectively it helps if the disconfirmation of the old behaviours and cognitions and the confirmation of the new culture is done as visibly and dramatically as possible (see Chapter 4, the integrative model of Lewin, Beyer and Trice, and Isabella). Reliance on internal motivators is useful because it does not allow employees the escape route of arguing that they have been coerced or bribed into changing their behaviour.

In coming to any firm conclusions concerning the possibility of managing organisational culture we are faced with the problem of how little we really know about the dynamics of collectively shared beliefs, values and assumptions. As Fitzgerald (1988) has argued, as yet we have no comprehensive theory to account for the process by which values and beliefs are relinquished and replaced. We also lack agreement on a theory about the conditions that support the formation of cultural values and that account for the hegemony of one competing set over another. There is also little certainty regarding how patterns of behaviour, rites, rituals and ceremonies influence and are influenced by values, beliefs and assumptions, and the relationship between these cognitive and behavioural orientations on the one hand and stories, myths and legends on the other. While there is consensus that mature organisational cultures are stable and self-reinforcing systems, there is little agreement on how long it takes to alter a culture, though most commentators suggest that we need to think in terms of years rather than months (Williams *et al.*, 1993). Reading the literature on organisational culture, massive though it is, rapidly leads one to the realisation that the case studies available, combined with the occasional anecdotes (mostly concerning famous or infamous American businessmen) and a few snippets of theory is an insufficient basis on which to draw any very firm conclusions. An indication of the sorts of opinions held by a wide spectrum of theorists and commentators in this field is provided by Exhibit 5.3.

Exhibit 5.3
Can culture change be managed?

For all the hype, corporate culture is real and powerful. It's also hard to change, and you won't find much support for doing so inside or outside your company. If you run up against the culture when trying to redirect strategy, attempt to dodge; if you must meddle with culture directly, tread carefully and with modest expectations. (*Fortune*, 17 October 1983)

Notice that I have not said 'manage the culture', because it is not clear whether that is possible or even desirable. But the consequences of culture are real, and these must be managed. (Schein, 1985b: xii)

Because some of the consequences of managing culture are often unanticipated, the process of working with organisational culture involves some risk. The challenge is magnified by the presence of multiple subcultures in a single organisational setting. Therefore, the management of culture ought to be carefully and cautiously undertaken. (Krefting and Frost, 1985: 156)

There has been a tendency for some researchers to treat organisational culture as a 'variable' that can be controlled and manipulated like any other organisational variable . . . . The basis of the argument presented in this paper is that culture should be regarded as something that an organisation 'is', not as something that an organisation 'has': It is not an independent variable, nor can it be created, discovered or destroyed by the whims of management. (Meek, 1988: 469)

According to the corporate culture perspectives, the culture *as* a culture (as a whole) – whether it is referred to as culture, clan, tribe or community – can actually be managed! (Alvesson and Berg, 1992: 148)

Cultural change is a slow process, it can be assisted rather than controlled but, in given circumstances, its pursuit might be worth while as long as it is not sought as a facile, cosmetic and transitory change. (Anthony, 1994: 5)

SUMMARY AND CONCLUSIONS

This chapter has elaborated seven main themes.

1 It was suggested that there is broad scope for disagreement concerning whether culture can be managed, depending on how the term 'culture' is understood. Most authors do, however, admit that cultures can be modified and most arguments centre on the extent to which it can be managed and the constraining influence of contextual variables such as the environment and various change resources like leadership, finance and mechanisms for co-ordination, communication and control.

2 A general framework for accomplishing culture change was provided. This suggested that the actual culture should be identified, the ideal state culture sketched in theory, and then practical steps taken to align the two. While not presenting any great advances in culture change theory the framework does at least remind us that successful change management requires that we know where we are starting from and to where we are hoping to travel.

3 A number of means of influencing culture through human resource systems, policies, programmes and procedures were identified. It was argued that by adopting a consistent cues approach, recruitment and selection procedures, induction, socialisation and training programmes, the performance appraisal and reward system can all play a role in a strategy for managing culture.

4 The role of leadership in the management of culture was discussed. This discussion had two main components: first, the scope for managing culture through symbolic means was illustrated; and second, the potential for managing culture through the use of organisational rites was considered.

5 Bate's four basic strategies for dealing with culture (conforming, deforming, reforming and transforming) were outlined. Some of the dominant symptoms of cultural stagnation were then identified, and Bate's four principal strategies for implementing culture change (aggressive, conciliative, corrosive and indoctrinative) discussed.

6 Silverzweig and Allen's normative systems model for managing organisational culture change was described and commented upon. It was suggested that despite some drawbacks it nevertheless provides a useful starting point for practical action.

7 Some of the many difficulties associated with arriving at firm conclusions concerning the possibility of culture management were exposed. If there is a conclusion to be drawn it is that it is too early to draw any definite conclusions.

KEY CONCEPTS

Resistance	Training	Use of meetings,	to culture change
Actual culture	Performance appraisal	agendas and	Confirming strategies
Ideal state culture	Transfers and	minutes	Deforming strategies
Culture gaps	secondments	Rites of passage	Reforming strategies
Consistent	Opportunities for	Rites of enhancement	Transforming strategies
cues approach	participation	Rites of degradation	Aggressive strategies
Human resource	Formal communication	Rites of conflict	Conciliative strategies
management	Counselling	reduction	Corrosive strategies
Recruitment and	Employee relations	Rites of integration	Indoctrinative
selection	Symbolic leadership	Rites of renewal	strategies
Induction	Use of time	Managers as actors	Normative
Socialisation	Use of language	Leaders as barriers	systems model

QUESTIONS

1 What is meant by resistance to change? Why do people resist culture change?

2 Why have some theorists suggested that organisational culture cannot be managed? Are they right?

3 What factors affect the relative ease (or difficulty) of managing organisational culture?

4 Of what use is the general framework for managing organisational culture as expressed by Wilkins and Patterson (1985) and Kilmann (1984)?

5 What is the consistent cues approach? How does it work in practice with human resource programmes and systems?

6 What are the main advantages and difficulties associated with attempts to manage culture using human resource programmes and systems?

7 In your opinion which individual human resource programme, policy or system is most important for leaders attempting to manage their organisation's culture? Explain your answer.

8 How can leaders manage culture through symbols?

9 What are the most effective symbolic means that leaders can use to manage their organisation's culture? What are the least effective symbols that leaders may choose to employ?

10 In what sense are organisational leaders actors? Does the idea that leaders are actors provide us with any new insights into how culture change might be accomplished?

11 Assess the strengths and weaknesses of the normative systems model.

12 With reference to an organisation you know well, suggest why organisational cultures are so difficult to manage?

MANAGING CULTURE AT DIGITAL EQUIPMENT CORPORATION (UK) LTD

Introduction

By the end of the 1980s senior personnel in the human resource function at Digital Equipment Corporation (UK) Ltd had become concerned that the explosive growth in staff numbers the company had experienced in the 1980s had led to an unwanted alteration in its corporate culture. This concern was bolstered by independent research which concluded that there was a growing divergence between the culture desired by the company and the culture as experienced by its employees. A strong culture was (and is) prized at Digital as a means of ensuring employee commitment and product quality. Moreover the strength and uniqueness of its culture were thought to be significant reasons for the company's commercial success from the very beginning. This fear that the culture was changing for the worse coincided with a downturn in the company's profitability, which served to focus still more attention on the health and strength of Digital's culture. One of the solutions the company adopted was to attempt to manage its culture through human resource systems and programmes, including recruitment and selection, reward and compensation, performance appraisal, and induction, training and development.

Digital: a brief overview

Digital Equipment Corporation is the world's second largest computer manufacturer after IBM (measured in dollar revenues) and the world's largest producer of minicomputers. Founded in 1957 by Kenneth Olsen and three employees in a converted wool mill in Maynard, Massachusetts, the organisation launched its first computer in 1960. Two generations of successful computer developments later, the organisation is internationally renowned as a producer of relatively inexpensive yet high-quality products. A few statistics give a feel for the scale of Digital's success: in the decade to 1982 the company recorded average annual growth revenues of 36 per cent per annum; in the early 1980s its operating revenues were well over £6 billion and in 1991 these had risen to nearly £14 billion; in 1990 it employed over 100 000 people

worldwide. Furthermore, Digital invested heavily in research and development (approximately 10 per cent of operating revenues) to maintain its position as market leader in the production of minicomputer systems. Interestingly, it was the company's policy not to pay dividends on its shares, but rather to reinvest profits. Employees, however, could purchase shares at 15 per cent discount.

Digital set up its UK operation in 1964, and by 1976 this employed just over 1000 people. By 1985 this had grown to just over 5000 people and by 1990 this figure had more than doubled. In 1990 Digital had its headquarters in Reading, its manufacturing plant in Ayr (southern Scotland), and its 12 sales and service centres were scattered between Edinburgh and London. In the early 1980s Digital's sales in Britain were around £450 million per annum, and by 1990 these had grown to £936 million. In 1991, however, operating revenue fell back to £877 million, a fall of 7 per cent and the first in the company's history. A deep recession and rapid change within the IT industry were blamed for the company's problems, which quickly led senior executives to initiate a 10 per cent reduction in the workforce. Additionally, attempts were made to increase the entrepreneurial drive of employees by making individual managers in charge of accounts responsible for their own profit targets. According to Geoff Shingles (the chairman and chief executive) this was 'a serious effort to regain the spirit and initiative of a small company while retaining the strength and resources of a worldwide organisation'.[1]

The desired state culture

It was universally acknowledged that Ken Olsen was the main driving force behind the desired culture of Digital. As a 1981 report[2] stated, 'Ken had strong ideas about what kind of company he wanted to have, a very strong disposition to what kind of environment he wanted to work in'. Unlike many other organisations *culture* was a topic of ordinary conversation in Digital, and was also evidently used instrumentally as a means of enforcing self-discipline and control by senior executives. One result of this preoccupation

Fig. 5.2 Digital (UK) Ltd: summary overview of desired state culture

Assumptions	Values	Desired norms
People are important	Caring – for employees, customers, other stakeholders and society	All employees should: • treat people justly • respect the rights of others • respect people's differences
Trust is the basis of quality relationships	Honesty	All employees should: • be honest with people • make only those commitments they can keep • be candid, open and truthful
Profitability is necessary for existence	Profit	All employees should: • understand and communicate the necessity of profit • understand how their work contributes to Digital's profitability
Quality is our competitive edge	Quality	All employees should: • produce quality results • value quality performance more than credentials, seniority or status symbols • hire the best-qualified people • demand and reward excellence
Success depends upon flexibility and responsiveness to environment	Open communication Simplicity	All employees should: • communicate all significant information to the appropriate people • be direct, say what they mean • have clear work goals and regular measurements Managers and supervisors should: • be accessible, listen to and help employees with work-related problems • share information within the group and across organisational lines • give usable feedback, both positive and negative • avoid overlap in work goals
People perform best when they 'own' their work	Taking responsibility	All employees should: • take responsibility for their own work • take initiative • stand up for what they are convinced is right Managers and supervisors should: • delegate authority • provide opportunities for individual and team contributions • encourage and reward initiative • hold employees accountable for proposals once accepted

Fig. 5.2 *continued*

Assumptions	Values	Desired norms
There is always more to learn and do	Continual learning and development	All employees should: • strive for improvement • seek opportunities for development Managers and supervisors should: • provide challenges for employees • provide opportunities for learning • tolerate mistakes which occur as part of learning and taking risks
The best ideas succeed	Competition	All employees should: • challenge and confront one another for positive results • take the risk that comes with presenting new and different ideas • fight proposals, not each other Managers and supervisors should: • encourage innovation, creativity and risk taking • make conflict productive
No one can know or do everything by him- or herself	Co-operation Teamplay	All employees should: • ask for and offer help and support • be team players • accept modification of their ideas • act in the best interest of Digital as opposed to protecting 'turf' Managers and supervisors should: • create the climate for teamplay and collaboration

with culture was a vast array of internal company documents and reports detailing various aspects of the cultural ethos that all in Digital were expected to subscribe and adhere to. A summary overview derived from several such documents is contained in Fig. 5.2.

In practical terms the desired culture at Digital was task-oriented: the overriding priority was to accomplish the task or finish the project in hand. To do this required teamwork. Consequently, role models and heroes were unashamedly team players who believed in the unifying power of the group. These groups were supposed to work according to peer-enforced organisational norms such as 'get it right first time', 'the customer is always right' and 'do the right thing'. Open communication and consensus were equally essential. Senior managers were expected to manage by walking around, to know the names of their subordinates, be available for discussion, and be good consensus-builders and facilitators. Conforming to such norms was essential. No one could achieve much without the help of an extended network of friends, confidantes and allies, and networking was thus key to personal success. As one employee noted:

This support orientation bonds people to the organisation through the formation of close and warm relationships with fellow employees. We became like an extended family, highly supportive and harmonious. You become part of the network. Entering the network enables the individual to become known as someone with a contribution to make. Few people can achieve anything by themselves without the support of the network. Everybody in Digital knows the process. You work within the process.

Control over who entered Digital was recognised to be vital, and considerable care seemed to be exercised to recruit and select people who were compatible with the desired state culture. In deciding to fill a vacancy or a newly created position the post would first be advertised internally. Internal job posting was an integral part of Digital's human resource strategy, as were internal promotions, job rotations and transfers. This meant that employee morale was generally high, that expectations of being promoted were the norm, and that personal development was at the top of many employees' agenda. When it was considered necessary to recruit externally, great care was exercised to ensure that the advertisement projected a positive corporate image. One side effect of this was that Digital always placed its own advertisements, and never used any intermediaries. Having sifted through the responses the HRM department then called some applicants for a series of interviews. Once at Digital the typical applicant could expect three interviews: with a representative of the HRM department, with a senior member of the function in which the job was located, and with the individual relinquishing the position (or someone who performed a similar role). Candidates who passed through these interviews were then called back for a second day of interviewing still more rigorous than the first. Depending on the level of entry (interviewing for more senior positions was most rigorous of all) interviews were likely to be conducted by the three people who had interviewed him or her last time, the line manager for the position, up to three managers from outside the function and two other people from human resources. If the vacant position was for a staff manager then a large number of extra interviews with existing senior managers could also be anticipated.

During these interviews three types of selection criteria were employed: those pertaining to the job, those pertaining to the function in which the job was located, and those concerning the organisation as a whole, including culture. As a matter of fact it was not unusual for applicants who were recognised to be good quality individuals who met the organisational criteria to be offered a position other than the one that had originally been advertised. This flexibility in the recruitment and selection procedures was much prized by Digital staff, who thought that it enabled them to offer employment to any useful and compatible people who made themselves available.

The actual culture

Digital UK's Reading headquarters consisted not of one large self-contained building, but a number of fairly widely spread complexes. Of these the largest was DECPark, with approximately 2000 employees. A vast car park, the spaces of which were available on a first-come-first-served basis, flanked the building. Given the sheer size of the operation those employees who did not arrive sufficiently early found they had a lengthy walk to one of the entrances. At the functional and unostentatious reception, security was taken seriously: my contact had to be called down to sign me in to a register, and I was issued with my own security pass. The building itself resembled a large aircraft hanger, and was pleasantly open and spacious. Office furnishings were standard throughout, and comfortable rather than luxurious. While there were large numbers of vending machines and a cafeteria that served good-quality lunches, these facilities were not free, though not exorbitantly expensive either. Smoking was confined to designated 'smoking rooms'. The building was mostly open-plan, though offices were reserved for more senior staff. It is worth noting that executive staff were housed not at DECPark but in another building several miles down the road, which was far more beautifully furnished. Unsurprisingly, in all DEC buildings, PCs and printers littered the desks.

A long and broad corridor ran the entire length of the DECPark building, and this served as a conduit not just for people but for ideas. As one senior manager explained: 'Walking down there I have just fixed up three meetings!' There seemed to be no informal norms as regards dress, with the number of people wearing a shirt and tie or smart dress equally matched by those in casual clothes. Everyone I could see appeared to be busy, and the building as a whole could aptly be described as a 'hive of activity'. On the surface it was difficult to distinguish senior from junior staff, though it soon became evident that Digital employees were highly adept at this. Indeed, I was to learn later that an ability to discern who had power over what was a necessary facility for survival within the organisation. More than one employee confided that the workings of Digital were more than a little arcane, and easy for the new recruit to misunderstand and misinterpret. It was not unusual for new recruits to the company to experience considerable problems adjusting to a culture in which the 'real' meanings and significance of ideas and actions required considerable understanding of the history and nature of the organisation.

Whereas the desired culture stressed the importance of individual self-actualisation and organisational support for employees, a recent independent consultancy report suggested that people were experiencing a culture that emphasised power and role. When asked, employees asserted that visibility was more likely to make someone successful than good performance, that individual freedom had become restricted, that political machinations dominated organisational processes, and that decision making was very much top-down. Furthermore employees complained that rules and procedures were often both inflexible and inappropriate, and that the organisation was becoming a highly complex web of systems, controls and structures which was difficult to understand. For example, one senior manager I spoke to was dismayed that he was unable to attend an advanced IT course because he had not attended some basic courses first, even though he obviously had no intellectual need to attend the introductory sessions. People were also becoming bitter about the increased incidence of verbal abuse and ill-considered rejection of ideas by senior colleagues. Others complained that while in the past the building had been full of people until well after office hours, it was now virtually deserted after 6.00 p.m.

A document written by a recent Digital recruit in 1988 and that was still circulating in Digital in the early 1990s is highly instructive:

DEC, the culture, is spoken of in tandem with Core Values, in the same tone as one might speak of Moses coming down from the mountain carrying the stone tablets or in the same way Australian aborigines chant about Dreamtime. This tells me something about where Digital is, historically, in its cultural self-reference. We are at a time when the precepts of the Founders are harder to discern. There was a time when everyone heard, shared, and created the precepts at the same campfire, so to speak. (In this case, it was the same parking lot, the same bar, and the same woods meeting.) Then they were transmitted by word of mouth, oral tradition, legends, parables, folklore, [memos] that served to elaborate, refine and reinforce the Message. This was the culture. And fewer of us are carriers of the culture.

There are the elders of the tribe, those of the First Generation, who have known no other way of life than the one of Digital. They are the Original People. There are the people who were close to them, like those who went on the Long March with Mao. They lived it and lived to talk about it. There are those who don't know if they lived it or heard stories so vivid and appealing that they might as well have been there. At any rate, they have joined their history and memory to those of the Original People, and by extension they have perpetuated the stories. This went on for some years. I don't want to overdo it, but I don't want to minimize it either. But something happened, as it does to any culture that cannot remain self-contained. Its points of contact with the barbarians increased, and it became subject to the influence of forces beyond its control. Its culture became a hybrid as other influences intermingled. For the last three years or so, Digital has been making new Badge-holders of some 25,000 people a year, or 100 a day. I call these people immigrants. I am one of them. And it is increasingly the luck of the draw as to whether these newcomers subscribe to the tenets of the Original People.

What this means is that the culture is not being transmitted in any particular way. The transmission is increasingly two-way. It is my contention that Digital's culture (taken as the Founding Way) is subject at least as much to the Other Ways of the immigrants as they are subject to it. This means that there are more people very new to Digital than there are who were part of the Long March. Digital's culture is increasingly not that of a little New England mill town company, and there is no way of cycling enough people through the Mother Church (the Mill) to inculcate in them the feel, and the spirit, of bygone days. All of this adds up to a review of Digital's culture that recognises its new reality. Some would say that the culture has been watered down, that hallowed traditions are in danger of being lost. Some would say it is more dynamic and pluralistic, which is a fancier way of saying the same thing. Many of the cliches about Digital no longer hold, and yet we hear people saying them.

I happen to believe in some of the features of Digital that are parts of its culture and I want them preserved and perpetuated. I put it in different ways perhaps, but you must allow for my immigrant dialect. I think Digital (the collective super-ego) fosters what I call distributed autonomy . . . . It suggests a degree of self-direction, initiative, ability to contribute to an interdependant relationship, honesty, openness, trust, mutuality, self-knowledge, self-respect, generosity: it is a protection of the Founder's ideal. Not everyone is ready for this, or the consequences of it. People who can't function effectively in a setting of distributed autonomy are dysfunctional to basic premises of the company, not only to the premises of its internal organisational behaviour, but also to the premises of its external product strategy. Yet there are such people. How are they acculturated? And how do they act, dialectically, to acculturate others? There are many examples that could be used. My point is that this is a two-way street. What rubs off is a reversible equation. The culture needs to figure out how to preserve itself even while it is changing.

Managing culture

Digital is an unusual organisation in that large numbers of people see human resource management as being at the heart of the company. Some employees even ventured the comment that 'personnel runs Digital'. Working within a matrix structure of multiple reporting relationships HRM staff liaise closely with line managers about human resource issues. This reflects a philosophy which states that people are part of Digital's strategic or competitive edge. The result is that the human resource department has considerable influence and is overtly responsible for managing culture.

In 1990 senior personnel in the human resource function at Digital's headquarters in Reading commissioned Manchester Business School to advise them on how to manage organisational culture. After much deliberation it was decided that, given the prevailing constraints, the most effective action that could be taken would be to formulate tools for evaluating existing (and future) human resource programmes in terms of their likelihood of promoting the desired culture. The result was a series of organisation development matrices that could be used to structure discussions concerning existing and prototypical human resource programmes, policies and systems, one of which is shown in Fig. 5.3. On the left-hand side can be seen various adjectives describing elements of Digital's desired culture, while across the top are the four principal components of an HRM programme as employed in this piece of research. The *modus operandi* of the matrix is extremely simple. Each desired cultural trait is discussed in terms of each of the four HRM programme components for the structure or system under consideration. By using the matrices it was hoped to modify existing programmes (and structure developing programmes) to ensure their support for the desired culture.

Authority in Digital is, however, unusually diffuse for a commercial organisation, and by the time this research had come to an end there was little evidence that the 'buy-in' from all interested parties that was required in order to proceed with these tools had been achieved. Those who knew Digital well suggested that this in itself provided more insight into the organisation's culture than many of the expensive reports that had been commissioned by senior executives . . .

Epilogue

By the early 1990s Digital's commercial problems had, if anything, intensified. Ken Olsen was personally

	Objectives	Language	Methods	Total programme concept
Openness				
Empowerment				
Achievement				
Equal opportunities				
IT-oriented				
Person-centred				
Co-operation				
Competence				

Fig. 5.3 Cultural matrix for the evaluation of human resource programmes

blamed for a number of poor business decisions*, and on 16 July 1992 the world's press announced that he had stepped aside as head of the company, ending his 35-year-reign. Analysts summed-up recent events with statements such as: 'A giant of the industry, the 66-year-old Olsen was also known as an autocrat who failed to let Digital change with the times and then eventually drove the company into chaos' (Reuters News Service, 17 July 1992). Pier Carlo Falotti, President and Chief Executive of DEC Europe, and the man who had grown DEC's European business from 25–50 per cent of the supplier's worldwide revenues in ten years, announced that he was leaving on the same day. Olsen's departure had two immediate effects: morale within Digital nose-dived, and Wall Street analysts put a positive face on the news, raising the share price by $3. The UK reaction was summed up by Geoff Shingles (Chairman and Chief Executive of DEC UK), who asserted that 'We expected Olsen to step down sometime, but we were taken completely by surprise by his decision last week. My first reaction was one of sadness. It's a major change – the end of the era.'

Before departing DEC, Olsen ensured that his hand-picked successor Bob Palmer would take over. The press described his task of re-building Digital as 'monumental'. Not only was the company in a poor financial state, but a staff already demoralized by instability, lay-offs, and management bickering, had to be dramatically cut if the company was to be turned around. The announcement of a $2.8 billion loss in mid-1992 further de-stabilized the corporation. Five traumatic years later and with 60 000 people cut from Digital's payroll the company was again profitable, but only just. While overheads had been slashed by a third since 1992, profit margins had declined by a quarter. By the end of 1997, commentators reflecting on Digital's fortunes were suggesting that the only reason Digital had survived so long was that an established customer base were still using old Digital systems. Headlines in the business press such as 'Is Digital over the hill at forty?' and 'How are the mighty fallen?' were symptomatic of analysts' expectations of further decline.

Note

*Digital had missed the personal computer revolution of the 1980s, entering the market only in 1991. By that time, its rivals were beginning to produce more powerful workstations using a new microprocessor called RISC (Reduced Instruction Set Computing). There was a further delay (which analysts blamed on Olsen) before Digital embraced this technology. Some industry observers also blamed Olsen for failing to respond positively to John Scully's overtures that might have led to an alliance with Apple Computer Inc.

Questions

1 Give a brief description of Digital's culture-in-practice.

2 How does Digital's culture-in-practice differ from its desired culture?

3 Compared with other organisations with which you are familiar how unique is Digital's desired culture?

4 What are Digital's desired culture's strengths and weaknesses?

5 Why were some people at Digital so concerned that the company's culture was changing? Was their worry justified?

6 Should the responsibility for managing organisational culture be left to human resource professionals? Who else might usefully be involved and why?

7 What advice would you give to senior executives at Digital UK?

Sources: Reuters Business Briefing 14 May 1992, 17 July 1992; *Computing* 23 July 1992, 13 November 1997.

NOTES

1 *Digital Review,* 1991.
2 'Shaping Values', written for Digital by McKinsey Consultants in 1981.

CHAPTER 6

Organisational culture, strategy and performance

OBJECTIVES

To enable students to:

- understand the relationship between culture, strategy and performance;
- distinguish what is meant by the terms 'strategy' and 'performance';
- comprehend how culture influences the formulation and implementation of strategy;
- examine the idea of strategy as a 'cultural artefact';
- evaluate the importance of culture as an influence on organisational performance;
- appreciate how high- and low-performance cultures can evolve;
- assess the cultural implications of mergers and acquisitions;
- consider the difficulties and complexities of providing general guidelines for action in this field.

INTRODUCTION

This chapter discusses the complex relationships between culture, strategy and performance. It has six major sections. First, a brief overview of what is meant by 'strategy' and 'performance' and how they relate to notions of culture is provided. Second, the influence of culture on the formulation and implementation of strategy in organisations is considered. Third, the importance of taking cultural considerations into account when planning and executing mergers and acquisitions is discussed. Fourth, some conclusions concerning the interdependence of culture and strategy are drawn. Fifth, the work of Kotter and Heskett (1992), Denison (1990) and Gordon (1985) concerning the relationship between culture and performance is reviewed. Finally, some general conclusions regarding the nature of the linkages between culture, strategy and performance are sketched.

CULTURE, STRATEGY AND PERFORMANCE

In recent years the concepts of *strategy* and *strategic* management have received increasing attention from scholars and practitioners (Dobson and Starkey, 1993). The supposed importance of strategy has been magnified by suggestions that it is somehow related to both the culture and the success of organisations. The connection between culture and strategy is considered critical because of the wide range of competitive challenges that currently face corporations around the world. All the evidence suggests that these pressures will accelerate in the immediate future, with technological advances, the increasingly global nature of markets, and trade legislation all playing significant roles. The point is that in the face of such pressures, a vital concern for managers will be to minimise the time span required to evolve new and effective strategies, and this requires an understanding of the influence of organisational culture. Importantly for us, there are a variety of different views on what strategy is and how it should be defined.

Strategy is a plan

According to some, strategy refers to a plan for interacting with the competitive environment in order to achieve organisational goals. Such plans are generally characterised as formal, explicit, devised by senior executives, long-termist, and having a significant effect on how the organisation behaves in its environment. Strategy in this sense has been derived from military strategy (the art of war), which in a business context translates into how an organisation seeks to survive and prosper in a hostile and dangerous world.

Strategy is a system of management

An alternative view of strategy suggests that it can be less structured, and more informal and implicit in its formulation. The idea here is that strategy is something intrinsic to the process of leading and managing. Rather than being a set plan, strategy is a set of principles or heuristics for managing that are encoded in a system of management and which allow for considerable flexibility and adaptability in dealing with the exigencies of a changing environment. In fact, most organisations seem to have an identifiable strategy both in the sense of a plan and a system of management.

Strategy is a craft process

Drawing on the traditions of strategy as a plan and a system of management Mintzberg (1987) argues that the formulation of strategy is a craft activity akin to the crafting of pots and plates by a lone potter. Managers then are craftsmen and strategy is their clay. Organisational strategies are patterns of decisions, events and activities that need not be consciously pursued (they may just emerge) and in some instances may never be identified by those who put them into practice. Consider, for example, how the National Film Board of Canada (NFB) came to adopt a feature-film strategy. Some years ago it funded a film maker on a project that unexpectedly ran long. In order to distribute his film the NFB turned to theatres and so inadvertently gained experience in marketing feature-length films. Other film makers then caught on to the idea, and over time the NFB found itself pursuing a feature-film strategy, that is, a pattern of producing such films. This strategy emerged craftlike from unanticipated events and unplanned responses in an *ad hoc* manner.

While these notions of strategy are very different from each other it is clear that they share some commonalities with mainstream views on culture. This is especially true of the approximations of strategy as a system of management and a craft activity. Indeed, Weick (1985) has suggested that for many researchers there is no real distinction between culture and strategy to be made at all. In other words, the terms culture and strategy describe the same sets of organisational phenomena. For example, both culture and strategy are said to guide expression and interpretation, they are retrospective, summarising patterns in past decisions and actions, they are embodied in actions of judging, creating, justifying, affirming and sanctioning, they summarise past achievements and practices that work, and they provide continuity and identity and a consistent way of ordering the world. Given these similarities, Weick suggests that, in many instances, culture and strategy may be substitutable for one another, that they serve a common function, that of imposing coherence, order and meaning, and that they may both be a liability because their tenacity makes it harder for organisations to detect changes in their environments and adapt to them.[1] Most commentators nevertheless accept that there is an important distinction to be made between culture and strategy. Certainly, strategic planning documents may be thought of as cultural artefacts, but there seems little point in expanding our already inclusive definitions of culture to include long-term plans or patterns of competitive activities. This would just make our notions of culture still more complex and more difficult to apply with precision or to use analytically to explain behaviour. Similarly, there seems equally little to be gained from expanding our usual ideas of strategy to include artefacts, values or beliefs, though these may of course influence the development and implementation of strategic patterns. The concern of this chapter is to elaborate the nature of the relationship between culture and strategy, and to discuss the implications this has for organisational performance. To avoid problems of meaning in this chapter 'strategy' will generally be used to refer to those long-term plans devised by senior executives in order to meet the challenges of the external environment and accomplish organisational objectives.

The strategic objective of many organisations is to achieve a *sustainable competitive advantage*. Sustainable competitive advantage is the unique position of a firm in relation to its competitors that allows it to outperform them consistently (Porter, 1990). While achieving a sustainable competitive advantage involves acquiring the right number, type and mix of tangible assets, it also requires appropriate beliefs, values and assumptions which specify efficient and effective patterns of behaviour. Furthermore this mix of assets and culture, if it is to lead to superior performance in the long term, must be imperfectly imitable. A pattern of tangible assets is far easier to imitate than a culture, leading some to suspect that if sustained competitive advantage can be obtained by organisations, then it is most likely to be through developing a strategically appropriate culture that facilitates high performance.

What, then, are we to understand by 'organisational performance', and what constitutes 'effective' and 'non-effective' performance? As with our attempts to define organisational strategy, there are no hard and fast rules here. The first thing to realise is that effectiveness is a relative concept, and therefore that the level of organisational effectiveness represents the degree of accomplishment compared with the best that can be hoped for, given the organisation's particular situation. In any given instance, when it is asked how effective an organisation has been, it is necessary to find answers to at least two questions. First, who is asking the question, and second, what measure of effectiveness is most significant given the nature of the organisation, its environment and the concerns of the person asking the question? Who asks the question is clearly important because different constituents have different interests. For instance, while shareholders may be interested in dividends and regard these as the prime indicator of good performance, executives usually regard these as costs. Another example makes the same point: managers might see improved technology, restructuring and cost-cutting as evidence of improving organisational performance, while those employees made redundant because of such measures may be less convinced of their efficacy. So in discussing whether a particular organisation is performing well or not we must always recall whose perspective is being taken.

The answer to the second question very much depends on the answer given to the first, in that each stakeholder group will have its own set of preferences for measuring organisational effectiveness: for instance, shareholders (who may concentrate on dividends), managers (who might be more interested in profitability) or unions (whose focus could be on how many workers are employed). Nevertheless there are other considerations to be taken into account here. For example, if the organisation is a public body, such as the civil service, or a charity like Oxfam, the usual financial indicators will not be readily applicable. Alternatives can be found, though. In the case of charities, profit, turnover and market share might not be relevant, but the percentage of revenues spent on administration might be. There are, however, still more complexities here. Some commentators have argued that 'stability' and 'equilibrium' can be good indicators of organisational effectiveness. In the very long term or in the short term during periods of severe economic downturn survival may be thought of as a good criterion for effectiveness. Some sophisticated views on organisational effectiveness suggest that many of the normal financial measures of effectiveness can be misleading as they give little indication regarding how the organisation will perform in the future and may be the result of fortuitous circumstances rather than intrinsic features of the organisation itself. In a similar vein some commentators have made the point that an organisation's ability to extend its control over its environment may be a better criterion of effectiveness than traditional economic indicators.

The definitional complexities and ambiguities which affect our attempts to understand strategy and performance are a source of both difficulty and inspiration for us. They are a source of problems because different authors have defined these notions in different (and sometimes even contradictory) ways. This can often make it difficult to understand how the concepts of culture, strategy and performance relate to each other. Yet this vagueness and these uncertainties, which in part reflect how little is actually known in this field, are also a source of fascination. Certainly we must always be sure what we mean by these words every time we see them written or hear them used in conversation. But having realised that their meaning is not something cast in stone but open to interpretation opens up a whole new world of possibilities for understanding and for managing.

Culture and strategy formulation

An organisation's culture may well exert an influence over the strategies it pursues (Beach, 1993). Strategic analyses are never value free. Moreover people are often locked into traditional or habitual ways of doing and seeing things, and this undoubtedly affects their ability to contemplate new options and new solutions. For example, organisations typically exist in highly complex and dynamic environments in which trends (in competitive forces, technology, the labour market and so forth) are difficult to discern. Under these conditions selective perception can mean that organisations in the same market but with different cultural assumptions can interpret their environment significantly differently, giving rise to radically opposed strategies. Of two large clearing banks one might interpret the competitive environment as favourable to an expansion of its international division, while the other might decide on retrenchment. The decision regarding which strategy to follow will depend in part on what information has been selectively focused on, how this information has been interpreted, the values and assumptions of the organisation, and the power relationships between subcultures. The influence of culture on strategy is manifested in at least six distinct ways.

1   Strategy formulation is crucially dependent on an organisation's *scanning behaviour*, that is, how it gains information from the environment. Cultural assumptions which lead strategy formulators to believe that the environment is *uncertain* but *controllable* will tend to lead to time and resources being devoted to environmental scanning. Conversely, where an organisation's assumptions suggest to strategists that the environment is either stable and known or impervious to control, they may be less inclined to devote time and resources to scanning activities. According to Schneider (1989) environmental scanning may be conducted not just in an active or passive way, but across a broad or narrow range, and either more or less systematically. In each case the cultural assumptions of organisations are likely to be important influencers of the scanning behaviour adopted.

2   In the conduct of scanning procedures prevailing assumptions can act as perception filters which naturally focus attention on some information and away from other data items. Thus in scanning their environment and in assessing their own internal capabilities organisations collect some but not all of the available information. This *selective perception* of internal possibilities and external exigencies tends to lead an organisation to make particular strategic choices, namely, those which respond to what are for them the more salient facts and trends. For example, of two organisations in the same industry with a similar approach to scanning (say, active, broad and systematic), one may collect information on market opportunities in south-east Asia and the other may not. In such a case the scope for different strategies being formulated is obvious. A large number of further differences in the ways in which organisations undertake scanning are noticeable, many of which are linked to their assumptions regarding the nature of truth and reality. For instance, some organisations prefer statistical evidence and other quantitative measures because they believe that facts and figures are the best way of reducing their uncertainty about the environment. In contrast, other organisations (such as Sony and Honda) tend to rely on more qualitative information often gained by reading newspapers and popular magazines, which provide valuable information concerning socio-political issues. A third category of organisations rely not on information but on ideology. It is also worth noting that different organisations tend to value different

sources of information. Japanese organisations, for instance, place a far higher value on the personal and subjective opinions of specialists than do many Western organisations, which often show a preference for objective measures.

3   Once information has been collected it must be interpreted, and the methods of interpretation used by organisations will also vary according to the demands of culture. This is seen most clearly with regard to national cultural differences. For example, rational analytic modelling tools such as forecasting systems which rely on empirical evidence, hard facts and linear deductive reasoning are very popular in the West. Even within the Western world, however, considerable differences in approach are evident. Thus while the French are keen to apply Cartesian logic and engage in theoretical discussion of business issues, American organisations are generally more pragmatic and action-oriented. In marked contrast to both the French and the American orientations, Japanese companies like to rely on intuition and inductive incremental reasoning, and accuse the West of using techniques and models which naively simplify reality (Pascale, 1984).

4   Once information has been interpreted and cause–effect relationships agreed, an organisation has to decide how it is going to react, and this often involves an ethical component. Strategies are not formulated just with reference to logic and reason; issues of morality which touch on an organisation's dominant value set can also play a crucial role. For example, of two chemicals companies one may choose to pursue a strategy of maximising profit at the expense of some environmental damage, while the other might accept reduced profitability in order to avoid despoiling its local area. In both instances, strategic considerations have been influenced by their different cultural values, with the result that divergent strategic plans have been devised. Another example of moral issues playing a role in strategic decision making occurred at Volvo-Kalmar and Saab-Scania, where concern for the quality of employees' working lives (rather than efficiency or profit) led to the restructuring of assembly line and automobile assembly plants.

5   Agreement on how information is interpreted does not necessarily imply consensus on what strategy should be developed. Most commentators agree that there will be a tendency for managers to rely on those beliefs and assumptions that have served them well in the past, whether or not those beliefs and assumptions are now valid. For instance, in the 1970s a UK-based food manufacturer invested in several overseas operations which ultimately failed, giving rise to the view that its distinctive competence was restricted to the UK. For the next ten years the firm turned down every opportunity to extend its operations abroad, despite evidence that due to changing circumstances it could make considerable profits from a number of the ventures. Senior executives were unable to respond adequately to changing market conditions because of deeply held cultural convictions. Lorsch (1986) calls this phenomenon *strategic myopia*. Much business information is incomplete and ambiguous, and consequently provides great scope for different interpretations.

6   Issues of power are extremely important here, with different subcultures within an organisation tending to offer different solutions to agreed problems based on their own interests. Such conflicts can be still more intense and intractable when the subgroups define the problem in different terms using specialist vocabularies, or disagree concern-

ing the nature of the problem to be tackled as a result of selective perception and inter-pretation processes conditioned by their own subcultural assumptions. For instance, it is not unusual for production, R&D and marketing departments to offer radically opposed solutions to agreed problems based on their own expertise and desire for resources. In response to greater competition production departments often argue that output should be maximised, R&D departments that an attempt to differentiate products on the basis of technical expertise should be made, and marketing departments that customer-focused solutions are required. In such cases the strategy pursued may well depend on the power resources available to each subculture and the extent to which power is employed effec-tively by senior decision makers in each subcultural group.

This is a problem of *validation*, and it is most easily illustrated with reference to organi-sations in different national cultures. South-east Asian organisations tend to enshrine autocratic leadership principles, for example, and thus often rely on the boss to make a final decision concerning strategy. The situation is similar in France, with the added complication that bureaucratic rules (most usually written into operating manuals) are also sometimes significant. In many European organisations *historical precedent* (what has been done in the past) is generally a more important factor in strategy formulation than in the USA, where organisations are less constrained by tradition. Organisations around the world often strive for consensus in strategy formulation, though the form this consensus takes and the processes by which it is reached differ greatly between, for instance, the USA and Japanese firms (see, for example, the work of Maruyama, 1984).

From what we have learned about culture in the first five chapters of this book the powerful effect of cultural assumptions on strategy formulation will come as no sur-prise. A brief example illustrates the point. The recently appointed chairman of a large oil corporation sought to modernise his organisation by bringing in outside profes-sionals, investing in strategic planning, focusing on profit contribution rather than volume (as had previously been the norm), and diversifying outside the energy field. To the chairman his actions were not just rational and coherent but necessary to over-come the restrictions placed on strategic planning options by the firm's culture, but for many employees his acts were a violation of cherished beliefs. Needless to say, as soon as the chairman resigned the organisation's leadership group resorted to the old pat-terns of action that had served them and the company well in the past. Thus the strategy which was supposed to change the culture was itself modified to fit the pre-vailing culture (Schwartz and Davis, 1981).

This account of the influences of organisational culture on strategy formulation is less relevant to some public organisations, whose strategy is often determined (or at least influenced) by outside forces, namely Government policy. An account of how a Chinese organisation's strategy was influenced by both organisational culture and Government is provided by Mini Case 6.1.

IMPLEMENTING STRATEGY

There is a widely held view that organisational culture is the key to understanding why some firms succeed in implementing their strategies while others fail. For example, according to Lorsch (1986) all twelve of the successful companies he studied had a cul-

Mini Case 6.1

Strategy formulation at Regional Industrial Bank (RIB)

In 1990 RIB was a regional industrial bank situated in a relatively large province in south-eastern China. It employed approximately 400 people, 300 of whom were based in a headquarters in the provincial capital, and the rest of whom ran eight local branches distributed throughout the province. The RIB had originally belonged to one of the five Chinese national banks, and had previously operated as a regional development agency. In 1988, however, it was re-created as an independent entity, the staff were moved into more luxurious buildings, local people were encouraged to purchase shares in the bank, and the RIB opened amidst a blaze of publicity.

The mission of the RIB was to help develop the local industrial and commercial base of the province by providing low-interest loans to businesses and entrepreneurs. These loans were generally to enable private firms to purchase capital goods (such as new equipment and buildings) and retail outlets, or to set up distribution networks. Officially all requests for loans were evaluated against objective risk–return criteria and a final decision made on the merits of the application. Indeed, in keeping with the new spirit of *market socialism* the RIB was to be run as a commercial venture. In theory at least there was considerable scope for the bank to pursue any strategy it chose so long as it was commensurate with its twin goals of promoting economic development and satisfying its shareholders.

The reality of strategy formulation in RIB was, however, rather more intricate. Almost all the staff of the bank had been appointed by the Government, mostly from the more prestigious universities, and the overwhelming majority of senior managers were also Communist Party officials. What is more, a relatively small percentage of the bank's equity had actually been sold to the public, and the view was expressed that this was largely a symbolic act indicating that this sort of economic reform was now acceptable. The result was that while the day-to-day operations of the bank were under the direct control of senior managers, and the strategy pursued reflected their concerns, these were also the concerns of the Communist Party which exercised influence through them.

Strategy was then implemented in a top-down manner, with middle and junior ranking employees mostly unaware of what was going on in other departments within the organisation. Employee acquiescence can partly be explained by the fact that working for the RIB was considered to be a great privilege, which brought above-average accommodation with gas cookers (a great luxury), and decent wages. It should, though, also be recalled that while dismissals were rare (and difficult for senior managers to accomplish), once expelled there was little chance of ever finding another job. Strategy formulation and implementation at RIB appeared, therefore, to be a process uncomplicated by the need to be market-focused or customer-sensitive, and undisturbed by the need to develop new products, show a profit, or the threat of competition.

Questions

1 Do you think that there is any scope for a unique culture to develop at RIB and influence strategy? Why or why not?

2 What similarities between strategy formulation at RIB and Western public organisations are you able to discern?

ture which supported the strategy they pursued. According to this perspective, if we could only understand how to evaluate culture we would then be in a position to manage organisations through periods of strategic change. Culture, then, is both the means to effective organisational performance through the medium of strategy, and a potential barrier inhibiting required strategic realignment which can adversely affect strategy implementation. The conclusion drawn has often been that: 'If the culture is not fully synchronized and consonant with the favoured strategy, then cultural resistance to change has to be eliminated' (Green, 1988: 7).

The idea that even cultures which have been associated with success can become serious obstacles to continued good performance is often illustrated with reference to the case of American Telephone and Telegraph (AT&T). In 1978 the chairman, J. D. deButts announced that AT&T was making a significant strategic shift from a service-oriented telephone utility to a market-oriented communications business. Then in late 1981 and early 1982 the US Government passed legislation which effectively broke up the company into independent regional concerns. In the view of commentators both within and external to AT&T the biggest challenge was to alter employees' beliefs, values, behaviours and assumptions in order to accommodate the new commercial reality, a challenge that is still being undertaken (Tunstall, 1983). The case of AT&T aptly demonstrates that strategy implementation is an administrative process rooted in people, and that even the most brilliant strategy is worse than useless if it is not socially accepted and so cannot be implemented. A more detailed example of how a prevailing culture can interfere with strategy implementation is provided by Mini Case 6.2.

Assessing cultural risk

Organisations such as Smith Electronics and AT&T illustrate that while culture exerts an influence over both strategy formulation and strategy implementation, there is nevertheless scope for organisations to develop strategies which are incompatible with their cultures. In fact, a certain degree of cultural risk is associated with any organisational strategy, and the implementation plans involved in pursuing it. Schwartz and Davis (1981) have suggested that the level of cultural risk implied by a given strategy can be evaluated using a simple graph (see Fig. 6.1). The graph has two dimensions: importance to strategy and level of culture compatibility, both of which are divided into three (high, medium, low) categories. The result is a figure which depicts three levels of risk, namely, unacceptable, manageable and negligible. Use of the tool is relatively straightforward.

Importance to strategy	Level of culture compatibility		
	High	Medium	Low
High	Manageable risk	Unacceptable risk	Unacceptable risk
Medium	Negligible risk	Manageable risk	Unacceptable risk
Low	Negligible risk	Negligible risk	Manageable risk

Fig. 6.1 Assessing cultural risk
Source: adapted from Schwartz and Davis (1981)

Culture, strategy and innovation at Smith Electronics

Smith Electronics was set up by Mr John Smith in 1950, and by 1985 had grown to employ 300 people in three major divisions, and turn over $30 million a year. Until the mid-1970s Mr Smith, who was chairman of the board, retained direct control of product innovation. At this time he realised that the complexity and size of the organisation made delegating control of the company to his top management necessary. This was part of a strategy designed to realise ambitious growth and profit targets. However, within a few years it was obvious that the cultural influences which dominated the firm were undercutting the organisation's ability to cope with the strategy of decentralisation.

From 1950 to the late 1970s the number of people working for Smith Electronics was small enough for everyone to know Mr Smith personally, and he dominated the dynamics of the organisation. He was a dedicated employer who provided not just job security, but a pension plan and various recognition schemes including 'employee appreciation days'. In return employees not only trusted and felt affection for Mr Smith, but in 1964 had even lent him money to help him retain control of the company. Mr Smith's authority was unquestioned, and his comments, criticisms and jokes were carefully analysed by his subordinates for clues regarding his preferences for what they should do. The cultural milieu that evolved thus encouraged employees to be sensitive to, and to follow, Mr Smith's lead.

Two of Smith's central concerns (which were also explicit company goals) were product quality and customer service. In the context of Smith Electronics the result was an internal focus on product engineering at the expense of an external focus on market dynamics and customer needs. Part of the reason for failing to develop a marketing orientation was that the senior management team had a strong engineering background and lacked the requisite skills and knowledge. A complementary reason was that the ideals of product quality and customer service were defined technologically (i.e. as technological problems) by senior managers, while marketing perspectives on these issues were ignored. Culture thus undermined strategy.

The internal focus of Smith and his management team together with certain elements of Smith's personality led to seven further strategy-related problems:

1 The internal focus led to the development of a conservative, risk-avoiding decision-making style that precluded fast growth of the organisation.

2 Customer needs were not systematically identified because most managers thought of customers only as users of Smith technology (rather than entities with highly individual requirements), while the marketing managers, who did appreciate customers, were not taken seriously because they did not understand the technology.

3 The objective of improving the quantity and quality of innovations (new product developments) was undermined by Smith's inability to deal with creative, self-confident managers, who, faced with the stifling culture of the organisation and the anxieties of Smith himself, tended not to stay with the company.

4 Smith was uncomfortable dealing with difficult matters like firings, which he delegated to the personnel department. The result was that Smith institutionalised an emotional buffer between himself and his organisation which in turn led to problems of jealousy, conflict, communication and alienation.

5 Smith tended not to listen to 'insiders', and had an extraordinary faith in consultants, hiring everyone from technologists to psychologists, labour relations experts, marketing specialists, accountants, strategic planners and general management consultants.

6   Smith was not in business primarily to make money, but to build an organisation that would bring him recognition from society. For example, when asked whether he would prefer to run a $70 million company with $5 million in profits or a $160 million company with no profits, Smith chose the latter, a choice his subordinates interpreted as his wish for more visibility and recognition as a leading industrialist.

7   The way the strategic management process was carried out at Smith Electronics led to the establishment of a culture riddled with internal contradictions. On the one hand Smith himself was a self-confident, strong-willed entrepreneur who set ambitious goals for the company. However, because he did not show confidence in his employees' judgements or tolerate ambitious, self-confident managers, his staff felt neglected, lacked confidence and relied heavily on the opinions of consultants. The result was a senior management team unable to create and implement the sort of strategy required to fulfil Smith's growth and profit objectives.

Further problems derived from the fact that Smith did not look at customers and competitors as a source of money and competition so much as a source of recognition. For instance, on learning that his salesmen were telling customers that a competitor was going out of business Smith demanded that they thenceforward stop talking about the competition, and ordered his sales manager to call the competitor and apologise. Needless to say, the salespeople, who knew their tactics to be used by many other firms in the industry, regarded this action as exaggerated and inappropriate.

To conclude, the innovation that Smith wanted to occur in his organisation was effectively precluded by the culture that he had himself evolved. By the mid-1980s the company was dominated by employees who wanted to please either Smith or themselves rather than pursue a new strategic direction. As Feldman noted: 'there was no one left with the passion and determination to set up their own sub-organisation, fight off innovation-stifling organisational procedures and preferences, and concentrate on doing something new'.

Questions

1   Describe the culture which predominates at Smith Electronics.

2   How is the culture at Smith Electronics influencing the organisation's ability to implement strategy?

3   What should Smith do to solve the problems his organisation is experiencing?

4   What learning points are there here for other organisations facing difficulties relating to strategy implementation?

Importance to strategy

First, the importance of each individual objective of the strategy must be evaluated in terms of its importance to the overall strategy. The authors suggest that two key question areas are explored when attempting to make this assessment: (1) What specific behaviour is the objective designed to encourage, and how will it affect management tasks and relationships? (2) How is this behaviour linked to critical success factors (for example, as regards customer needs, costs, the unions, etc.)?

Level of culture compatibility

Second, the compatibility of elements of the strategy with the prevailing culture must be determined. In order to accomplish this assessment the authors recommend the use of questions such as: How much change is involved in key tasks and relationships? How adaptable is the culture? How skilled is the management?

In addition to providing a means of understanding something of the relationship between strategy and culture the model also implicitly suggests two courses of action to strategists keen to minimise risk. On the one hand, attempts should be made to make implementation plans compatible with the culture, and on the other, any scope for reducing the strategic significance of the new behaviours sought should be taken advantage of. Depending on a variety of contextual variables some options available to the strategist include:

1   *Ignoring the culture* This is not usually a viable alternative, except where the organisation is relatively young and has not yet developed a strong sense of identity or has suffered a major haemorrhage of employees.

2   *Managing around the culture by changing the implementation plans* If the strategy is vital to the success of an organisation but its culture cannot accommodate the implementation plans designed to realise it, then there is a good case for managing around the culture. For example, Schwartz and Davis cite the instance of an organisation that needs to focus its marketing on the most profitable market segments. While the most obvious means of pursuing the strategy involves developing a reward system which encourages such behaviour and adjustment of the management information systems, cultural barriers in the form of diffused power, highly individualised operations and a relationship-oriented ethos preclude these measures. However, by dedicating full-time personnel to each key market the organisation can bypass cultural constraints and maintain its strategic intent.

3   *Modifying the culture to fit the strategy* This is an extremely difficult, time-consuming, expensive and uncertain option. For further information refer to Chapter 5.

4   *Adapting the strategy to fit the culture* This needs to occur in certain situations, notably after a merger, when particularly complex and involved cultural situations are likely to emerge. A strategy suffering greatly from cultural blocks and pressures may require that other action be taken, including managing around the culture in order to bring cultural risk into the manageable zone (see Fig. 6.1).

So far we have considered the relatively simple case of a single business unit. In reality, though, executives managing large corporations will need to assess cultural risk throughout a portfolio of businesses, each with its own strategy, culture and implementation plans. Such executives require answers to questions such as:

- how much cultural risk is there in the corporation as a whole, including all the subsidiaries?
- how is this risk spread across the businesses?
- what are the specific sources of cultural risk? Are there any detectable patterns of risk in the business portfolio?
- given the level of risk identified is the total corporate strategy in danger?

In order to answer these (and related) questions strategists can apply the Fig. 6.1 framework across the corporation.

Quality at CSL

Communication Systems Limited (CSL) is a wholly owned subsidiary of Siemens and GEC, both of which have a 50 per cent stake in the company's equity. CSL is primarily concerned with selling, installing and maintaining business telephone communication solutions in the UK, and in order to maintain its customer base effectively, employs approximately 1500 people on 11 sites. From 1987 onwards CSL became interested in the idea of quality as a means of competing in an increasingly hostile global market. A focus on overall quality was recognised by CSL management as a potential solution to the problem the organisation faced of distinguishing itself from competitors selling essentially similar products.[1] As the senior executives at CSL saw it, differentiating on the basis of quality was a means to an end: better-quality products and services meant more satisfied customers, and happier customers meant an increase in market share and profitability.

The first step towards creating a quality-oriented culture was, from July 1992, to embark on the process of becoming BS 5750[2] accredited. While still not widely recognised in other parts of the world, BS 5750 is a well-known and highly regarded UK quality specification that encourages organisations to formally define procedures, create job descriptions, and invent formal systems for dealing with work activities in a rational and coherent manner. In order to facilitate the acceptance of the new quality standards the quality programme director at CSL customised them to suit the organisation's culture and work patterns. As the quality director said, 'we put it into more friendly terms, made it more meaningful for our people'. Such was the success of the programme of change that 15 months later the firm attained accreditation to BS 5750, and so became only the twelfth company to gain the standard across the whole organisation.

Crucial to the success of the enterprise was the support of the managing director, who not only had a good knowledge of the quality programme but visibly demonstrated his commitment to it by visiting customers on a regular basis and chairing a monthly 'quality council' meeting in which he probed senior managers for detailed information regarding issues of quality and customer satisfaction. The quality programme director himself was another key player, who was expected not just to regularly update other members of the organisation concerning progress towards agreed quality and service targets, but also to visit customers and suppliers and to foster long-term partnerships with CSL. In this way it was hoped to mirror the success some Japanese corporations have had in forming close alliances with main suppliers and important customers, and involve them in the process of quality improvement and service enhancement. A visible demonstration of CSL's commitment to the ideal is its decision to base engineers on the sites of some big clients, such as IBM and BP: now, if there is a problem, CSL can offer these corporations an immediate solution.

The attempt to create a quality culture did not always run smoothly. There was some initial resistance to the burden of documenting systems and formalising procedures needed to achieve BS 5750, and building the internal partnership relations within CSL that are required to make it work. Such were the advantages which emerged, however, and the determination of the managing director and quality programme director, that resistance to the programme quickly withered. The change in the relations between marketing and sales amply demonstrates the kind of practical benefit which emerged from this process. Before BS 5750, marketing had always considered itself exploited and made a scapegoat by other departments, especially sales, which landed all sorts of product-related problems at the marketing door. Sales, on the other hand, thought that marketing did very little and was poor value for money. But with the introduction of the quality specifications both sides had to come together to agree what they wanted from each other, to allocate duties and responsibilities, and define these in written documents. With the sorting out of all

▶

the old grey areas around which disputes used to emerge a more professional working relationship has evolved in which marketing receive adequate information from sales and know what is expected of them, while sales can now see clear deliverables emanating from marketing. Thus greater formalisation has resulted in a general reduction in interpersonal and interdepartmental conflict and a greater willingness to work collaboratively to solve mutual problems.

The pursuit of quality and the alteration of employees' beliefs, values and assumptions in order to support this strategic pattern is, of course, an ongoing process. Moreover the quality system needs to be kept under regular review to ensure that it continues to be appropriate and to be followed. There are, therefore, continual reviews of procedures and periodic assessments of what is being achieved. These internal assessments are engaged in at two levels. First, each department conducts a self-appraisal on an annual basis using a checklist of questions covering all aspects of quality and work activities. Second, there is regular peer appraisal, in which managers (and more junior employees) from other departments audit the quality of a department other than their own. The quality consequences have been dramatic: for example, customer complaints are now answered within a matter of a few hours and have shown a hefty reduction in volume. Certainly there are still problems. For instance, no one has yet figured out how adequately to predict lightning strikes, one of the main causes of maintenance backlogs. Terrorist attacks on London's financial centre also initially caused a few headaches, as finance organisations often need a lot of telecommunications equipment (and they need it immediately) once their offices are destroyed. CSL overcame the problem of the huge costs of storing spare equipment by developing a Disaster Recovery contract (a form of insurance for financial organisations under threat), thus tackling a thorny problem with an imaginative customer-focused solution.

With the reduction in conflict, mutual blame and finger-pointing has come the opportunity to enhance quality still further. Despite obvious advantages BS 5750 is not a perfect measure of quality, being far more concerned with formal systems than intangibles like leadership, human resources and culture. Significant improvements in quality, then, were going to require the pursuit of a more subtle strategy. To ensure that the company was 'doing the right things' as judged by the customer as well as 'doing things right', an additional strategy was required. A little over a year ago CSL management adopted the 'Baldrige Award' criteria.[3] With IBM, one of CSL's biggest customers, also pursuing this quality award, it is little wonder that CSL are in the vanguard of GEC/Siemens's quality accreditation efforts. Under the generic name of *Market Driven Quality* a new phase in the quality journey has been announced, with Areas For Improvement (AFIs) now routinely identified and neutralised by senior management on a six-monthly cycle. This is currently being cascaded downwards to involve the whole organisation. While full accreditation to Baldrige is recognised to be some years away, there is now a confidence about CSL that the cultural shift required will ultimately be achieved.

Questions

1 What do you think is meant by phrases such as 'a quality strategy' and 'a quality culture'?

2 What are the keys being used by CSL in its pursuit of a quality strategy and its attempts to create a quality culture?

3 What else could CSL be doing to create a culture of high reliability as advocated by Weick?

4 Are there limits on the extent to which CSL will be able to use its culture to foster high reliability?

Notes

1 In fact, CSL was formed in 1991, and it was the antecedents of CSL that first flirted with quality in the late 1980s.

2 This quality standard has now been superseded by BS EN ISO 9001 or 9002.

3 The Baldrige Award is an American quality award.

Source: compiled from information supplied by Ralph Morris, Quality Programme Director, CSL

Realising strategic intent

In order to be effective, organisation strategies require the participation not just of the senior executive team, but of the organisation as a whole. For example, Xerox's pursuit of total quality necessitates that all organisational members adopt standardised procedures and a *quality mentality*. Without this organisation-wide embracing of a quality orientation the pursuit of a quality-led strategy in which things are done right first time would be impossible. The same is true at CSL (see Mini Case 6.3). The realisation of such a strategy will be more likely where the cultural inclinations of the organisation support it. As a matter of fact most organisational attempts to emphasise quality are normally represented as a form of culture change, blurring the distinction between strategic intent and culture. The important point being made here should, however, be clear: an organisation's culture can be a useful source of high reliability in the pursuit and realisation of strategy.

Weick (1987) has argued that the significance of culture as a source of high reliability is seen most clearly in those organisations which cannot afford to make mistakes, such as NASA and nuclear power plants. In these sorts of organisations technology has become increasingly complex to the point where the humans who operate and manage it are not sufficiently complex themselves to sense and anticipate the problems generated by the technological systems. Accordingly, it is suggested that if humans can be made more complex, then disasters such as Bhopal, the Challenger and Three Mile Island will be less frequent. While individuals can be brought to a higher level of sophistication through training and education, the complexity of the social system itself is a further potential source of solutions, and thus reliability. The suggestion that Weick makes is that a homogeneous culture can impose order on a social situation in much the same way that rules and operating procedures do, but that culture also provides scope for interpretation, improvisation and unique action based on shared beliefs, values and assumptions. Furthermore, culture co-ordinates action through vicarious experiences expressed in the form of stories and other symbolic representations of technology, and its effects can be a valuable reservoir of knowledge for participants in the culture. In other words, a culture which values stories, story tellers and story telling will be more reliable than an organisation that does not. In Weick's terms:

> A system that values stories and story telling is potentially more reliable because people know more about their system, know more of the potential errors that might occur, and are more confident that they can handle those errors that do occur because they know that other people have already handled similar errors. (Weick, 1987: 113)

MERGERS, ACQUISITION AND CULTURE

While merger and acquisition activity once used to be conducted with little regard to the human consequences, this blinkered strategic approach is no longer tenable. Too many mergers have been attempted on the basis of what looked to be good strategic and financial arguments only to founder on the rock of cultural resistance. Where two organisations with very different cultures seek to merge there can be extreme problems of integration, co-ordination and control which in turn often lead to a lower level of post-merger performance (Marks and Mirvis, 1986; Mirvis and Marks, 1985a, b). This failure to take culture adequately into account can mean that 'synergy' is a strictly pre-merger concept (Denison, 1990). One company that has made a large number of successful acquisitions, and which attributes this in part to its careful consideration of cultural fit, is the Dana Corporation, based in Toledo, Ohio. According to Dana's philosophy, firms should not only be prepared to walk away from potential acquisitions which do not fit their culture, but having acquired a company should honour its traditions and heritage (Sathe, 1985a, b). An example of the sorts of culture-related problems that can emerge post-merger is illustrated with reference to the Acme Advertising Agency (AAA) and Equatorial Advertising Agency (EAA) described in Mini Case 6.4.

UNDERSTANDING CULTURE AND STRATEGY

The Miles and Snow typology

As long ago as 1978 Miles and Snow suggested that the strategy of an organisation tended to reflect the dominant managerial ideology or culture. Their finding, that organisational strategy may be as much (or more) influenced by internal factors as the nature of the environment, has fed interest in organisational culture *per se*. They identified three basic types of organisation distinguished according to prevailing culture and strategic pattern: *defenders, prospectors* and *analysers*. The Miles and Snow typology is summarised in Exhibit 6.1. Their conclusions once again illustrate the intimacy of the relationship between culture and strategy, and make it clear that the managerial culture of an organisation is 'likely to be the product of past strategy, a moderator of current strategy and a determinant of future strategy' (Williams *et al.*, 1993: 34–5)

Exhibit 6.1
Organisational culture and strategy: the Miles and Snow typology

	Culture/strategic type		
	Defender	Prospector	Analyser
Environment	Stable	Dynamic growing	Moderately changing
Strategy	Specialisation, cost efficiency	Growth	Steady growth
Objectives	Secure the market	Seek new opportunities	Expand and protect
Systems	Centralised, emphasises efficiency	Decentralised, flexible, *ad hoc*	Mixed, co-ordinates, loose–tight

Source: derived from original material by Miles and Snow (1978)

The Acme and Equatorial advertising agencies: a clash of cultures

Introduction

The Acme and Equatorial advertising agencies (henceforward referred to as AAA and EAA) were both based in Singapore. AAA was a relatively small branch of a large international ad agency which employed about 1000 people worldwide. AAA had 35 employees, turned over approximately 15 million Singapore dollars, and always returned healthy year-end profits. EAA was half the size of AAA and an independent organisation. The two organisations were dominated by ethnic Chinese, though some Malays and Indians were also employed. Within AAA and EAA English was the main medium of written communication, though in conversation Mandarin, Cantonese, Malay, and Hokkien were also spoken. Having staff who were fluent in the four official languages of Singapore (English, Mandarin, Malay and Tamil) was an advantage, as many Government publications had to be produced in all four languages.

Both companies had to survive in an extremely tough and competitive market where the poaching of staff and lucrative accounts (by both fair means and foul) was commonplace. While the market was expanding, so was the number of small ad agencies. Further, the market was a heavily regulated one, with strict censorship laws, a total ban on cigarette advertising, and intimidating consumer protection legislation. As all the TV and radio stations and the newspapers came under the influence of the Government, so these laws were strictly enforced. It was in this climate, in the late 1980s, that the possibility of a merger was voiced.

The merger

The managing director of AAA, who was the only Asian MD in the worldwide company's network, clashed with a new regional MD based in Hong Kong. As a result he decided to leave AAA and join EAA taking two-thirds of its staff with him, including many of his senior as well as some more junior colleagues. While not a merger in the

legal sense of the term, this move nevertheless represented a *de facto* merger of the two organisations. In the end 20 AAA people joined forces with EAA, the idea of senior executives being to fully integrate the two sets of employees. In addition to some talented staff, EAA also gained a large number of highly profitable accounts which the MD of AAA had cultivated over a number of years. Furthermore, both AAA and EAA staff were used to handling very similar types of work, were typically used to a fairly autocratic regime, embraced the Singaporean ideal of promotion based on merit, and were used to working a 10–12 hour day. As a result of these synergies and compatibilities the future of EAA as a significant force in the Singaporean advertising market seemed assured.

It was not long, however, before problems emerged. Despite attempts to integrate the old AAA staff and the existing EAA staff along functional lines, they in fact formed two quite separate cliques. For the first six months a noticeable 'them and us' mentality pervaded the organisation to such an extent that the quality of the organisation's work was affected. Focusing on the ex-AAA staff it was evident that they were generally older, better qualified, and more willing to accept the authority of senior managers than the pre-existing staff of EAA. The staff of EAA were not just younger (the average age was only 25), but more energetic, vociferous and rebellious. They were by and large a highly cohesive group who regularly socialised together. However, their loyalty to the organisation was more questionable, many were individualistic and ambitious, and possibly as a result of this they thrived in an organisation where politics and personal antagonisms dominated working life.

The ex-AAA staff had not just entered EAA, they had also taken on some senior roles in Accounts Service, and the Creative and Media departments. The existing EAA staff were obviously alarmed by the sudden increase in the

▶

number of managers that effectively demoted some, and made advancement for them all more difficult. In the status-conscious world of Singaporean ad agencies this was a cause of serious frustration. To make matters worse the newcomers had brought with them their own rules, procedures, and even some forms which they insisted that everyone use. The EAA staff naturally already had well-developed systems of their own, and felt that the newcomers should comply with existing regulations and ways of doing things. While it is not part of the Asian tradition to air grievances in public, tensions were evident. Where conflicts that could not be contained did occur, it was normal to refer these up to the departmental heads for their views.

Consolidation of EAA culture

Recognising that there were problems, the senior executives organised a weekend-long 'company retreat' featuring a series of team-building and training exercises. During this time senior managers regaled their employees with the message that they were 'one company now'. They also decided to try to break down the cohesiveness of the original EAA staff by promoting one of them to a more senior level within the Creative department. However, what was supposed to be a symbol of the organisation's willingness to promote talented staff and upset the dynamics of the clique had limited effect. The retreat too was only partially successful, and the internal problems only really came to an end more than 12 months later, by which time the dozen most resistant EAA staff had left, and newcomers to the business, who had no shared history in the merger, had joined. Thus in the end, it was the high staff turnover of EAA (rather than attempts at organisation development) which resolved the tensions between the two cultures and allowed a consolidated EAA culture to develop.

Questions

1 Why was there a clash of cultures between AAA and EAA staff?

2 What steps could senior executives have taken before the merger in order to ensure that the organisation ran more smoothly post-merger?

3 Once culture-related problems had emerged, could senior executives have done anything that would have been more successful than the weekend retreat, or did they just have to wait for staff turnover to have its effect?

Strategy as cultural artefact

As we saw in Chapter 1 artefacts are the products of human action, and are visible expressions of a culture. Such artefacts often have symbolic value. That is, they have extra meaning for organisational participants over and above their normal associations. While the traditional view holds that strategy is little more than an economic means of matching internal resources to meet environmental opportunities and threats, from a cultural perspective such a characterisation is massively incomplete. Strategy can in fact be thought of as a cultural artefact, and within an organisation any given strategy is likely to have symbolic associations for employees. Some of the many functions that strategy plays in its role as artefact and symbol include the following.

1 *A focus for organisational and individual self-understanding* It allows individuals to formulate answers to questions such as 'Where is the organisation going?', 'How is it going to get there?' and 'What is my role in the life of the organisation?'

2 *A focus for identification, loyalty, and motivation* It provides individuals with goals and longer-term objectives with which they are able to identify and value, and in the pursuit of which they are prepared to exchange energy and enthusiasm for material gains.

3 *A means for comprehending social phenomena* An organisation's strategy is often encoded in various written statements and reports and plays a key role in general conversation between employees. From these sources individuals gain the information they require to understand and classify people, businesses, markets and events. It provides a context and a vocabulary for understanding the past and making guesses about the future state of the organisation and its markets. Indeed, it has been argued that the creation of such knowledge, understanding and faith through the strategic management process transforms strategy from a sophisticated economic plan into a potent social symbol signifying change (Green, 1988).

Final thoughts

While it is tempting to think of strategy as a dependent variable determined and constrained by the culture in which it develops, such a view is not sustainable. Strategy does not merely reflect or externalise culture, but influences and modifies it. An organisation's strategy makes visible its culture, expressing it in much the same way that speech creates meanings from language (Green, 1988). This is an important point.

It is vital to remember that organisational strategy is not just a reflection of organisational culture. The formulation and implementation of strategy is generally influenced by a wide variety of non-cultural environmental factors such as the activities of competitors, customers and suppliers. Certainly the resulting trends, activities and events will be interpreted through the perception filter of culture, but this fact does not make a new technological breakthrough or a reduction in the number of supplier companies any less real. This means that it is impossible to accurately predict an organisation's strategy from knowledge of its culture alone. It also means that when we observe an organisation it is possible for its strategy to appear not to match its culture because of the influence of external exigencies. For example, Hewlett Packard was effectively forced to follow the IBM standard when manufacturing personal computers, even though its natural cultural inclination was to create its own specification: to have done anything else was to have risked disaster. If it is true that as a general rule strategy gives voice to a culture, then in analysing the relationship between any particular culture and strategy we should expect to find a number of coughs, splutters and hiccups that distort the pattern.

Given the commercial importance of understanding the links between culture and strategy, many commentators have chosen to offer their advice to executives. This advice usually takes the form of imperatives to conduct culture audits in order to render the dominant beliefs and values visible. In this way it is suggested that the restrictions that culture places on strategy formulation and implementation can be overcome. Another popular recommendation is to build flexibility and adaptability into the organisation, perhaps by appointing managers without portfolio, by involving outside directors, and bringing in new managers from outside the business, all of whom can challenge beliefs and question ideas. Just how valuable such advice is, is questionable. The most obvious problem is that senior executives, imprisoned by their basic assumptions that have evolved over the years, are likely to find it extremely unpalatable to follow. The most likely scenario is that only those managers already convinced that culture can be a source of disadvantage, and that they personally have a lot to learn, will take much notice of these academics and consultants.

CULTURE AND PERFORMANCE

While a large number of authors have addressed this topic, little rigorous research has actually been undertaken. Indeed, most of the evidence which suggests a link between organisational culture and organisational performance consists of stories and anecdotes. Very few studies start by outlining a theory of culture and then 'test' it by applying it to successful and unsuccessful organisations to see if it is in fact applicable. A notable example of the less than convincing approach is Peters and Waterman's (1982) *In Search of Excellence*, which attempted to identify the factors that made firms successful: within a very short space of time it has become apparent that there are many firms which possess these characteristics but which do not perform well (*Business Week*, 1984). Two recent books that do attempt to address this crucial issue in a rational and coherent manner are *Corporate Culture and Organisational Effectiveness* by Denison (1990) and *Corporate Culture and Performance* by Kotter and Heskett (1992). Much of the rest of this chapter will be taken up by a consideration of the findings of these two works, and some influential papers by Gordon (1985), Barney (1986) and Saffold (1988). It is noticeable that by 'performance' is generally meant 'economic performance', and given the scarcity of data concerning other indicators of effectiveness, unless otherwise stated it is high and low economic performance which is referred to in the following sections. One point that needs to be made explicit at the outset is that under certain conditions an organisation can prosper despite, not because of, its culture, and that therefore there is no simple correlation between the sorts of culture that promote success and success (however this is defined) itself (see Mini Case 6.5).

From his detailed quantitative and qualitative research studies Denison (1990) has suggested that there are four different aspects of an organisation's culture that have an impact on organisational effectiveness. He discusses these aspects in the form of four *hypotheses*, which he labels *involvement*, *consistency*, *adaptability* and *mission*. These four hypotheses conjointly implicate those cultural variables that, according to Denison's research, influence an organisation's performance. Kotter and Heskett's (1992) work builds on the ideas of Denison, and the findings of the two books are strikingly similar. Kotter and Heskett argue that performance-enhancing organisational cultures are those that have many shared values and practices, are able to adapt to change, are strategically appropriate, and which value both large stakeholders and effective leadership at all levels. Let us examine these findings in more detail.

Culture strength and performance

One of the most widely cited hypotheses is that a strong culture enables an organisation to achieve excellent performance. Deal and Kennedy (1982: 15), for example, have argued that: 'The impact of a strong culture on productivity is amazing. In the extreme, we estimate that a company can gain as much as one or two hours of productive work per employee per day.' 'Strong' is usually used as a synonym for consistency. Thus the phrase 'strong culture' is frequently employed to refer to companies in which beliefs and values are shared relatively consistently throughout an organisation. Such strong culture firms are also often identified as possessing (or having possessed in the past) an exceptionally gifted and charismatic leader. Examples of organisations generally recognised as having strong cultures include Tandem Computers and IBM. Precisely how a strong culture leads to exceptional performance is not always spelled out by commentators, but three key arguments are discernible here.

1   A strong organisational culture facilitates goal alignment. The idea is that because all employees share the same basic assumptions they can agree not just on what goals to pursue but also on the means by which they should be achieved. As a result employee initiative, energy and enthusiasm are all channelled in the same direction. In these organisations there are few problems of co-ordination and control, communication is quick and effective, and resources are not wasted in internal conflicts. This all means that organisational performance is likely to be healthy.

2   A strong culture leads to high levels of employee motivation. There are two main arguments here. First, it has been suggested that there is something intrinsically appealing about strong cultures that encourage people to identify with them – in short, that employees like to be part of an organisation with a distinctive style and ethos with its own peculiarities and idiosyncrasies, and with others who share their view on how an organisation should work. Second, it is sometimes thought that strong culture organisations incorporate practices which make working for them rewarding. These practices tend to include employee participation in decision making and various recognition schemes. High levels of motivation among employees, so the argument states, translate into high organisational performance.

3   A strong culture is better able to learn from its past. The idea is that strong cultures characteristically possess agreed norms of behaviour, integrative rituals and ceremonies, and well-known stories. These reinforce consensus on the interpretation of issues and events based on past experience, provide precedents from the organisation's history which help decide how to meet new challenges, and promote self-understanding and social cohesion through shared knowledge of the past (see Chapter 1). The suggestion here is that an organisation which is able to reflect on its development and which is able to draw on a stock of knowledge encoded in stories, rules of thumb and general heuristics is likely to perform better than competitors unable to learn from their past successes and failures.

The first two of Denison's hypotheses elaborate the strong culture thesis further, and merit close attention.

The involvement hypothesis

This states that organisational effectiveness is a function of the level of involvement and participation of an organisation's members. The involvement may be either informal and spontaneous or formally structured and planned as in the case of *ad hoc* task teams, cross-functional product teams and quality circles. According to Denison both voluntary, bottom-up involvement and structured approaches for achieving involvement have a positive impact on effectiveness. The argument here is that high levels of involvement and participation create a sense of ownership and responsibility. The result is greater employee commitment to the organisation, reducing the need for formal systems of control, and leading to performance enhancement.

Culture and performance at National Petroleum Company (NPC)

National Petroleum Company (NPC) was a state-owned, Middle Eastern oil company. It employed approximately 8000 people to service three oil refineries, a gas treatment plant, a fleet of tankers, its international export dealings, and a chain of domestic petrol stations. NPC's culture and working practices were highly distinctive, fed as they were by its multiracial workforce and, most importantly, the laws and traditions of the Arab country which was its host and owner.

NPC was a highly stratified and hierarchical organisation. At least four distinct 'classes' of employee could be distinguished. The most privileged of these were the Americans. The approximately 80 American employees were not only the highest earners (from $100 000 to $200 000 per annum), but also enjoyed the most luxurious life styles: superb villas with their own swimming pools, servants, chauffeur-driven cars, and every conceivable benefit an organisation could provide. Second in status were the Europeans, of which there were approximately 700. These were mostly British nationals, though there were also people from Italy, Canada, Australia and France. This strata of employee were also provided with free housing (though not up to the standard of the Americans), tax-free incomes up to $100 000, and a range of fringe benefits. Third in terms of pay and benefits came the locals, which were about as numerous as the Europeans. These people were often either wealthy or from wealthy families. Interestingly, their salaries were typically low (under $20 000), and they were not provided with free housing. Finally, there were the Third Country Nationals (TCNs), of whom 2000 were Asian (from Sri Lanka, India and Pakistan) and the rest Arabs from neighbouring and nearby countries. While a few of these had managed to attain the status of the Europeans, most of them were employed as secretaries, clerks and labourers, and paid only $1000 a year: it should, however, be noted that these sums were often very substantial by their own national standards.

NPC was, thus, extremely culturally diverse. These racial and cultural divisions found their most obvious expression in linguistic and religious divides. The dominant religion was naturally Islam, with Christians considered as being 'of the book' and so acceptable, and Sikhs the least well regarded of all. As English was the general language of business but Arabic was the language of the host country, all documents had to be prepared in both languages. As a result, agreeing the precise phraseology of contracts could be a long and tortuous affair, with various people noted for their linguistic ability being asked to scrutinise them clause by clause to ensure that the two versions effectively meant the same thing. So heterogeneous was the workforce that employees considered their only bond to be their mutual desire for money. As people were working purely for financial gain, so they were prepared to put up with racism, affronts to dignity, and other little insults from arrogant bosses.

The working day at NPC started at 8.00 a.m. and finished at 2.00 p.m. During this time work was punctuated by two prayer sessions, both of which generally lasted between 20 and 25 minutes. Although the offices were not open-plan, they were always open, closed doors being taboo: this was arguably a reflection of the Islamic notion that everyone is equal in God's eyes. The offices themselves were well furnished with couches and other comfortable chairs in order to facilitate 'diwanna', that is, social/business gatherings of men. Diwannas were the mainstay of working life at NPC, with people dropping in and out of each other's offices drinking coffee and engaging in loosely work-related conversation. During these meetings employees 'peddled in wasta' (influence), the outcomes of which determined everything from minor interpretations of rules to company strategy. In these meetings the locals held the upper hand, and the foreign workers relied on their assistants (who were often of local origin) to get things done and explain what decisions had been taken.

The general attitude of the locals was relaxed, and the foreign workers soon learned that in order to survive you had to 'play the culture', not fight against it. During Ramadan, a month-long Islamic religious festival during which believers were forbidden to eat from dawn to dusk, the pace of work dropped still further, with the working hours limited to 9.00 a.m. until 12.00 p.m. The summer months were also a quiet time, with many of the rich locals leaving for holidays in Europe, and a strict labour law (which proscribed labouring work if the temperature rose above 120°F) frequently resulting in the workforce being sent home. These casual attitudes towards work were matched by a highly intricate and bureaucratic system of control, 'invented by the British and run by Egyptians', which required between 10 and 15 signatures in order to sanction the most minor activities.

This male-dominated (the only women employed were secretaries), status-conscious and tension-ridden organisation was, nevertheless, highly economically successful. People were content to conform as required and put up with their lot because of the phenomenal financial advantages of working for NPC. Damaging internal conflicts between Sunni and Shiite Muslims, and between Muslims, Christians and Sikhs were effectively bought off with money. Thus no one talked politics and overt attacks on people's religious beliefs were rare. Everyone was intent on preserving the stability of NPC at a time when there were increasingly frequent border attacks and political activities in the country generally. What is more, at this time oil was selling at $20 a barrel, with production costs at approximately $1–$5 a barrel, the result of which was that the company's profits soared.

Questions

1 Some observers noted that NPC was successful despite, not because of, the organisation's culture and questioned what might occur if the price of oil ever fell dramatically. How do you think NPC would cope with a downturn in its revenues?

2 If money was the solution to all internal conflicts within NPC, could money be the solution to the sorts of internal conflicts faced by organisations in (a) the UK, (b) Japan and (c) Hong Kong?

The consistency hypothesis

This states that a shared system of beliefs, values, and symbols is an effective basis for reaching consensus and achieving co-ordinated action. In consistent cultures communication is a more reliable process for exchanging information because there is general agreement on the meaning of words, actions and other symbols. Organisational effectiveness can also be facilitated by consistently held value-based principles which prescribe action in unfamiliar situations.

Consistency, though, can be a double-edged sword. There are two main points to note here. First, whether these value-based principles do in fact enhance performance largely depends on whether they are appropriate to the business environment; and second, where there is inconsistency between the espoused culture and the culture in practice, integration and co-ordination within the organisation may tend to break down.

Given the apparent plausibility of the 'strong culture equals high performance' equation, it is unsurprising to find that many practising managers subscribe to it. The popularity of this view has been massively reinforced by books such as Peter and Waterman's (1982) *In Search of Excellence*, Pascale and Athos's (1981) *The Art of Japanese Management* and Deal and Kennedy's (1982) *Corporate Cultures*. However, serious questions can be raised concerning the validity of the argument.

1   A strong culture may facilitate goal alignment, but the goals set by a culture may not always be positive in two senses: they may not be ethical, and they might not encourage good economic performance. In the first case we can imagine an organisation such as a political or religious sect that brainwashes its members into pursuing violent ends, or an economic organisation that pursues environmentally catastrophic objectives. An example of the second case would be an organisation with a culture which dictated that care for employees was of greater value than profitability or market share, with the result that economic objectives were made subservient to human resource objectives.

2   It cannot be assumed that all strong cultures are associated with high levels of employee motivation. Many UK public services have well-developed and strong cultures, but it is at least questionable whether all these organisations are populated by highly motivated individuals. Certainly the customers of organisations such as British Rail, the Post Office and the civil service are not all fully convinced. The point is that strong cultures may encourage many different attitudes toward the organisation and to work other than the purely positive. As regards motivation, therefore, strong cultures can work both ways.

3   It is probably true that an organisation which appreciates its past and which encodes information about past decisions in stories and anecdotes is advantaged compared with similarly placed organisations which do not. However, it is also true that organisations can become too wrapped up in the past and fail to focus on the present and the future. It is also possible for organisations to reapply lessons learned in the past to current situations where the old rules no longer apply, perhaps because of technological innovation or increased competition. In other words, there is a thin dividing line between being able to learn from the past and being a prisoner of the past.

4   There are in fact quite a few well-known examples of organisations with both strong cultures and strong economic performances. Yet even these companies do not necessarily lend credence to the strong culture argument. The reason for this is the problem of determining causality. After all, it may be that good economic performance is the cause of a strong culture rather than a strong culture being responsible for high performance. We saw in Chapter 5 that organisational success often consolidates cultural beliefs and values. It therefore seems more than reasonable to suggest that economic success can strengthen a culture.

5   The strong culture argument fails to take account of the fact that few organisations have a single, unitary culture. Most scholarly commentators suggest that not only do organisations tend to have multiple subcultures, but that there are often highly complex operational and power relationships between them. Certainly some or even all of these subcultures may be strong in the sense of being cohesive, but this may mean that they function to undermine the initiatives of other subcultures rather than to support them. This was found to be the case at an automobile plant where the managerial and worker subcultures subscribed to very different value systems, and vied with each other for organisational control.

So much for the theory, but what evidence is there? In their book Kotter and Heskett present the results of four studies on the relationship between culture and long-term economic performance. Their findings led them to suggest that there was a positive correlation between corporate culture and long-term economic performance, but it was extremely weak. Moreover they found a number of organisations with strong cultures yet which performed poorly, and organisations with weak cultures which nevertheless performed extremely well. Kotter and Heskett's analysis of these organisations thus suggests not only that strong cultures can lead an organisation into decline (for example, Citicorp, General Motors and Proctor & Gamble), but that weak cultures are not necessarily economically disadvantageous (for example, at McGraw-Hill and SmithKline). These results should not surprise us. It has long been recognised that companies such as Kodak, Polaroid and Xerox once held seemingly unassailable positions, and were supposed to be bolstered by their strong cultures, yet all have experienced significant performance difficulties in recent years. The same is true of the pioneers of strategic planning, General Electric and Texas Instruments, while Digital Equipment Corporation, once held up as a model of how to combine growth, flexibility, profits and humanism, currently finds itself struggling to come to terms with its own intricate bureaucracy and fiscal problems (Davis, 1984).

Culture fit, adaptation and mission

The problems associated with the strong culture hypothesis have led other commentators to suggest various alternative perspectives on the link between culture and performance. One of the most interesting of these is the idea that high economic performance is correlated with a strategically appropriate culture. This view suggests that those organisations that have cultures which 'fit' the environment and the business strategy will perform well relative to those whose fit is poor. Obviously, different cultures will be appropriate in different competitive environments and for different strategies, so there is no one best culture that always breeds success. However, it may well be that the culture has to be strong (at least in certain respects), as well as contextually suited, in order for an organisation to attain excellent performance.

This perspective is certainly worthy of consideration, neutralising as it does one of the key problems with the strong culture theory, namely, that strong cultures may take organisations in the 'wrong' direction. For commercial organisations a 'strategically appropriate' culture will almost always involve a commitment to optimise economic performance indicators. Most schools, hospitals, the police and other public bodies are, though, likely to have less interest in profitability and market share than, for example, maximising the potential of students, the quality of patient care and reducing levels of crime. More specifically, what constitutes appropriate beliefs, values and assumptions will depend on factors such as the nature of the industry sector operated in, the technology employed, geographical location, strategic goals, and the personalities of the employees. In practice, the list of variables that affect the internal and external contexts of an organisation, and thus which specify the type of culture appropriate to that organisation, will be vast. This means that engineering a culture to fit the context is always going to be a phenomenally complex and difficult thing to achieve, even if it is desirable.

Testing this perspective in any objective sense is rather difficult. Again, the work by Kotter and Heskett provides the most insight. From a detailed study of 22 firms they concluded that cultures which fitted their market, competitive, technological and other environments were likely to perform better than those whose fit was less good. Yet the same study also provided suggestive evidence that the 'appropriate culture equals high performance' equation is itself problematic. The difficulty is, what happens when an organisation's environment changes? Looking at their evidence Kotter and Heskett discovered that all of the lower-performing organisations they studied had in the past enjoyed a significantly better culture-environment fit. This fit had worsened as a result of environmental changes to which the organisations had not effectively responded. The conclusion that can be drawn is that for any given organisation a good culture–environment fit will be associated with short-term high performance, but that this does not guarantee the success of the organisation in the long term. A large number of commentators have dismissed even this weak claim as misguided, arguing that what little research that has been conducted has been methodologically questionable (see, for example, Siehl and Martin, 1990, Alvesson and Berg, 1992).

In order for an organisation to be continually successful it must have more than just a strong and appropriate culture, it must be able to continuously adapt to its environment. An adaptive culture is generally characterised as one in which people will take risks, trust each other, have a proactive approach to organisational life, will work together to identify problems, share considerable confidence in their own abilities and those of their colleagues, and have enthusiasm for their jobs. While the specific qualities associated with adaptive cultures vary from author to author the organisations most frequently cited as possessing exemplary adaptive cultures are corporations like Digital Equipment Corporation, Honda and 3M. The third of Denison's hypotheses (adaptability) concerns these issues. The adaptability hypothesis states that a culture which allows an organisation to adapt to changing demands and circumstances will promote effectiveness. Adaptability aids organisational effectiveness in three ways. First, it allows an organisation to recognise and respond to its external environment. Second, it means an ability to respond to internal constituencies, such that different functions, departments and divisions interact positively with each other. Third, in response to either internal or external prompting it requires the capacity to restructure and reinstitutionalise behaviours and processes as appropriate.

In its most general form the 'adaptive culture equals high performance' equation is open to criticism. Not only can it not account for those organisations which are not obviously adaptive but which are successful because they fit the relative stability of their organisation's environment, but it is unconvincing in important respects. For example, risk-taking cultures may well go out of business if they take too many bad risks, and not all innovations are always good for the organisation. In fact, too much change can lead to instability and a loss of sense of direction. Refinement of the perspective is, therefore, required.

Based on their research findings Kotter and Heskett argue that a more coherent formulation of this perspective would emphasise two further points. First, the culture must be one which values and supports all the large stakeholders in the organisation. In the case of commercial organisations these will be customers, stockholders and employees, and in the case of public organisations may well include the government, regulatory agencies and the general public. Second, the culture must also value excellent leadership from its managers at all levels. So for Kotter and Heskett adaptive cultures which provide effective leadership aimed at satisfying the legitimate and changing interests of stakeholders will be more (economically) successful than those organisations whose cultures are not so oriented. According to the findings of their study over an eleven year time span, those organisations which emphasised leadership and key stakeholders increased revenues by an average of 682 per cent against 166 per cent for those which did not, expanded their workforces by 282 per cent versus 36 per cent, raised their stock prices by 901 per cent against 74 per cent, and improved their net incomes by 756 per cent as opposed to 1 per cent.

The truly stunning results of Kotter and Heskett's research merit careful attention. Perhaps the main point to note is that much of their data were collected from industry analysts and senior individuals in the organisations themselves, whose views on the content of an organisation's culture may have been influenced by knowledge of that organisation's performance. In short, if individuals know that a company has performed poorly over the past decade they may well be inclined to state that the firm suffers from a lack of good leadership and fails to pay attention to the needs and requirements of key stakeholders. This does not, however, prove that the organisation was lacking in these respects. The converse also holds. It may well be that industry analysts and prominent employees of the organisations concerned attribute success *post hoc* to good leadership and attention to stakeholders. Again, this does not constitute overwhelming evidence that such organisations actually did possess these cultural characteristics. Moreover, there is the same problem of deciding on the direction of causality which afflicts so many of the theories linking culture and performance: does emphasising leadership and stakeholders bring success, or does success lead to a culture in which leadership and stakeholders come to be valued? Further research is required before any definitive answer can be provided.

The last of Denison's hypotheses, the mission hypothesis, is in one sense closely related to these ideas of Kotter and Heskett, in that it emphasises the need to consider an organisation's culture in the context of both internal factors and its external environment. The mission hypothesis states that a culture which provides a shared definition of the function and purpose of an organisation will be positively associated with effectiveness. There are two arguments here. First, a sense of mission provides employees with non-economic reasons for investing their efforts in the wellbeing of the organisation, efforts which can surpass those normally expected of organisational employees; and second, a sense of mission provides both a direction and end goals which make it easier to identify appropriate courses of action for the organisation.

Summary

Many commentators have in fact questioned whether there is a 'single best culture' that will bring success to all commercial organisations. Kotter and Heskett's response is to suggest that there are in fact some general features of organisational cultures which are likely to be associated with economic success. In their view a culture in which there is strong consensus that (1) large stakeholders be valued and (2) leadership at all levels is important to success, and which (3) engages in practices that fit a sensible strategy for the organisation's context, will enhance economic performance. Interesting though such a conclusion is, we should always recall that it is speculative only. It is also as well to remember that Kotter and Heskett are interested only in commercial organisations, and that economic performance indicators are just not relevant to many not-for-profit entities such as charities, social and activity clubs, and religious institutions, which may nevertheless be very interested in the relationship between their culture and performance. We should also bear in mind that the research work of Kotter and Heskett is pioneering, and has yet to be validated by other researchers.

Seemingly in contrast to the 'one best' prescription of Kotter and Heskett, Denison adopts a more 'academic' approach, and suggests that his four hypotheses can be integrated into a single explanatory framework (see Fig. 6.2). He makes a number of points concerning this figure. First, it is pointed out that while involvement and consistency are primarily concerned with the internal dynamics of an organisation, adaptability and mission are focused on the relationship between the organisation and its external environment. Second, it is argued that adaptability and involvement emphasise the organisation's capacity for flexibility and change, while consistency and mission provide stability and direction. The framework is useful, asserts Denison, because it points out some of the inherent contradictions between the hypotheses. For example, a culture that is highly consistent might lack the flexibility required to deal with change. Both flexibility and consistency are, however, required for effective organisational performance. In fact, for Denison, an effective organisational culture must provide all the elements covered by the four hypotheses. The ideal culture is thus one which can simultaneously reconcile the conflicting demands of being adaptive, consistent, involving and directed. Thus the model does, therefore, implicitly contain a 'one best culture' formulation quite similar to that advocated by Kotter and Heskett. Such 'one best culture' formulations, are however, intensely problematic.

Some complications

While the 'single best culture' formulations of Kotter and Heskett and of Denison have great intuitive appeal, we should nevertheless be careful not to accept them uncritically. Many commentators have argued that a vast array of internal and external factors influence how cultures develop, and it is to be expected that different combinations of internal and external variables will conspire to determine the characteristics of relatively high- and low-performing cultures. This point is well illustrated with reference to different business contexts, concerning which Gordon (1985) has reported some interesting

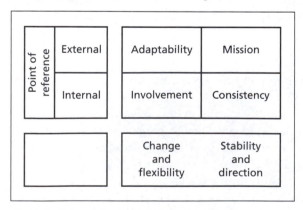

Fig. 6.2 Culture and effectiveness model
Source: reproduced from Denison (1990)

findings. Using data collected by the consultancy organisation Hay Associates, Gordon studied three broad groups of organisation: utilities (such as electric, gas and telephone companies), dynamic-marketplace companies and financial institutions.

Utilities

A comparison of high economic performers against low performers revealed very similar cultural profiles (see Chapter 2). There were, though, two major points of dissimilarity. First, higher performing organisations were oriented toward a higher degree of interdependence, with units encouraged to operate in a co-ordinated manner; and second, employees were more likely to receive clear communication and support from upper management. High-performing utilities were also more inclined to pay competitively and fairly, and provide opportunities for employees to grow and develop within the company. Interestingly, neither high- nor low-performing utilities were found to encourage individual initiative or to approach business innovatively.

Dynamic-marketplace companies

Gordon found that all the values which are associated with high-performing utilities were subordinate for the successful dynamic-marketplace companies. High-performing companies in these market sectors tended to value making the organisation bigger and different from what it was previously. Such firms had venturesome goals, encouraged individual initiative, were fired with a sense of urgency to get things done and were responsive to their marketplaces.

Financial institutions

According to Gordon's data high-performing financial institutions shared many of the cultural characteristics of dynamic-marketplace companies. They focused on enlarging themselves, had a bias for taking action rather than delaying through procrastination or poor co-ordination, and fostered employee initiative. Conversely, low-performing financial institutions appeared to have the dominant traits of utilities, that is, were highly conservative.

It is, thus, highly probable that the nature of the organisation's activities and its business context exert influence regarding which cultural characteristics are functional and which are not. In other words, it may not be the case that, for example, adaptability is always an economically desirable trait, even over the long term (decades). The argument here is that many utilities have not only survived but prospered in part because they stifled initiative and innovation, and valued stability and control because this is what their environment and operational activities required. For these organisations an adaptability-oriented culture may have seriously damaged their economic performance ever since they were formed. Indeed, it is only recently in the UK that utilities have been forced through Government legislation and industry watchdogs to become more adaptable, and a difficult process it has been for many of them. But it is only since the mid- to late 1980s that adaptability has become a desirable culture trait, bringing into question the assertion that adaptability is always a performance-enhancing characteristic. Similar questions can also be asked regarding the need for organisations to emphasise leadership at all levels and to the assertion that organisations should pay careful attention to large stakeholders. In other words, there are always likely to be exceptional organisations in which the general strictures of Denison, Kotter and Heskett do not apply.

It is suggested here that the relationship between organisational culture and performance is so complex, so dependent on large numbers of dynamic variables and human personalities, that no simple cultural 'formula for success' can be relied upon. We should remember that even if high-performing organisations do share some common cultural traits they may be benefiting from them in different ways (Barney, 1986). We would also do well to recall that low-performing organisations might share many of the same traits that characterise high-performing organisations, yet they might not possess these traits in performance-boosting configurations (Miller and Mintzberg, 1983). This means that it may not be advisable for less successful organisations to modify their cultures in order to emulate their high-performing competitors, because what works for one firm may not be useful for another. Indeed, it has been suggested that to be a cause of sustained competitive advantage a culture must be rare and only imperfectly imitable (Barney, 1986). If a culture is not rare then it is unlikely to be associated with uncommonly high performance over a sustained period of time because it does not differentiate an organisation from its competitors. If an organisation's culture is easily and perfectly imitable, then over time competitors will probably adapt themselves to match it and so obviate any competitive advantage that organisation may have once possessed.

Other commentators have argued that it is a mistake just to concentrate on organisational culture when considering strategy and performance. One suggestion is that particular industry sectors have their own cultures (sets of assumptions) that need to be studied in order for a complete picture of strategy formulation and organisational effectiveness to be revealed (Whipp et al., 1989b). Another group of commentators ascribe considerable weight to national culture, and attempts have been made to explain the long-term decline of the British economy and the rise of the south-east Asian economies by reference to national cultural differences. Perhaps most important of all is the realisation on the part of many scholars that culture itself does not provide a direct explanation of performance. Rather, it is but one component of a much more complex set of relationships contained within the process of competition. Without wishing to denigrate the work of commentators such as Denison, Kotter and Heskett it might prove wise to treat with caution those studies which: 'are based on a simplistic model of the link between culture and organisational outcomes, which [have] insufficient theoretical sensitivity to illuminate the complex, mutually causal interactions of cultural phenomena as they affect an organisation's outcomes' (Saffold, 1988: 550). An indication of the complex and dynamic relationship between organisational culture, industry sector culture, organisational structure, and performance is provided by Mini Case 6.6 which concerns Jaguar Cars.

Culture and performance at Jaguar Cars

Jaguar Cars is a Coventry-based luxury car manufacturer with a chequered history of success, decline and turnaround. The post-war performance of the company may be divided into three main periods.

1945–1968

Up to 1968 its market performance was generally strong. During this period it was dominant in the UK luxury saloon and sports classes of car, 50 per cent of its output was exported, costs were kept down and pricing was competitive. In short, Lyons, the founder and chief executive, achieved considerable success with the firm, which won major awards with its XJ6 and XJ12 models. Some of the hallmarks of his regime were a strong craft identification with the product, the pursuit of product engineering innovation, and a 'can-do' mentality which resulted in the meeting of many short deadlines. Lyons himself was noted for his authoritarian and interventionist style, his aversion to unnecessary expenditure, and his distaste for formal management techniques.

1972–1980

From 1972 until 1980 the strengths of Lyons's culture withered, and Jaguar Cars went into decline. Now owned by British Leyland, Jaguar was technically no longer a company but a manufacturing location. A succession of senior managers were imposed from corporate level, each of whom applied widely contrasting policies. Part of the problem was that BL's managers were from volume/mass production not specialist car backgrounds. On top of this came three substantial reorganisations, the dismemberment of Jaguar's finance, sales and marketing functions, and the development of divisional warfare. The result was that the 1979 Series III model was beset with quality and reliability defects, production fell dramatically, and losses for its main site were running at £4 million per month. In 1980 Michael Edwardes, the British Leyland chief executive, gave notice that unless the plant broke even within a year it would be closed.

1980–

Later in 1980 a new managing director and chairman of Jaguar, called John Egan, was appointed. There followed a remarkable turnaround in the fortunes of Jaguar, with vast increases in turnover, profitability and productivity. Jaguar re-established its market position by restructuring its retail operation and reformulating its relations with outside bodies both in the UK and abroad. Key to the firm's success was a new senior management team and the re-establishment of finance, sales and marketing, and purchasing departments. As a 'stand alone' company Jaguar was better able to reduce operating costs, raise quality standards and reliability, and improve communications. Meeting these objectives involved reducing the workforce from 10 000 to 7000, setting up company-wide task forces to tackle 150 specially targeted problems, and making operators and suppliers directly responsible for quality.

Five features of Jaguar's survival and regeneration programme touch on issues of organisational culture: leadership, the quest for quality, communications, project management and language:

1 *Leadership* John Egan provided a new mission for Jaguar, which suggested that it now aimed 'to become the finest car company in the world'. A strategic plan was produced which dictated that £1 billion was to be invested over 5 years, expenditure on R&D was to increase dramatically, and production was set to rise from 14 000 to 100 000 cars per annum. The new set of beliefs Egan sought to create clustered around the notion that Jaguar could produce world-class luxury cars by focusing on growth, quality, market sensitivity, learning and human development, and professionalism. Some observers have noted that what Egan has done is to merge the best elements of the Lyons culture (such as product excellence and craft pride) with new beliefs (such as market sensitivity).

▶

2 *Quality* The 'cult of quality' involved the devising of quantifiable standards and the establishment of new working practices. All managers were trained in statistical process control. In addition, American dealers were invited to talk directly to work stations responsible for faults, making workers immediately accountable for problems. Unlike many organisations Jaguar's quality programme was not used as a PR device, and its substantive impact was most noticeable in terms of the new types of stories that began to be told. Instead of stories of mercy-dashes to Jaguar car owners stranded in their new cars, directors and engineers began telling stories about the number of workers and relatives who attended the new XJ40 model launch days.

3 *Communications* Key to the success of the quality programme was a comprehensive communications structure. This involved not just a company newsletter and monthly management bulletins, but video programmes, briefing and discussions sessions, management conferences, 75 quality circles and a set of performance and review committees which linked the shopfloor with senior executives. External consultants were also brought in to mount surveys of employees' views of the communications scheme. Given the degree of cynicism among staff at the time, this extensive communications infrastructure was vital.

4 *Project management* The *ad hoc* though inspired methods of designing cars had in the late 1970s become a competitive liability. Throughout the 1970s they resulted in late, over-budget exercises and cars not acceptable to consumers. With Egan came a whole new approach to project management. Instead of supplying a car for marketeers to sell, engineers now ask 'What type of products do you want?' Cross-functional teams with 10-year product plan objectives have revolutionised Jaguar's approach to car design, manufacture and marketing.

5 *Language* Influential changes in language have accompanied Jaguar's programme of cultural reform. In addition to the new stories mentioned above, a whole new glossary of terms such as 'programme status reports' and 'business objectives' have been incorporated into the linguistic repertoire of engineers.

Finally, it is worth noting that Jaguar's competitive renaissance has been both assisted and constrained by the 'shared assumptions' of the automobile industry as a whole. In the 1970s the industry had a lack of faith in product planning, management training and marketing, and Jaguar's management adopted these beliefs with disastrous results. An enormous rise in the price of oil, massive increases in imports, and changes in Government policy conspired to shatter the industry's assumptions concerning the inevitable survival of domestic producers such as Jaguar. Similarly, Jaguar's adoption of a new set of assumptions has mirrored what is going on elsewhere within the industry. Industry sector culture as much as organisational culture may thus be used to explain how Jaguar has achieved so dramatic a turnaround.

Questions

1 How has Jaguar's culture changed since 1946?

2 How do you account for the development of a sectoral culture within the automotive industry?

3 Are you convinced that Jaguar's programme of culture change has been responsible for its improved performance, or do you think that other factors might also have been in play?

4 Why is Jaguar's current good performance not guaranteed to continue over the next decade?

5 How much support for the ideas of Denison and Kotter and Heskett does this case study provide?

Source: compiled from Rosenfeld *et al.* (1987); Whipp (1987); Whipp *et al.* (1989b); Williams *et al.* (1993); Goldsmith and Clutterbuck (1985)

The evolution of high- and low-performance cultures

How do cultures which undermine good performance develop? While no definitive answers have as yet emerged, Kotter and Heskett have suggested one possible pattern of organisational development that leads to low economic performance. Their account of how such cultures evolve was drawn from studies of twenty firms during the late 1970s and early 1980s, including Avon, Goodyear, PanAm and Xerox. The pattern they describe is as follows.

1 For some reason a committed group of people are successful at what they do. Possibly because of excellent leadership or maybe just sheer luck, a strategy is formulated and implemented which leads the organisation to command a dominant niche in the marketplace.

2 The dominance of these organisations over their market means that they are exceptionally economically successful. This is a period of sustained growth for these companies, and they become increasingly larger and more complex.

3 In order to cope with the size and complexity of the organisation, skilled managers need to be developed within the organisation or brought in from outside. These people understand structures, systems, budgets and controls, but are less comfortable with 'soft' issues such as vision, culture, strategy and inspiration. Over a period of years these individuals assume senior positions within the organisation. As this process occurs there is a loss of any collective sense of why the firm was successful in the first place. These unhealthy cultures tend to have three general components: first, managers tend to be arrogant; second, managers do not value all the key stakeholder groups; and third, the cultures no longer value leadership or other change-oriented structures and values.

4 Over time the environment alters, and because managers now tend to ignore relevant information and cling to outmoded strategies and practices, economic performance begins to deteriorate. Arrogance, insularity and poor leadership all combine to restrict the organisation's scope for, and ability to cope with, change.

How, then, do performance-enhancing cultures develop? In start-up situations Kotter and Heskett suggest that an entrepreneur initiates an organisation with an adaptive culture which values stakeholders and encourages leadership at all levels. In addition, a business strategy is developed which fits the organisation's context and brings success. The result is that the founder and his or her culture are highly regarded by employees, who adopt the central beliefs, values and assumptions. The perpetuation of the culture is, though, not guaranteed. Large-scale expansion of an organisation can lead to a gradual loosening of cultural ties, continued success can make managers complacent, and time can lead to a blurring of people's memories regarding why the organisation was successful in the first place. This can mean that by the time the organisation is mature there is a need to re-create a performance-enhancing culture.

According to many authors, including Kotter and Heskett, in these situations what is required is one or two unusually gifted leaders at the top. The new leadership team must then create a sense of crisis or need for change. They must then provide a new direction, which encompasses building an adaptive culture and an appropriate business strategy.

IKEA: evolution of a high-performance culture

Introduction

From its origins as a mail-order business set up in 1949, by 1991 IKEA[1] was a £2 billion retail furnishing empire with 96 stores in 24 countries. The company had opened its first warehouse-showroom in 1953 in Almhult and its second in Stockholm in 1965. Between 1965 and 1973 IKEA opened 7 new stores in Scandinavia and sales reached SKr 480 million. It was at this juncture that the company began its entry into Continental Europe, opened franchise operations in Asia, and then entered the Canadian and US markets. Most commentators agreed that the organisation had been phenomenally successful, and that its rapid expansion had been facilitated by its culture, which drew both on the personality of its founder Mr Ingvar Kamprad and the national culture of Sweden.

Kamprad's vision

According to his colleagues Mr Kamprad was driven by a wish to create a better life for people in Sweden and abroad. Quite how IKEA the company fitted in with this vision was unclear. What was more certain was that he had helped accelerate a fundamental change in consumer needs and a structural shift in the furniture retailing industry. Pivotal to the success of his vision were a series of simple organisational heuristics (some would call them 'norms', others 'rules'):

- *Cost consciousness* Some of Mr Kamprad's more memorable sayings included 'waste of resources is a mortal sin at IKEA' and 'expensive solutions are often signs of mediocrity'.
- *Informality* Not only were dress codes informal (jeans and sweaters were the norm), but the atmosphere in the offices was relaxed, forms of address were familiar, and status and hierarchy were played down.
- *Simplicity and attention to detail* IKEA employees would be heard to say that 'retail is detail', while Mr Kamprad maintained that 'complicated rules paralyse'.

- *Creative solutions and common sense* While creative solutions were much prized, so too was common sense. One well-known story made the point: when the original Stockholm store opened it could not cope with the rush of customers. In response, the store manager allowed customers into the warehouse to pick up their purchases. This was so successful that future warehouses were designed to allow self-selection by customers, resulting in reduced costs and a faster service.
- *Youth and enthusiasm* IKEA preferred to recruit young people without experience of another organisational culture, who were not just hardworking but had '*odmjukhet*' – a Swedish word implying humility, modesty and respect for others.

Sustaining the culture

As the organisation expanded overseas, so maintaining the unique IKEA culture was perceived as a potential problem. To combat this Mr Kamprad wrote *Testament of a Furniture Dealer*, which became an important means of spreading and reinforcing the company's values. In addition, there were training programmes steeped in Kamprad's ideology and several hundred specially selected 'IKEA ambassadors' assigned to key positions in all units to educate subordinates and act as role models for the culture. The maintenance of the organisation's internal cultural identity was matched by attempts to present a unified IKEA personality externally to customers. According to Kamprad, IKEA stood for domestic products that were simple, durable, well designed and competitively priced.

The rapid growth of the organisation meant that there were plentiful opportunities for top managers to assume positions of responsibility. It also allowed individuals to develop through varied experiences. For example, Anders Moberg, who rose to be IKEA's CEO, had worked in store administration, been a store manager in Austria and in Switzerland, and led IKEA's entry into France. Interestingly, the organisation's senior management remained overwhelmingly Scandinavian. Indeed, of the 65 senior executives in IKEA, 60 were Swedish or Danish. Many within the company argued that this resulted in certain distinct advantages: everyone instinctively followed the Scandinavian philosophy of simple, people-oriented, non-hierarchic operations, leading to efficiency gains and a high-trust environment. While some non-Scandinavians were disappointed that their career prospects with the organisation were limited, most realised that it was important to speak Swedish and understand the Smalandish[2] psyche to achieve a senior position.

Challenges to the culture

In the early 1990s IKEA still had ambitious expansion plans, with fledgling ventures in Russia, Eastern Europe and America all showing growth potential. The sheer size of the organisation combined with the absence of Mr Kamprad (who had retired to Switzerland as a tax exile) meant that change was inevitable. Anders Moberg, president since 1986, was already pressing for a more formalised and systematised organisation, and innovations like a formal budgeting and planning process, better integration of the various country business plans and the different product groups, and a three-year corporate plan to which the country units had to conform, were all evident. Cost-consciousness was still emphasised, but there were indications that the least cost route was chosen only if the more expensive options were not cost-beneficial.

There were also some potentially difficult decisions and damaging trends on the horizon. One of the principal causes for concern was the organisation's continued investment of huge sums of capital in new stores. Another worry was that demographic trends in most developed countries seemed likely to result in a shrinkage in IKEA's target market (young low- to middle-income families). Yet given IKEA's history of incremental and continuous improvements and relatively strong financial position, there were many independent observers who thought that there were good grounds for optimism. For many involved with IKEA, however, it was the difficulty of sustaining a high-performance culture in a large and geographically diverse organisation which was the primary source of concern. As Kamprad himself conceded:

> The IKEA spirit was easier to keep alive in former days when we weren't so many, when we all reached each other, and could talk with each other. Before, it was more concrete, the will to help each other, the art of managing with small means – being cost-conscious almost to the point of stinginess, the humbleness, the irresistible enthusiasm and the wonderful community through thick and thin. Certainly it is more difficult now when the individual is gradually being wiped out in the grey gloominess of collective agreements.

Questions

1 How well does Kotter and Heskett's theory of how high-performance cultures evolve explain the case of IKEA?

2 Is the biggest danger to IKEA's continued success the fact that Ingvar Kamprad is no longer a dominant player within the organisation?

3 What conclusions concerning Scandinavian culture can you draw from the culture of IKEA?

Notes

1 IKEA is an acronym formed from the initials of the founder Ingvar Kamprad, his farm Elmtaryd, and his county, Agunnaryd, in Smaland, South Sweden.

2 'Smalandish' refers to the Smaland county in South Sweden where Ingvar Kamprad lived.

Source: compiled from C. A. Bartlett (1990), *Ingvar Kamprad and IKEA*, Harvard Business School 9–390–132; Johnson and Scholes (1993)

The effective communication of key messages and the motivation of middle managers to take on similar leadership roles for their subordinates are also key. New structures may then be implemented to facilitate the new vision. Growing organisational success then encourages increasing numbers of people to adopt the tenets of the new culture and strategy. A virtuous circle has now been created: adherence to the leader's assumptions brings the success which broadens and intensifies adherence to the culture and strategy.

Once again, the problem is how to maintain and preserve a performance-enhancing culture. For Kotter and Heskett this is a difficult balancing act for which they make the following prescriptions: first, core values and beliefs must be rigidly adhered to; second, most other values and practices should be regarded more flexibly, and discarded if they become dysfunctional; third, leaders must always communicate messages consistent with the culture's core values; fourth, pride must not be allowed to degenerate into arrogance; and fifth, failings must be confronted in a practical and realistic way. An overview of how IKEA has developed and perpetuated a performance-enhancing culture is provided by Mini Case 6.7.

While these patterns of culture development identified by Kotter and Heskett are very interesting, some commentators have questioned whether they stand up to critical scrutiny. According to Martin *et al.* (1985), such rosy portraits of cultural evolution gloss over much of the detail to the point that they tell us little of worth. They suggest that because real organisational cultures are so complex many authors have chosen to stress the importance of leaders and focus on their contribution, omitting the impact of various other opinion-formers and subcultures. By emphasising the role of the leader, commentators like Kotter and Heskett can reduce the amount of complexity they are forced to deal with, and are able to present what appears to be a coherent narrative of culture development. Martin *et al.* point out that certain cognitive biases have played an important role in supporting these simplistic models of cultural evolution. Some of the most important of these are:

- *Attribution* Many employees tend to attribute powers to leaders that they do not possess or which they cannot exercise fully due to situational constraints.

- *Salience* When leaders speak and act, their words and deeds often make a greater impact on their audience than do the speeches and actions of others, and thus tend to be remembered more vividly.

- *Self-enhancement* Leaders themselves tend to think of themselves as being in command, and are in fact more likely to see themselves as responsible for successes than for failures.

Thus for all these reasons leaders may be given undeserved credit for having created or changed culture. That these biases are not frequently recognised is potentially dangerous. This is because it encourages us to adopt a massively incomplete view of how high- and low-performing cultures actually emerge, which in turn limits managers' scope for attempting to re-engineer them as they see fit. The argument being made here is that although Kotter and Heskett may have identified some leadership-oriented developmental patterns of note, we should not forget that in the case of any particular organisation the impact of environmental constraints, organisational technologies, and various subcultures and influential individuals (among others) may be no less significant.

UNDERSTANDING CULTURE, STRATEGY AND PERFORMANCE

The issues discussed in this chapter are highly interconnected. This section provides a summary and integration of some of the main ideas in very general terms. An overview of the conclusions of this section (and hence the chapter) is provided by Fig. 6.3. This illustrates that an organisational culture develops under the influence of its wider environmental context (business environment and national culture) and in response to the unique personalities, events, decisions and processes that have characterised its evolution. The result is an intricate web of rites, rituals, symbols and cognitions that we refer to as organisational culture, and which finds expression as a complex of cultural dynamics.

An organisational culture, or rather the dynamics it generates, thus directly affects strategy formulation in at least five different ways: culture acts as a perception filter, affects the interpretation of information, sets moral and ethical standards, provides rules, norms and heuristics for action, and influences how power and authority are wielded in reaching decisions regarding what course of action to pursue. The formulated strategy is a cultural artefact which helps employees understand their role in the organisation, is a focus for identification and loyalty, encourages motivation, and provides a framework of ideas that enables individuals to comprehend their environment and the place of their organisation within it.

An organisation's culture, then, influences how its strategy is implemented. It is suggested that the more consonant a strategy is with the prevailing culture the more effectively that strategy will be put into practice. It is further anticipated that the stronger and richer the culture (in the sense that there is agreement on beliefs, values and assumptions, and many relevant strategy-supportive stories) the more likely it is that the strategy will be successfully implemented. The idea that the process of strategy formulation and the dynamics of strategy implementation will also have an impact on culture is worthy of note. It should also be observed that environmental opportunities and constraints are significant here, influencing both strategy formulation and implementation. In fact, the resulting level of performance will depend as much on environmental factors as it will on culture.

This said, it is hypothesised that certain cultural features are more likely to be associated with high levels of economic performance than others. It is at least arguable that

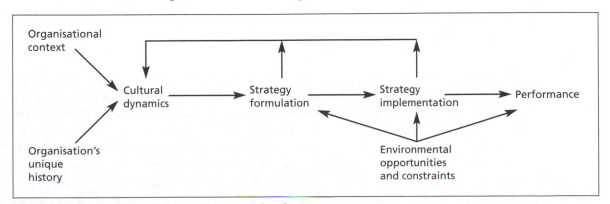

Fig. 6.3 Understanding culture, strategy and peformance

243

the most effective cultures are those which are not only strong (in the sense of being consistent), but actively involve large numbers of individuals in consultative and decision-making bodies. In addition, it seems reasonable to suggest that some cultures allow an organisation to exploit a given environment more effectively than others, and are thus more 'strategically appropriate'. If a culture is able to adapt to changing circumstances in order to maintain its strategic appropriateness over time, then this too may well be advantageous. There is also suggestive evidence that cultures which value large stakeholders and leadership at all levels are associated with superior economic performance.

Conclusions

In this chapter we have seen that an organisation's culture has a direct and significant impact on performance. Organisational strategies and structures and their implementation are shaped by the assumptions, beliefs and values which we have defined as culture. Furthermore, it has been suggested that this culture both constrains and presents opportunities for what an organisation is able to accomplish. Thus organisational effectiveness must, in large part, be interpreted as a cultural phenomenon, albeit mediated by various management systems, strategies and procedures. This does not mean that we can simplistically argue that culture causes good and poor performance, because culture is itself massively affected by, for instance, changes in strategy and to organisational structures. The complexity of the intercausal relationships between strategy, culture and performance makes hard and fast generalisations difficult to make.

SUMMARY AND CONCLUSIONS

This chapter has elaborated six main themes.

1 It was suggested that there are many different interpretations of what is meant by the terms 'strategy' and 'performance', and that in using these words we should always be clear to specify what we mean. This said, there is certainly considerable interest in how these aspects of organisational life interact, interest which has been fuelled by suggestions that the right combination of culture and strategy can massively improve organisational effectiveness.

2 Five different ways in which an organisation's culture can influence strategy formulation were identified: through its influence on scanning behaviour, selective perception, interpretation, the impact of values, the effects of assumptions and the power of various subcultures. The importance of culture to strategy implementation was then discussed with reference to Schwartz and Davis's framework for assessing risk, and Weick's suggestion that culture can be a source of high reliability in realising strategic intent. A brief account of the Miles and Snow typology which links particular cultures to specific strategies was then provided.

3 The functions that strategy performs as a cultural artefact (a focus for organisational and individual self-understanding, a focus for identification and loyalty, and a means for comprehending social phenomena) were considered. It was then concluded that it is inappropriate to see culture as the independent and strategy as the dependent variable, as culture and strategy mutually impact on each other.

4 The importance of taking cultural considerations into account when planning mergers and acquisitions was highlighted.

5 Some of the most significant work concerning culture and performance was reviewed. This research suggested that strong, appropriate, adaptable cultures which value stakeholders and leadership, and which have a strong sense of mission, are likely to be associated with high performance over sustained periods of time.

6 Some conclusions regarding the complex nature of the relationships between culture, strategy and performance were drawn. An account of how high- and low-performance cultures evolve was presented. Finally, a framework for understanding the linkages between culture, strategy and performance was presented.

KEY CONCEPTS

Strategy	Analysers	Mission hypothesis	Effectiveness
Strategy formulation	Culture strength	Selective perception	High-performance
Strategy	Stakeholders	Mergers and	cultures
implementation	High reliability	acquisitions	Low-performance
Competitive advantage	Strategic myopia	Goal alignment	cultures
Scanning behaviour	Strategy as artefact	Motivation	Cognitive bias
Validation	Leadership	Organisational learning	Attribution
Cultural risk	Involvement hypothesis	Strategically	Salience
Defenders	Consistency hypothesis	appropriate cultures	Self-enhancement
Prospectors	Adaptability hypothesis	Performance	Single best cultures

QUESTIONS

1 What do you understand by the terms 'strategy' and 'performance'?

2 In what ways can organisational culture affect strategy formulation?

3 What is 'cultural risk'? What implications does it have for organisations contemplating strategic change?

4 How can an organisation's culture promote internal consistency and reliability? Why are these characteristics desirable? What are the potential disadvantages associated with consistent and reliable cultures?

5 What functions does strategy perform as a cultural artefact?

6 Can strategy influence the development of a culture, and if so how?

7 Can mergers and acquisitions be managed so as to avoid cultural problems?

8 Are executives well advised to create strong organisational cultures in the pursuit of high economic performance?

9 Using your own ideas as well as those contained in this chapter, describe your ideal organisational culture working on the assumption that you want to maximise organisational effectiveness.

10 How can executives prevent a high-performance culture deteriorating into a low-performance culture?

CULTURE, STRATEGY AND PERFORMANCE AT SHELL CHEMICALS (UK)[1]

Introduction

In 1990 Royal Dutch/Shell reported a post-tax profit of $6.539 billion on a turnover of $85.412 billion for 1989, making it the most profitable publicly quoted company in the world.[2] This was the first time since the early part of the century that a European company had occupied this position, with IBM pushed into second place, and General Motors into third. While a world recession hit Group net income hard over the next few years, Shell remained (and remains!) one of the most economically powerful of all multinational companies. According to the Group's own literature, the objectives of Shell companies were to engage efficiently, responsibly and profitably in the oil, gas, chemicals, coal, metals and selected other businesses, and to play an active role in the search for and development of other sources of energy. Although Shell publicly contends that it operates in a wide variety of social, political and economic environments over the nature of which it has little influence, it has also been claimed that 'Shell is powerful in its own right – a countervailing force to Downing Street and other national capitals'.[3]

The Royal Dutch/Shell Group of Companies grew out of an alliance made in 1907 between Royal Dutch Petroleum Company and The 'Shell' Transport and Trading Company plc, by which the two companies agreed to merge their interests on a 60 : 40 basis while keeping their separate identities. As parent companies, Royal Dutch Petroleum Company and The 'Shell' Transport and Trading Company plc do not themselves directly engage in operational activities. They are public companies, one domiciled in the Netherlands, the other in the United Kingdom. The parent companies directly or indirectly own the shares in the Group holding companies but were not themselves part of the Group. They appoint directors to the boards of the Group holding companies, from which they receive income in the form of dividends. Shell Transport has some 300 000 shareholders and Royal Dutch some 325 000. The shares of one or both companies are listed and traded on stock exchanges in eight European countries and in the USA. Further information on the structure of the Group is provided by Fig. 6.4.

Introducing Shell Chemicals UK (SCUK)

SCUK is one of the operating subsidiary companies of Shell UK, and has head offices in Chester, and manufacturing operations at Stanlow and Carrington. In 1990 Shell UK made a profit of £414 million, a little higher than the 1989 figure of £363 million. For SCUK, however, which reported a £25 million loss, 1990 was a disastrous year. This followed pre-tax profits of £66 million the year before. Shell UK's annual report and accounts blamed a number of operational difficulties, which made manufacturing problematic, and adverse exchange rate movements for this poor showing (see Fig. 6.5). While SCUK was accountable to Shell UK in terms of its results, its product planning and operating activities were co-ordinated by a service company (Shell International Chemicals). SCUK conducted the downstream cracking and conversion of feedstock extracted from Shell UK's production fields, principally in the North Sea. Similar operational facilities were situated in the Netherlands, France, Germany, Belgium and Spain, with each national operation treated as a separate profit centre. In addition, Shell had chemicals subsidiaries operating in North and South America and in the Far East. Chemicals manufactured at the SCUK plants included plastics and resins, base organic chemicals, detergents and intermediates, additives and industrial chemicals. Products were transferred to and from other Shell Group companies in other countries as required. Plants were large and efficient and were designed to cope with a variety of feedstock in order to ensure continuous operation.

Some thoughts on SCUK culture

On arrival at Heronbridge House (SCUK head quarters) visitors are requested to register on a computerised system which generates a tailor-made name label. The entrance to the office area was

Parent companies

As parent companies, Royal Dutch Petroleum Company and The 'Shell' Transport and Trading Company plc do not themselves directly engage in operational activities. They are public companies, one domiciled in the Netherlands, the other in the United Kingdom.

The parent companies directly or indirectly own the shares in the group holding companies but are not themselves part of the group. They appoint directors to the boards of the group holding companies, from which they receive income in the form of dividends.

Royal Dutch/Shell Group of Companies

Service companies
Shell Internationale Petroleum Maatschappij BV.
Shell Internationale Chemie Maatschappij BV.
Shell International Petroleum Company Limited
Shell International Chemical Company Limited
Billiton International Metals BV.
Shell Internationale Marine Limited
Shell Internationale Research Maatschappij BV.
Shell International Gas Limited
Shell Coal International Limited

The main business of the service companies is to provide advice and services to other Group and associated companies, excluding Shell Petroleum Inc. and its subsidiaries. The service companies are variously located in the Netherlands or the UK.

Shareholdings
There are some 325 000 shareholders of Royal Dutch and some 300 000 of Shell Transport Shares of one or both companies are listed and traded on stock exchanges in eight European countries and in the USA.

The estimated geographical distribution of shareholdings at the end of 1990 was:

	Royal Dutch	Shell Transport	Combined
	%	%	%
United Kingdom	1	97	40
USA	37	2	23
Netherlands	36	*	21
Switzerland	17	*	10
France	5	1	3
Germany	2	*	1
Belgium	1	*	1
Luxembourg	1	*	1
Others	*	*	*

*Less than 1%

Group Holding Companies
Shell Petroleum N.V. and The Shell Petroleum Company Limited between them hold all the shares in the service companies and directly or indirectly, all group interests in the operating companies other than those held by Shell Petroleum Inc.

*Shell Petroleum N.V. holds equity shares in Shell Petroleum Inc which are non-controlling but entitle it to the dividend flow from that company.

Operating Companies
Operating comanies are engaged in various branches of oil and natural gas, chemicals, coal, metals and other businesses in many countries. The management of each operating company is responsible for the performance and long-term viability of its own operations, but can draw on the experience of the service companies and through them, of other operating companies.

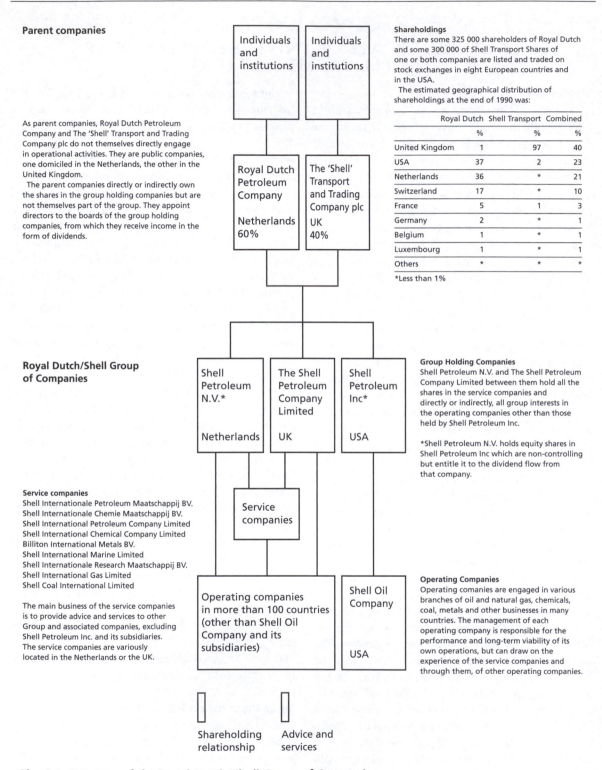

Fig. 6.4 Structure of the Royal Dutch/Shell Group of Companies

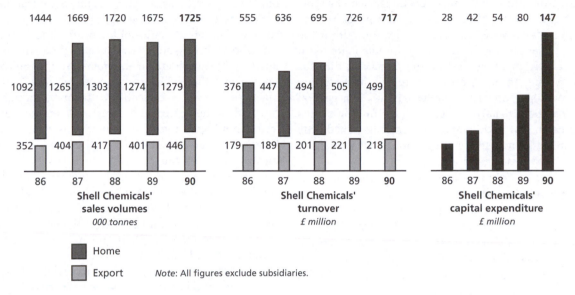

Fig. 6.5 Shell Chemicals, performance data

notable for its message screen, which was employed to make birthday announcements and welcome special guests. The work areas inside the head office were mostly open-plan and were well illuminated with both natural daylight and soft fluorescent lighting. All furnishings were of a standard design, highly functional and reasonably comfortable. A PC on every desk illustrated SCUK's commitment to IT. There were many plants, giving the working areas a pleasing 'green' appearance. Smoking was restricted to a specified area and permitted only at certain times of the day. Free drinks were obtainable from vending machines throughout the building, and a free staff restaurant provided healthy, attractively presented food. The corridors were decorated with fine art prints and bulletin boards containing information on sporting events and travel opportunities. In addition, several copies of the company's annual report and other company brochures were free for the taking. There were also display cabinets containing trophies won by members of SCUK at company-sponsored events, and a 'domesday' book of the local area. Individual employees had personalised the screens around their desks by putting up items such as family photos, posters and clippings from magazines or newspapers. A final point worth

noting were the considerable numbers of Shell 'quality' posters and Shell calendars on display.

A striking feature of Shell culture was the extent to which individual employees expressed a commitment to the organisation. Most people said that they were proud to work for Shell, that the organisation treated them extremely well, and that their colleagues were ambitious, intelligent, hard-working, rational, self-motivating, analytical, creative and team players. Such attitudes were linked to Shell's determination to recruit what it considered to be the cream of the annual graduate crop. While some had reservations about the quality of the training they had received and a performance appraisal system that provided bonuses only to the most outstanding performers, most claimed to be motivated by the challenge of hard work and the excellent career prospects offered by Shell. A few employees suggested that to get promotion at Shell one needed to play a political game in which satisfying one's immediate boss and your boss's boss was vital. Others claimed that Shell was a meritocracy in which the quality of an individual's performance and educational qualifications were of paramount significance in the decision whether to promote. It was noticeable that few staff seemed to remain in one job for long as broad experience was a criterion for promotion, and some questioned whether this led to an overemphasis on short-term goals. Vertical upwards/downwards communication within the organisation was held to be unproblematic, with quarterly meetings led by the managing director providing ample opportunity for two-way discussion of operational and strategic issues. This general perception disharmonised with the finding of this research that middle and lower managers had little detailed knowledge or appreciation of the organisation's strategic intentions.

There was near unanimous agreement that employees tended to work in groups (rather than as individuals), and some thought that this sometimes fostered bureaucracy and inefficiency. Indeed, complaints about 'red tape' which made even the smallest changes difficult to implement were frequently made. These issues were reflected in the decision-making apparatus, which placed great value on the expertise and opinion of every team member. While Shell liked to project an image of itself as a forward-looking entrepreneurial business, many employees thought that it was focused on the past and the present. More than one employee ventured the suggestion that Shell was still revelling in its glorious past, with a tendency to interpret the downturn in its fortunes as a function of the cyclical nature of the industry rather than anything to do with the company. The reactive (rather than proactive) character of the organisation was held to be linked to the essentially bureaucratic nature of its systems and procedures.

A number of other cultural traits were identified as being significant. Survey data collected using the BOCI suggested that those in the organisation were deeply conscious of the impact of their actions on the environment and the importance of cultivating a good press. The same survey discovered that intellectual ability was highly valued, especially as manifested in scientific and technical competence. Other results suggested that individuals were highly sociable, and indeed, many employees described their colleagues as 'friendly', 'sincere' and 'relaxed'. It was widely thought that the organisation was rules-oriented and configured to maximise administrative efficiency, while minimising the psychological distance between leaders and followers, and levels of interpersonal aggression were decidedly low. But in other ways Shell was a highly flexible organisation. For example, it invented the idea of planning by concocting alternate scenarios of the future. The Group was also relatively non-hierarchical, with operating units having considerable autonomy. All the indications were that SCUK attempted to pursue its business objectives ethically, with much thought devoted to the health and safety of its employees: 'the upholding of the Shell reputation is a common bond which can be maintained only by honesty and integrity in all activities'. [4]

The survey also concluded that most individuals considered Shell to have a strong organisational culture with which they identified intensely. This seemed to be a crucial belief (mentioned both by managers working for Shell and in the publicity material of SCUK), that is, that uniformity and homogeneity are required to be successful in business: 'Essential for commercial success, our coordinated business demonstrates throughout a uniformity of attitude and approach'. [5] The apparent de-emphasis of individual personality was reflected in the facts that no obvious corporate heroes could be identified, that people were recruited partly on the basis that they were good team players, and referral to people not by job title but by reference number. Shell is, however, more gently managed than US oil companies, and slower to cut back on its units making a poor return on capital.

SCUK objectives and strategy

In 1992 SCUK's mission statement boldly asserted that the aim of the organisation was to 'become acknowledged as industry leader in customer focus through total quality management, resulting in number one or two market position in all major products and consistently achieved profitability above the average petrochemicals in the relevant sectors of the UK chemical industry'. Other objectives defined by SCUK's senior management included: (a) to generate a cash surplus for shareholders; (b) to establish a cost base sustainable in economic downturns; (c) to pursue the highest HSE (health, safety and environment) standards; and (d) to drive the process of continuous quality improvements forward. Pressed more closely, senior managers would, however, admit that 'the objective is to survive! – we have to structure ourselves in a way, on an income-basis, where we break even, but cost-cutting must never result in losing quality . . . damn difficult'. Interestingly, most people in SCUK seemed to have a sophisticated appreciation of the mission statement, which some described as a 'form of consistent brain-washing'.

SCUK's strategy had been formulated to cope with a particularly severe recession, and consisted of three main elements:

1 A focus on core-business activities. By concentrating on what the organisation was best at (e.g. higher olefins, polymers, base chemicals, solvents and resins) and pulling out of more marginal areas (e.g. the wax business) SCUK hoped to maximise profitability and market share.

2 The reduction of costs without affecting the quality delivered. The short-term objective of breaking even while the chemical industry was in a downturn meant cutting costs dramatically.

3 The improvement of customer-focus and market-orientation within the organisation by introducing Total Quality Management (TQM) and Product Business Teams (PBT). SCUK recognised a need to be more customer- and quality-oriented. These programmes, combined with a restructuring exercise that emphasised decentralisation and business centre autonomy, were designed to help.

In summary, SCUK's strategy may be described as being primarily one of focused cost leadership, with some attempt made at differentiation through quality- and customer-focus. The extent to which this espoused strategy was likely to have any long-term positive benefit was hard to gauge: the directors of SCUK were narrowly focused on immediate operational needs and problems, and evidently found it hard to take a long-term perspective.

The future

According to Sir Peter Holmes, then the chairman of Shell Transport & Trading, an unpredictable economic and political environment required that Shell seek to consolidate its position in the marketplace. As this case was being written the Gulf War had not long ended, the world economy was in deep recession, the effects of the 1992 single market legislation were unclear, Eastern Europe was in turmoil, and an

environmental protection act that could cost up to £1.5 billion in capital investment and as much as £300 million a year in additional running costs appeared likely to find its way on to the statute books. Some commentators were already beginning to refer to Shell as 'complacent', while industry analysts attempting to explain the Group's good showing in 1989 spoke of the organisation's luck in not having had to deal with any major oil disaster,[6] and warned of the Group's dependence on an alliance with the Sultan of Brunei to export liquefied natural gas to Japan.[7]

Expectations for the future were difficult to read at SCUK. Most employees agreed that the 1992 Single European Act would have a crucial impact on the business, but no one could say what would change. While it was recognised that the industry was becoming more pan-European and that customers were looking for European rather than national deals, SCUK and its counterparts in Europe were still discussing how best to react to the new market. Senior managers in SCUK also recognised a need to conform with environmental legislation, but reflected that while 'green issues are important, so is the bottom-line in these difficult times'. Will SCUK be able to meet the challenges of the 1990s? The company's own publicity material leaves us in no doubt as to the senior management view of what was required:

In a world where something new is happening daily, ideas are not hard to come by. But selecting the ones which can be developed into successful business to augment the Shell Chemicals product portfolio calls for a mixture of astute judgement, hard-nosed logic and creative thinking: three qualities in high demand at our Business Development Centre (BDC). It is here, in this birthplace of business opportunity, that each fresh proposal is examined against a range of criteria. Of primary concern to the Business Development managers is the potential synergy that will develop between new opportunities and Shell Chemicals' existing activities. We need to know, is there a customer need? What about potential growth rate, competitor strength, likely market size? No one has the monopoly on innovation and in recognition of this, an invitation to all Shell Chemicals' staff has been issued. Entrepreneurial energy must be harnessed and all staff have received the call to action.[8]

251

Epilogue

As a matter of fact, many of the difficulties faced by Shell Chemicals UK wre also being experienced by the three other chemical companies in Europe (Shell Chimie in France, Deutsche Shell Chemie in Germany, and Shell Nederland Chemie in The Netherlands). Analyses of the trading environment conducted in early 1994 suggested that the European chemicals industry was suffering from too many small players, over-capacity, and a lack of competitiveness worldwide. This was reflected in Royal Dutch Shell's continued reported losses on its European chemicals operations (£409 million in 1993). Shell's response was announced on 24 February 1994, namely to restructure its European chemicals businesses with a single new company called EuroChem being created to oversee the European petrochemicals operations. This was recognised by analysts as an abrupt departure from Shell's traditional practice of granting full autonomy to local divisions. The policy was, it appears, forced upon the company by the need to cut the costs of supplying the market, and to deal with issues such as pricing and capacity on a Europe-wide basis. Some executive functions, such as sales and marketing, were to continue under the control of the four local companies. These events led some commentators to argue that industry and market forces are often more potent than those exerted by an organisation's culture.

Questions

1 Briefly characterise SCUK's organisational culture.

2 Give a concise overview of SCUK's objectives and strategy.

3 Use the Schwartz and Davis matrix to assess the degree of risk Shell's strategy implies.

4 What aspects of SCUK's culture will help, and which will hinder, the organisation's attempts to successfully pursue its strategy?

5 'However good and appropriate an organisation's culture is, environmental factors are always a more potent force affecting the formulation and implementation of strategy.' Discuss with reference to SCUK.

6 What short-term and long-term recommendations would you make (1) to the board of SCUK and (2) to Shell UK?

NOTES

1 The view that there is no real distinction to be made between *culture* and *strategy* seems to be attracting increasing support. Dalmau and Dick (1991: 4) for example, have suggested that 'strategy, and structure, and culture are part of the same package, and require simultaneous attention'. Hennestad (1991: 30) has argued that 'the organisational culture constitutes the existing strategy or the *strategy in use* (or realised strategy)'. Bate (1994: 22) has theorised 'that culture and strategy are substitutable for one another'.

2 *Independent on Sunday,* 17 February 1991, p.10.
3 Ibid.
4 L.C. van Wachem, Chairman of the Committee of Managing Directors of the Service Companies, RDS Pamphlet, 1990.
5 'Making the Difference', SCUK publicity document.
6 The *Exxon Valdez* disaster had cost Exxon about $3 billion.
7 The future of Brunei seemed uncertain at this time.
8 'Making the Difference', SCUK publicity document.

CHAPTER 7

Integrative cases studies

Background to the company

Situated a few miles from the city of Lyon in the Rhône-Alpes region of France, the Renault Véhicules Industriels (RVI) site in Vénissieux is rumoured to be the biggest factory in the country.[1] RVI not only dominates the landscape, but also the local labour market. Like many large companies, it has provided employment for entire families. Although this is less marked in the present day, given the length of service of many of its employees, its legacy is still felt. The operation of an internal labour market, characteristic of many large French companies, contributes to long service records. Originally built to house around 12 000 employees, production of buses and coaches at the Vénissieux site currently requires the employment of a workforce of little more than 5000. This is a marked change from the description of RVI thirty years ago as a hive of activity, a 'human ants' nest'.[2]

Formerly Berliet, the company was established by the Berliet family in 1915, and was nationalised in 1945. The name Renault Véhicules Industriels, arose from the merger of Berliet and another vehicle manufacturer, Saviem in 1978, at which point the company began to specialise in the production of heavy goods and transport vehicles. Today, the RVI Group is an international company with a turnover of more than 25 000 million francs worldwide. Across Europe, Renault VI has nearly 10 per cent of the market for heavy goods vehicles. In France, it has more than 50 per cent of the market for coaches and close to 60 per cent for buses,[3] although this represents a reduction over the past 15 years.

At the Vénissieux site two series of buses and coaches are produced. Other factories on this site and elsewhere in the Rhône-Alpes region serve these, producing motors, electrical circuits and other components. In 1992, 2072 buses and cars were produced and sold.[4] Between four and five vehicles are produced per line per day. Buses and coaches represent only some of the enormous range of heavy goods and transport vehicles produced and sold by RVI across the world. This extends from school buses to luxury tourist coaches, from small delivery trucks to 38 tonnes heavy goods vehicles, with customers including the military, state services and industry. Neither has the technology developed by Renault been restricted to road transport; it has, for example, been used in the Paris Métro.

To a British visitor to the site, some of the ways people treat each other at work are particularly striking. Work colleagues greet one another by shaking hands, and a brief walk around one of the factories may involve twenty or more handshakes! My host on the tour was a man with 26 years' experience of working at RVI, so he knew a lot of people from his time as an unskilled shopfloor worker to his present job as a training assistant, but his behaviour was not unusual.

The language people used to refer to one another and about the jobs they were doing was also significant. New terms seem to be used alongside instead of replacing the old descriptions. One example of this is the use of the new terms 'agent de fabrication' and 'collaborateurs', together with the older word 'ouvrier' to refer to shopfloor workers. Interestingly, 'ouvrier' has recently acquired a certain stigma, and some managers considered it to have negative connotations. Similarly, words meaning 'cells' and 'teams' were frequently mentioned and seemed to indicate a change in managerial style and a re-emphasis on co-operation and teamwork, while at the same time the more hierarchical terms 'foreman' and 'supervisor' were retained. This may reflect current changes at RVI as the company moves towards cellular manufacturing.

Of the 5143 people employed at the Vénissieux site, more than 60 per cent are shopfloor workers. A further 31 per cent are categorised as 'techniciens', some of whom may work on the shopfloor as supervisors, for example, while others hold administrative positions.[5] Although not surprising, the lack of women in the heavy assembly areas was noticeable. Only 1.4 per cent of the shopfloor workers are women. Most of these women work in the component factories, for example assembling electrical circuit boards. This was explained by reference to the 'natural dexterity' of women that makes them particularly good at this kind of work, so much of their work was not formally recognised as skilled. A relatively higher proportion of more senior positions are filled by women, who constitute 11.1 per cent of 'cadres'.[6, 7]

Current concerns at Renault Véhicules Industriels

RVI considers itself to be at the forefront of technological development and innovative employment practices. Occupying third place in the world market for heavy goods and transport vehicles, it promotes an image of dynamism, adaptability and responsiveness in an international arena. This is evident in the company's dealings with its employees as well as with its external customers and suppliers. One lunch time in the canteen at the training site, there were a large number of people watching the RVI promotional video continuously playing in the coffee area, impressed perhaps by the glossy image of the buses and coaches, and by extension the company.

The old problem for managers – how to get the workforce to do what managers want them to do – is as keenly felt today at RVI in the era of enlightened human resource management as it was in the time when the company was reputed for regular industrial action. As one of the personnel managers I met commented: 'The big problem we have today is how to motivate people to work.' In the present day, the source of the problem is viewed by many as being the nature of the workforce, and working conditions themselves.

The workforce at RVI is often described as falling into two distinct populations: those workers between 40 and 50 years old who have at least twenty years' service in the company, and more recently hired young people, many of whom are quite ambitious and are interested in pursuing further training. The latter group is described as 'raring to go' but held back by 'the inertia of the system', and as a consequence some of them have left the company. In fact the average age of the Vénissieux workforce is 45 years, and around three-quarters are over 40. The average length of service stands at 22.5 years, including a significant number of people with between 30 and 40 years experience in the company. According to some managers, a majority of these people are content in the jobs they are doing, and performing tasks they know well. This reflects their motivation for their current work but some managers perceived an unwillingness on their part to develop and learn new skills. However, it is worth noting that the company has achieved very significant changes in production with its existing workforce. In many ways RVI already has the kind of commitment from its more established workforce that it tries to develop in its newer recruits. Most long-serving people expect to work at the company until they retire; they are loyal to Renault and proud of the high-quality buses and coaches they produce.

Of the two factories where each series of buses and coaches are assembled, one has been radically reorganised according to some of the principles of cellular manufacturing. Cells of around six workers are positioned at the six or so workstations along the line. The line is organised so that almost all of the work carried out on each section of a vehicle is done before that section is assembled onto the main body of the bus or coach. Ergonomic design has particularly contributed to the improvement in working conditions, and production time is reduced with the new cellular system, aided by training interventions. This contrasts with the way in which work is organised in the other factory, which has not yet been modernised. In this factory, the frame of the vehicle is assembled, after which everything else is fitted onto it. Consequently, fewer people can work on a vehicle at any one time as there is limited room inside it. Current plans to replace the series currently manufactured here will mean that all the vehicles will be produced on the same lines in the other factory, where the workstations can be modified according to the specifications of each vehicle, and superior working conditions can be provided for all those directly employed in production.

The idea of there being two distinct populations (or cultures) at RVI extends to cadres. There is a tension here between the younger cadres who have been accorded this status through formal qualifications (usually five years full-time higher education) and those who have perhaps twenty or more years company experience and have achieved the status of cadre through internal promotion. This tension was frequently commented on by interviewees. It is not just a feature of RVI but arises from the education system in France and the operation of an internal labour market in large companies. The average age of cadres is 41 years, although the age distribution is less skewed than in other categories of the workforce, with one-third of cadres under the age of 40.[8] However, such a tension is not always a negative experience for those working alongside colleagues from a different background. It frequently offers opportunities for fruitful and enriching collaboration.

There are particular aspects of the French employment system which may exacerbate the tension between the different populations identified above. Pay is calculated according to each person's 'coefficient', a figure which corresponds to the skills and competencies necessary for the job. These coefficients are established by the collective conventions for the metallurgy sector in the Rhône-Alpes region of France. Formal qualifications as well as skills and competencies are considered, which then determine a person's position in the employment hierarchy. There are five formal levels in the hierarchy, some with a range of coefficients within them. In the case of cadres within the same grade, there is some limited scope for the reward of individual performance, that is above the minimum salary which is determined by the national conventions pertaining to the employment of cadres. Exhibit 7.1 sets out the employment structure at RVI.

There are many problems associated with this system including the comparability of jobs, the recognition of skill, and more generally, the interpretation of the conventions. At all levels men earn more than women. This may in part be explained by the concentration of men in more senior positions at each level, coupled with the definition of certain jobs as skilled or unskilled. The Loi sur l'Egalité Professionnelle de l'Emploi requires the publication on an annual basis of the respective positions of men and women in the company, in terms of their jobs, salary and training. This serves as a useful mechanism to expose inequalities.

Exhibit 7.1
Employment at RVI

Level	Job	Qualifications	Coefficient
I	Unskilled worker	Primary education	175
II	Semi-skilled worker	Secondary education to age 16	185
III	Skilled worker/supervisor technicien	Secondary education to age 18	195–240
IV	Technicien	2 years' full-time higher education	260–290
V	Technicien	3/4 years' full-time higher education	305–365
Cadre	e.g. Engineer	5 years' full-time higher education	Minimum salary set by conventions

Training and human resource management

Training is a means of preparing people for change. (Personnel Manager)

Central to the model of human resource management are training and development. In 1992 RVI committed 4.3 per cent of the total salary bill on continuing education and training of the workforce, totalling more than 500 000 hours. In France large companies are legally obliged to spend 2 per cent of their salary bill in this way. RVI's spending far exceeds the average in companies in the metallurgy sector in France, which was 3.3 per cent of salary bills in 1992. At the Vénissieux site 3144 people had some kind of training in 1992, which represents just over 60 per cent of the workforce.[9] Of several companies visited in France, RVI had the most sophisticated training policies and practices, and offered the best opportunities for development and progression to its employees.

Training initiatives such as the 'Learning to Learn' programme have been aimed at unqualified workers to enhance their understanding of the tasks they perform. Many of these are long-serving employees. The merging of production of the two lines of buses and coaches into one factory means that assembly workers will need to know how to assemble more than the current range of vehicles, hence an emphasis on multi-skilling. Some of this training is obviously skills-based and the Learning to Learn initiative does result in a recognised qualification. According to the comments of interviewees, the training provided by RVI is impressive in terms of its range, content and outcomes. As one interviewee commented: 'It's true that Renault VI offers better training than other companies' (Designer). At the same time, RVI makes use of training interventions to foster the commitment of the workforce to management-led policy and cultural changes. That attitudinal changes are sought is not surprising in the context of the current emphasis in companies generally on the effective utilisation of human resources, and does not detract from the impressiveness of the training opportunities the company offers.

In discussions with a training assistant who organised training for 1000 shopfloor workers, I was impressed by the systematic evidence he showed me concerning the identification of training needs. With a quality manual open on his desk showing a flow diagram of the needs identification process, and the training record of each employee available on his computer screen, his commitment to developing the workforce was unquestionable. An example of similar commitment is of a manager reputed to say, 'I have succeeded when my colleagues move to another department'. For him, training and development were an integral part of daily work. However, problems do arise, as reflected in the following comment:

> It [training] depends on the goodwill of the boss. I have several bosses, a line manager, his line manager, etc. It's a lot of people to persuade when you want some training. It's the most senior who makes the decision. He knows us but he's not someone we have a lot of contact with in our work. (Designer)

Furthermore, as part of human resource management initiatives, line managers have been made responsible for the training and development of their staff. Some of the managers consider that they have not been adequately trained to advise and make decisions about other people's development, something they must do as part of the annual appraisal system. Appraisals are very important as they are not only concerned with the evaluation of performance and decisions about training, but are also formally linked to salary.

Overall, RVI has achieved an average of thirty hours training per person per year. Newly recruited cadres may receive 100 to 150 hours off-the-job training per year, including personal and professional development, from communication skills and time management, to personnel management courses. Senior positions in the company are filled by highly qualified people, many of whom have an engineering qualification (based on five years' full-time study). These people are then trained to perform personnel as well as technical functions, hence the high levels of investment in training. This compares favourably to similarly high levels of training for other categories of new recruits: for example, those working as apprentices, on courses leading to a formal qualification and/or recognised skills, or retraining for a change of function. In all functions and levels, the need for such high levels of training is most acute upon initial employment or at a time of major change within the company. It therefore varies according to the different stages of a person's working life.

Training and total quality

The idea is to motivate people, to involve them in their work. (Personnel Manager)

Total Quality Management (TQM) has been given a high profile recently at RVI. Quality initiatives are promoted by the quality division which is separate from Direction des Affaires Sociales where the personnel and training functions are located. For the introduction of total quality management, company-wide meetings of up to 200 people at a time were used as a forum to familiarise the workforce with some of the principles of total quality. For example, the idea of customers and suppliers within the company has been emphasised. TQM has been cascaded throughout the company with reference to two concepts. The first, referred to as QDC, is based on a model represented by a triangle with a letter at each of its points: Q for quality, D for deadlines, C for cost. This is intended to make people aware of the relationships between quality, time and money. Secondly, the 12-stage model of total quality is what it suggests, an attempt to promote total quality through 12 defined points. The way in which some of these initiatives are translated into everyday activities was evident during a tour of one of the factories. By each workstation there was a quality chart where the number of mistakes found in each assembled section was noted next to the name of the person responsible for finding a solution to them. Introduced in 1981, the ongoing success of quality circles is evident in the creation of an average of 400 new ones each year. In 1992, 500 quality circles and around 750 Continuous Improvement Groups were in existence. The opportunities these groups offer are valued by many employees: 'The Continuous Improvement Groups allow group cohesion to develop and offer them [participants] the chance to work on something that involves them' (Cadre).

Total Quality Management is notoriously difficult to implement, and at RVI it has not yet involved all employees, as the following comment suggests:

> As far as cadres are concerned total quality is integrated. On the other hand, the problem of Renault VI is there are people in high positions who reflect on policy initiatives who make decisions about them and who set things in motion . . . I think that at Renault VI today we're going too quickly, it goes down to a certain level then at the bottom . . . people don't know anything about it. (Cadre)

Clearly, issues of quality and the implications for working practices such as enhancing motivation and commitment, and facilitating communication, are high on the agenda at RVI. Widespread support for such measures and a genuine transformation of labour relations is not yet secure. However, in the context of an average failure rate of two out of every three TQM projects in work organisations, Renault VI is making much progress.

Into the future

At the time of going to press, media attention has focused on the failed merger plans that Renault has developed with Volvo. The breakdown in merger proceedings has massively increased the uncertainty concerning the future of the Renault Group, including RVI. A further complication is that it has now become clear that the French government is serious about privatising Renault in the near future. Thus not only has RVI lost the opportunity of becoming the world number one producer of heavy goods vehicles (by allying with Volvo), but its medium and long-term prospects are as difficult to predict as the intentions of French politicians.

RVI has developed a number of prize-winning vehicles in recent years, yet some argue that the company does not utilise its workforce to the full. It needs to find a way of maintaining the commitment of its established workforce while continuing to transform itself into the more dynamic and responsive company its management would like to see, to develop its competitiveness.

Questions

1 Provide an overview of RVI's organisational culture.

2 Is there anything 'typically French' about RVI's culture? Illustrate your answer with information from both this case and your general knowledge.

3 What subcultures are evident within RVI? Are they supportive, conflicting or orthogonal?

4 Is motivation of the workforce a substantive problem for RVI?

5 How successful do you think RVI's quality initiatives have been so far?
  How do you account for any problems you have detected?

6 Are you confident about RVI's long-term future prospects? What recommendations for change would you make to the board of RVI?

Acknowledgement

This case study was composed by Ms Dawn Lyon, School of Continuing Studies, the University of Birmingham.

RENAULT AND VOLVO: A BROKEN ENGAGEMENT

Introduction

In early September 1993 the financial press reported that a merger between the French and Swedish vehicle groups Renault and Volvo was imminent. These press reports generated considerable excitement within the automotive industry, with analysts suggesting that the merger would create one of the four biggest car groups in Europe and the continent's second-largest truck group. Even at this early stage, however, some cautionary notes were sounded, not least by those who predicted that reaching an amicable decision concerning the division of ownership might prove 'a thorny problem'. Three months later, on 6 December 1993, the *Financial Times* reported that: 'Volvo and Renault are like two lovers who cancelled their wedding on the eve of the ceremony. Now they have to pick up the pieces of their broken relationship and see what can be salvaged.'

To many observers the failure to achieve a deal was perplexing: after all, there had seemed to be an overwhelming strategic case for merger. Other commentators suggested that what had been witnessed was the power of national and organisational cultures to undermine and overwhelm the dictates of commercial logic and strategic need.

Volvo in France

In 1982 Volvo sold 10 000 cars in France. In 1986 Volvo's sales had climbed to 21 000 despite a 20 per cent fall in the size of the national market. This success, led by Goran Carstedt, may have infused Volvo with the belief that French culture was sympathetic to co-operative Swedish working methods. Before Carstedt it had been argued that France, being a hot-blooded, passionate, Latin nation would not purchase Volvos – the product of cerebral, melancholic Scandinavians. This simplistic analysis was soon discredited.

According to Carstedt Volvo incorporated much of the spirit of Swedish culture, which embraced individualism but tempered it with a concern for the welfare of others. This translated into an insistence on the decentralisation of authority and initiative in the workplace and a preoccupation with building safe products. Research conducted for Carstedt showed that, contrary to popular belief, reliability and safety were in fact the two most important factors for the French in deciding what car to purchase. The problem of low car sales was thus not one of cultural incompatibility but of communicating the message, to both French car dealers and the general public. Carstedt responded to the challenge by introducing a regional organisation which allowed Volvo France to build up close relationships with dealers while initiating a major marketing campaign to entice the French public to buy Volvos. Within the organisation, French attitudes to authority were also considered to be part of the problem by Carstedt, and managers were encouraged to be more flexible, less deferential, more inclined to share information, and encouraging of subordinates to shoulder responsibility.

The stunning impact of Carstedt on Volvo's fortunes in France was, however, short-lived. Once he left to head up the American division in mid-1986 market share fell back to the level of 1983, and commentators suggested that under 'normal' conditions organisational cultures may have a tendency to revert to the form most typical of their macro-culture. This said, it nevertheless seemed that Carstedt had provided ample evidence that French and Swedish organisations could work together for their effective mutual benefit.

Renault and Volvo: a history of co-operation

Co-operation between the two groups began in 1990, and was followed in 1991 by an exchange of sizeable (but minority) cross-shareholdings: AB Volvo gained a 20 per cent holding in Renault SA, and Renault obtained both a 25 per cent stake in Volvo Car and a 45 per cent interest in Volvo Truck. During the three years of their alliance a considerable number of joint projects were initiated. For example, work was undertaken to develop a common platform to replace the Renault Safrane and Volvo 900 series, Renault's Laguna model was designed to accommodate Volvo engines, and Volvo made use of Renault engines and gearboxes in its 400 series. Joint quality and purchasing bodies were also established, based jointly in Paris and Gothenburg. The purchasing body was set up in January 1993, and aimed to increase joint procurement from 20 per cent of the estimated FFr 85bn ($14.4bn) of combined total purchases to 80 per cent. Both the purchasing and quality control organisations were designed to achieve substantial cost reductions. Other areas of co-operation included joint distribution agreements.

Co-operation, however, had a price. Towards the end of 1993 industry analysts became increasingly alarmed that the advantages of co-operation were being lost due to the cumbersome bureaucracy of Franco-Swedish joint corporate committees, which seemed to be running the alliance. In addition, there were indications that disagreements concerning how savings and profits should be allocated between the two organisations had developed. Furthermore, factional in-fighting had become a way of life. Some of the many powerful committees included the joint policy general committee (JPGC), joint car technical co-ordination committee (JCTCC), the joint truck technical committee (JTTCC), and the economic interest groupings (EIGs) for purchasing and quality previously mentioned. This commercial sluggishness had alarming bottom-line implications, leading Louis Schweitzer, the chairman and chief executive of Renault, to argue that: 'The advantage of a complete merger is simplicity and speed. Agreement between two companies does not go as fast as managing a single group. Speed is of the essence, we must go beyond the limits of the co-operation to date.'

The impetus for merger

In the early to mid-1990s the European motor industry was in a depressed state. Part of the reason for this was that Europe had become the battleground of the world auto industry, as the Japanese car makers followed their dramatic incursion into North America during the 1980s by building another regional production base in Europe during the 1990s. Even before the Renault–Volvo deal was mooted there had been a restructuring of the industry along national lines, with smaller producers picked off by larger players: in cars, Jaguar by Ford, Saab by GM, Seat and Skoda by Volkswagen, and Alfa Romeo by Fiat; in trucks, Pegaso and Ford Trucks by Iveco, Steyr by MAN, and Leyland by Daf. A further pressure on European automotive manufacturers was the threatened expiry of the transitional period to a free car market by the end of 1999, when all restrictions on Japanese car and light commercial vehicle imports were supposed to be removed.

Given the nature of the competitive environment, the motives behind Renault and Volvo's original decision to forge an alliance are clear: both were driven by the need to survive. While Volvo had struggled back into the black in the first six months of 1993 this was only after three years of painful restructuring that included a cut of nearly a fifth in the workforce of its car operations, the planned closure of two car plants in Sweden and the closure of a truck plant in the US. In 1990 the company had made a small loss. This was followed by meagre profits in 1991 and yet another (this time hefty) loss of SKr 3.3bn ($406m) in 1992. By contrast, Renault had performed rather better, having returned profits of just under FFr 2bn in 1990, just over FFr 4bn in 1991, and FFr 6.6bn ($1.13bn) in 1992. These gross figures, however, disguise as much as they reveal. In the first six months of 1993 it was clear that Renault had suffered an 87 per cent year-on-year drop in pre-tax profits, and had been in loss in the final quarter of 1992.

The advantages of a full merger were most usually expressed in terms of economies of scale and reduced costs. Continually updating a product range in the automotive industry is not just commercially essential but time-consuming and expensive. For example, in September 1993 Volvo launched its new flagship heavy truck range, which took seven years and an investment of SKr 6.6bn (£530m) to develop. Smaller companies, squeezed by intense competition, were predicted to find it increasingly difficult to sustain this level of investment. A new Renault–Volvo group with a combined turnover of about $41bn and complementary positions in the car market thus seemed an attractive proposition.[10] Within the European market such a group would move into fourth place, leap-frogging both Fiat and Ford, with 12.1 per cent. In the commercial vehicle industry the merged group would be even more powerful, with the capacity to challenge Mercedes Benz for world leadership in heavy trucks. Furthermore, Volvo and Renault publicly proclaimed that the merger could generate savings of about FFr 30bn (£3.4bn) before the year 2000 as costs would be shared over a larger volume of production.

Storm clouds gather

On 6 September 1993 the shareholding arrangements for the proposed new group were revealed. What had begun in 1990 as a 50–50 alliance between equals emerged as a 65–35 per cent arrangement in favour of Renault. This corresponded to the relative worth of each partner as valued at the time.[11] Initially there were some encouraging signs. Volvo's head, Mr Gyllenhammar, had kept the Swedish prime minister, Mr Bildt, abreast of the negotiations, and Sweden's centre-right government soon gave its blessing to the full merger, with a senior official asserting that: 'Volvo is very important to the Swedish economy, but this is a market-oriented government . . . . Our view is that Volvo as a private company must do what it thinks is right for Volvo.' Most independent analysts in Stockholm also viewed a 35 per cent share for Volvo as a reasonable outcome. The French government, which owned a 79 per cent stake in Renault, also seemed happy with the merger, though probably only because French interests would be dominant. By this time Renault and

Volvo were embarked on a publicity campaign designed to smooth the way forward for the deal. Volvo's position was that 'if people look at this in a neutral way they must see that it is the best deal for shareholders, given the alternative of a future on our own'.[12] Mr Schweitzer of Renault succinctly expressed the French view as being 'we have offered a fair deal'.

Opposition to the merger and doubts about its long-term future were quick to emerge. Those dubious about the deal employed two different sorts of argument in their attempts to block it.

What is a Renault share worth?

Swedish shareholders (mostly institutional investors) were acutely aware that Renault was one of 21 state-controlled enterprises that the French government intended to sell. The French view was that the merger was a necessary precursor to privatisation. The Swedish shareholders objected that as the company was to be sold after the merger, so it was not currently possible to assess the market value of Renault. This was considered important because Renault was seen as effectively making a bid for Volvo's cars and trucks, a bid that was to be funded by offering Renault shares. Furthermore, the French government intended to retain a golden share in Renault. This was interpreted by Swedish investors as a 'poison pill' which would lead to a discount in the share price of the merged company, devaluing the worth of the deal to Volvo shareholders.[13]

Would a full merger work?

Industry analysts were quick to point out the scale of the difficulties involved with the merger. First, it was argued that it took the Peugeot group more than a decade to rationalise and integrate its Peugeot and Citroën ranges, that Renault and Volvo had already experienced problems trying to win synergy gains from their truck operations, and that therefore more problems could be expected. Second, basic cultural problems were anticipated. It was pointed out that when Peugeot and Citroen merged they at least spoke the same language, but that Volvo and Renault would be forced to resort to English as the group's common language. More thoughtful commentators argued that as French and Swedish attitudes to basic management variables like authority, delegation and uncertainty were very different, so a whole new organisational culture that spanned national divides would have to be created.

Outcomes

Volvo and Renault originally hoped that the merger could be officially announced before the start of the Frankfurt motor show on 7 September. However, it soon became clear that the agreement would not be signed in time when Volvo shareholders forced a postponement on the vote. Swedish investors then continued to demand more information on the French timetable for privatisation and the golden share, arguably in an attempt to force the French government to make concessions. Evidence of the importance of the deal to the French was Mr Gerard Longuet's (the French industry minister) telephone call to Mr Per Wersterberg (his Swedish counterpart) in order to clarify the French position: privatisation of the merged group would be quick and the golden share would not be abused. As far as the French were concerned Swedish opposition was the result of a lack of information. Armed with such reassurances, and promises that changes to the deal could still be made, Volvo's leaders sought to talk their shareholders round.

A 'difference in emphasis' was now apparent between Renault and Volvo, with Renault insistent that the agreement would not be renegotiated and Volvo aware that some new concessions would be required for the merger to succeed. Both sides faced severe difficulties. Renault and the French government found it politically impossible to be seen to bow to Swedish pressure, while Mr Pehr Gyllenhammar, whose flamboyant style had won him enemies as well as friends among shareholders, was being portrayed as selling-out Sweden's industrial crown jewels to foreigners. Some elements in the French press did not help by talking about 'L'absorption par Renault'

rather than 'fusion' (merger). Mr Schweitzer was also criticised. It was argued that he did not help matters by failing to offer to relocate the merged group's headquarters rather than maintain it at Renault's existing HQ in western Paris. It was further suggested that he should have offered to staff the HQ using people chosen on merit and from a wide range of nationalities in order to quash fears that it would be dominated by the French. Neither suggestion was adopted.

If the merger was to proceed, then it was apparent that much depended on Mr Schweitzer being able to convince Swedish shareholders that Renault would be a benign senior partner. Having been educated at the Ecole Nationale d'Administration,[14] and with a training in logic and debate, Mr Schweitzer seemed likely to possess the required skills. But faced with what was obviously a difficult situation, in which the negotiations were clouded by emotion and national sensitivities, it was questionable whether a training in logic and his treasured belief in the power of reason were sufficient. One definite overture he did make was to assert that: 'It is in everybody's best interests that Volvo should not lose its identity, nor its homebase. That would be crazy, that would not be sound management. You must keep a strong base in Sweden, technically and in manufacturing.'

However, it was evident that he found it difficult to appeal to his crucial audience (Volvo's shareholders) direct, claiming in a report published on 29 November that 'I have no reason to say I know Swedish shareholders better than Volvo does'. A few days later the proposed merger had been cancelled with little hope that the deal would ever be resurrected. Mr Soren Gyll, the chief executive of Volvo had led a management revolt that not only doomed the merger but led to Mr Gyllenhammar's resignation.

Looking back to the future

With the plans for merger finally scrapped a large number of issues became open for wider debate. Some observers argued that the failure to reach an agreement was symptomatic of Sweden's national self-doubt and uncertainty about joining the European Union. The *Financial Times* considered that the fiasco illustrated the dangers of mixing national politics and legitimate business matters, and recommended that if both parties could keep politics out of business, then a union would still remain the best way forward. Mr Gyll revealed that there had, in recent weeks, been growing dissent within Volvo among engineers, white collar workers and a number of senior managers. He further disclosed that he had held a meeting with senior managers at his home at which it had become clear that a successful merger was unlikely, and that he had received a letter signed by 25 senior managers which advised him that the merger should be abandoned. With emotions still running high Mr Gyll gave his thoughts on the way forward:

> Now we are back in the position where we should consider if we can build the alliance for the future. I mean we could create some joint structure if we want – with 50–50 ownership, for example. It's a question of whether Renault still have a trust in Volvo, because we know we have failed to deliver.

Epilogue

In the aftermath of the failed merger, Volvo made a net loss of $434 million, largely due to the huge costs involved in dissolving the ambitious cross-ownership scheme with Renault. With sales surging, however, the company soon began reporting respectable profits, and by mid-1994 Volvo was becoming increasingly attractive to foreign investors who then owned 28 per cent of the equity. The almost universal feeling among industry analysts was that Volvo could expect to perform well in the medium-term (5–6 years), but that eventually it would need to find a partner or purchaser. Rumours in the press sought to link Volvo to companies like Chrysler and Mitsubishi. Indeed, Volvo did become involved with Mitsubishi in a car factory located in the Netherlands, and in 1995 formed a joint venture with the British engineering company TWR in order to produce convertibles and coupes. Despite a strong financial performance, speculation tinged with a fair degree of concern regarding the long-term prospects of Volvo continues to reappear in the business press.

With the proposed merger with Volvo no longer an option, resurgent French nationalism threatened to undermine the government's privatisation programme ('why should we – the French – relinquish control of Renault, one of Europe's most profitable volume producers?'). Related to this, corporate policy at Renault now asserted the need, not for a marriage, but for a series of partial alliances with other car makers. Meantime both Renault and Volvo began disposing of each others' stock, a process that did not end until August 1997 when Renault finally sold its remaining 3 per cent stake in the Swedish company and Volvo cashed-in its 11.4 per cent in Renault. Both companies made significant amounts of money from these and other sales of their ex-partner's shares. In 1994 a partial privatisation of Renault was accomplished, with the State's holding reduced from 79.02 per cent to 50.1 per cent. However, with the maket for Renault products becoming ever less friendly, full privatisation, despite constant rumours, was put on hold.

Questions

1 How do you account for the dominance of the myth that Volvo could not do business in France?

2 From the information contained in this case and your own general knowledge compare and contrast the national cultural characteristics of France and Sweden as they relate to management practice. You may find it useful to refer to the case studies of Renault Trucks (see p. 251) and IKEA (see p. 238) in answering this question.

3 How do you account for the failure of Volvo and Renault to merge? How important were (a) national culture; (b) organisational culture; (c) politics; (d) leadership?

4 Using the Schwartz and Davis model (see p. 213) for assessing the degree of cultural risk associated with a strategy, in which quadrant would you place the merger strategy for (a) Volvo and (b) Renault?

5 What lessons can you draw from this case that may be of use to executives contemplating cross-national mergers?

Acknowledgement

This case was compiled from the following published sources: *Financial Times*, 3 Sept. 1993, 17; 6 Sept. 1993, 26; 7 Sept. 1993, 19; 10 Sept. 1993, 13; 3 Nov. 1993, 24; 29 Nov. 1993, 14; 6 Dec. 1993, 1, 13, 17; 29/30 Jan. 1994, 9; and Hampden-Turner (1990).

TUDOR ROSE: A GLIMPSE OF ORGANISATIONAL CULTURE

On managing an old company

Change, reflected Robert Cecil, was sometimes disconcerting. Looking back over the last 18 months in Tudor Rose Insurance Company, Cecil was aware of frenzied activity and a dramatic upheaval in the operations of the company. Sometimes the new management policies had gone to plan, at other times unexpected consequences had occurred which in turn had demanded fast response.

Yet there was also something else. While Tudor Rose had clearly changed dramatically in several senses, Cecil was vaguely aware that in certain respects long-standing and deeply rooted elements of traditional management style in the company remained powerful and indeed even found expression through what were ostensibly efforts to refocus the culture of the organisation. Change, it seemed, could mask continuing traditionalism.

This was of direct concern to Cecil, since as an associate director to the main board, he had been appointed to manage strategic change in Tudor Rose, to foster management styles and operations which would allow the company to meet rapidly changing market conditions. Looking through his files now, Cecil remembered once more the circumstances which had prompted this attempt at organisational transformation.

Background

For several decades, Tudor Rose had operated as a large, well-established company in the UK financial services sector. With a nationwide branch network, powerful underwriting facilities and a large range of commercial clients, Tudor Rose generated reasonable profits and had emerged as one of the largest insurance players in the market. Despite this stability, or perhaps because of it, Tudor Rose had gradually evolved systems of working and management which were strongly conservative and occasionally monolithic.

Centralised control, centralised power had been the dominant motif. Careful and minute sanctioning of underwriting and policies from central headquarters at Hampton Court had been normal. One standing company joke had been that branch offices and regional management had autonomy over the paper clip budget granted to them on completion of 25 years' service.

The atmosphere and management style of the branches and regional offices reflected this theme. Managers and staff were organised in a fixed hierarchy of rewards, status and sanctions. Emphasis was upon the formal, with managers addressing subordinates by surname, and promotion based on length of service (usually depicted as 'experience' by senior managers) and conformity to the views of existing established office holders. All employees worked on mounds of detailed paperwork in sombre surroundings, with individual efforts daily checked and counterchecked by an army of supervisors. For years, ideas and orders came from the top. Others merely scribbled.

Catalyst

Two events, one immediate and dramatic, the other part of a larger change in the whole industry, had prompted the dissolution of this picture. In the first place, Tudor Rose had become the subject of a hostile takeover bid from Panillo and Panolli, an aggressive holding company bent upon asset stripping and rapid resale of the company. This bid had been discreetly rejected by the financial institutions, and in any case, analysts had argued that the existence of severe underwriting losses in the engineering sector of Tudor Rose's portfolio had acted as a 'poison pill', deflecting a serious bid.

Secondly, various legislative changes in the late 1980s had opened up previously unrecognised opportunities in the financial services market. Galvanised by panic generated by the Panillo and Panolli bid, senior management in Tudor Rose had realised that stable profits were inadequate to retain market share over the medium term. If the company was to avoid decline – and the dangers of another acquisition attempt – much less take advantage of the emerging market opportunities, the whole management policy of Tudor Rose needed radical review.

A plan . . .

Various steps were taken to encourage this process. The incumbent chairman, Sir Walter Raleigh, was encouraged to retire (a large retirement fee and a collection of mounted butterflies had been provided) and four other Directors had followed him. Replacement Board members had been appointed from internal candidates, with the exception of the new chairman, Thomas Cromwell, who was appointed from a multinational background, and Cecil himself, who had been given responsibility for marshalling the forthcoming changes.

Working closely together, the revitalised senior management had taken a first step of commissioning a consultancy review of all the company's operations. The report had been undertaken by The Drake Consultancy Group (DCG), an international consultancy specialising in 'dawn raid' acquisition tactics. The DCG report had advocated two major steps:

1 a focusing of the company's attentions onto specific segments of the market, to ensure higher profitability;

2 a rationalisation of operations, with decentralisation of previously centralised administrative functions into regional branch centres.

. . . and its implementation

Over the last 18 months, Tudor Rose management had moved to implement the DCG report. Through a series of project briefs, glossy leaflets and video mission statements in which various directors engaged in question and answer sessions with pop stars and various media luminaries, senior management emphasised the need for change and adaptation, under the project title 'Sticking With It'.

The key themes in these policies had been a mix of decentralisation and specialisation. First, the company's sales and marketing efforts had been reorganised into 'channel focused' business units, concentrating in specific markets. This had required some transfers of staff and resources throughout the organisation. A much more drawn out process had been the effort to decentralise operations and reduce costs. This had involved several steps:

1 the creation of regional branch centres in important locations throughout the country;

2 the concentration of all administrative and support functions – MIS, accounts, underwriting and claims, training, and so on – within these regional centres;

3 the transfer of functions and some staff into the regional centres from local branch offices (some small subbranch offices were to be closed);

4 the devolution of various operational responsibilities from HQ at Hampton Court into the new regional centres. Important decisions on staffing levels, underwriting proposals, sanctioning levels and development within the region were now to be left to the new regional management cadres;

5 the new regional management teams – carefully selected for the task – were now directly responsible to an individual board director, who in turn had responsibilities for that specific region and some company-wide areas of management policy. Thus the regional team from south-west England, for example, reported direct to Richard Grenville, a director with board responsibilities as well as for computerisation throughout Tudor Rose.

The implementation of these policies had involved enormous effort and considerable logistical organisation. Some management staff had been transferred around the country to form the regional teams. Some staff, especially the more hidebound managers of the old guard, had been encouraged to retire, while redundancies had occurred in other groups. The formation of the regional teams had required the purchase of new premises in some cases, the closure of offices in others.

Overall the picture had been mixed and implicated by local circumstances. Nevertheless the objectives had been clear; in a recent video discussion with one well-known media personage, which had been widely distributed throughout the company, the chairman had declared these to be:

1 the concentration of commercial efforts onto profitable sectors of the market;

2 the reduction of operational costs by reducing administrative duplication;

3 the creation of the conditions whereby the new regional units and supporting branches could respond more effectively to localised market conditions;

4 the freeing of the central HQ for strategic, as opposed to tactical and administrative, management functions.

Reading the tea-leaves

Many of the steps entailed in 'Sticking With It' were still in process and unresolved. Nevertheless, at this point into the project, Cecil had felt it to be useful to undertake a progress review. He had been encouraged in this step by two factors: his specific reponsibility for stimulating and encouraging change in Tudor Rose, and the comments of senior managers which he had picked up as he travelled around various parts of the emerging network. As part of this review, Cecil had utilised the services of Ed Young, a confused academic from a major busi-

ness school, and reports from small management teams which he had set up to review the local effects of 'Sticking With It'. At the same time, Cecil kept up his own visits and sought information wherever he could find it.

The information from these sources had proved complex and sometimes contradictory. However, some recurring themes were evident, which suggested to Cecil that the implementation of 'Sticking With It' was raising some awkward issues. These varied in intensity and type, of course. Although Cecil was still unclear about how precisely to order the materials now available to him, he had made a provisional listing of the common themes into two categories: short term (operational) and long term (strategic). These lists – drawn from Cecil's confidential files – are recorded below.

Short-term (operational) issues

1. Variations on a theme

The total of the reports indicate that there are considerable variations in the markets and local social conditions across different regions of the new structure. These variations have had considerable impact upon the precise implementation of 'Sticking With It'.

Despite differences of detail, two extreme situations are evident in the reports. On one hand, the formation of the regional branches has entailed new premises, and the expansion of one branch into a regional centre. On the other hand, the transfer of branch staff into what is in effect a new 'greenfield' regional branch is not always possible, so that redundancies occur in the local branches, while the regional branch must very quickly recruit large numbers.

Where the regional branches are made up of new recruits it appears easier for management to instil the aims and objectives of 'Sticking With It'. Morale and commitment appear to be higher in these regions, with managers reporting few difficulties of motivation. With the opportunity to 'start from scratch' – new structure, new premises, new jobs, new staff – the traditional values of the old Tudor Rose are more easily replaced.

Outcomes are different at the other extreme. Here the regional branches are already located in what was previously the main office for the area. Few transfers of staff are necessary, so traditional social attitudes and values remain largely in place. Although management personnel may have been changed in these locations, the new teams are frequently made up of those with a background in the region and hence influenced by the old values, or they must work with established staff well rooted in that background. It is notable that managers report lower interest, less commitment, even mild indifference and hostility to the changes inherent in 'Sticking With It' in these branches. These managers themselves are more frequently traditionalistic and lacking in new ideas.

These are the two extremes. Most of the new regional branches and the local branches display a mix of these characteristics. Finally, there are the impacts of local socio-economic circumstances. The degree of commitment to 'Sticking With It', the levels of motivation among all staff, the speed and efficiency with which the operational changes are implemented, are strongly conditioned by:

1 *Buoyancy of local labour markets* Influencing labour supply to the new regional branches and/or influencing the extent that existing branch staff will transfer into the regional branches.

2 *Buoyancy of local market conditions* Where this is high, the marketing and business development role of the branches is easily undertaken. Where it is low, negative and dispirited responses are common. (For example, in one of the new 'greenfield' regional branches, located in an expanding city centre, decisions were taken to organise a sponsored programme through local radio networks, advertising company products and services through a competition. Interest and practical involvement in this scheme were very low from three outly-

ing branches of the region. Each of these branches was in a depressed local market, where business is extremely thin and difficult to attract.)

These points appear to have the following implications for the immediate implementation of 'Sticking With It'.

1 Although in retrospect it is obvious that different regions of Tudor Rose would face different market and operational conditions, this perhaps raises doubts about the wisdom of the blanket model of regionalisation in the DCG report. Is it feasible to have one more or less standardised operational network throughout the company?

2 If a standardised new model is the objective, there is a need to address the issue of pace. Some regions will be able to move fast down this road; others will lag. It is important to identify the causes of lag, assess their implications for performance, and act accordingly.

3 Over a period of time – without action – we may see the emergence of 'advanced' and/or 'backward' regions. What will be the implications of this for motivation, career structures, payment systems, and so on?

2. On ambiguity and uncertainty

Across all the new regions, one objective is the division of Service functions from Underwriting and Development. Different regions presently vary in their degree of advance toward this outcome, but ultimately the Underwriting and Development tasks will be separated from the Service roles. In some regional offices the division is also geographical, with the Service functions characteristically located in separate offices.

All reports suggest that there is expressed uncertainty about this step from several sources. The main concerns are threefold.

1 The separation of Service functions means a loss of control over complex and intricate cases by Development and Underwriting staff. Case

details may become easily 'scrambled'. Clients are faced with Development contacts for new policies and liaison, but a different set of contracts for Service queries. There may be communication and information processing delays. It is widely recognised that a separate Service function reduces duplicated effort, but there are fears that there are hidden costs of delay, internal communication and customer dissatisfaction. (Note that these views are usually put by Development and Underwriting staff.)

2 The new Service functions are sometimes regarded as likely to generate staffing problems. Respondents frequently comment that the new functions are 'paper factories', with routine and high volume work tasks likely to induce boredom and indifference among employees. The advocates of this view argue that these circumstances may well reduce commitment and – where labour markets are buoyant – a continuous staff turnover. Among Development managers especially, there is some feeling that the Service functions will be permanently hampered with semi-trained and changing staff, which will further slow down processing of documents.

There are also opposite views. Some senior managers and training specialists argue that Service tasks must be carefully designed to offer personal interest. Opportunities for customer liaison are the most frequently mentioned. Similarly, Service staff may need to be selected on criteria of their suitability for routine work.

3 The increasing emphasis throughout Tudor Rose on profitable growth and development is sometimes viewed as importing glamour and rewards to certain functions rather than others. The role of attracting and capturing profitable business for instance is viewed as putting the broadly developmental and underwriting functions into the spotlight, while some support and income retention functions (Claims, for instance), are viewed as lower in the prestige hierarchy. Some characteristic comments are:

> In summary, their job is to bring money in. Our job – my job – is more negative. I have to control

money going out. It's a different ethos if you like. Not so glamorous, but critical in insurance. And that's got to be recognised. (Claims Manager, Kent)

> Despite all the videos and all that, all the business development, there are other groups who do the quiet backroom work. Without that you couldn't survive. You couldn't generate profit. So the worry is that we might fail to reward the foot soldiers . . . (Asst Claims Manager, Wales)

In summary, there is uncertainty about the operational viability of separating the Service functions in terms of maintaining client satisfaction. Development and Underwriting personnel view the separation as reducing their control over functions which have an impact upon the performance of their own tasks. The actual jobs in the new Service functions will need to be carefully designed.

There is little firm evidence for any of these views at present. Regional branch reviews of documentation show only a rising trend of outstanding items, but many branches are at present still transferring functions into the regional branch, and the sheer logistics of moving may well cause delays which are only temporary.

3. On managers and their style

The management teams in the regional branches vary considerably in ability, history and preferred management style. As noted earlier, situations facing managers range from new 'greenfield' sites with virtually an entirely new personnel, to situations where new teams operate what are effectively the old autocratic styles associated with the company. In other cases, sustained efforts are made to ensure a dialogue with employees and to generate wide commitment.

Neither style is necessarily effective in all circumstances. However, the reports suggest that there is growing pressure upon the more open and participative styles at the regional branch level. As the regional branches expand; as new staff arrive or are transferred into these centres; as they increasingly take on the servicing of the outlying branches, senior managers are faced with maintaining contact with growing numbers and under the constraints of high work volumes.

In these cases, contact between senior managers and their staff in general becomes progressively fleeting, and the sense of team identity sought as one element of 'Sticking With It' declines. There appear to be several symptoms of this process. From leading a small unit – usually hand-picked, especially in the 'greenfield' branches – regional branch managers find themselves distant from very large numbers of new staff. Unable to have a full knowledge of the team, senior managers are dependent upon their assistants to manage staff effectively and to generate involvement and high effort. One example captures the theme:

> When we started here, you could integrate the whole team. It was possible to keep in touch easily with anyone, whatever their position or whatever they did, as individuals. You could know them as people. But over the last 13 months we've grown from 60 to over 240 people . . .
>
> There's no way I can keep a personal touch going with that number. It's a problem for me. I think we need to keep a good sense of team effort, everyone pulling together. But I see people in the corridor now, and you can see in their eyes something's wrong. I really wonder whether to intervene. I don't, increasingly I don't. I contact lower management and warn them. They do react; we're lucky, I have a good management team, but when I meet that person again, I can tell that somehow it still isn't right . . . Yes, it's a problem. I'm trying to switch off about it. (Archie Wolsey, Regional Manager north-east England)

This is a recurring issue across several of the reports. As the regional branches grow, the managerial style appears to be confronted with a classic 'span of control' problem. Increasing numbers, increasing tasks, prompt distance between managers and employees, militate against concerns to reduce the hierarchies of the earlier Tudor Rose, and prompt wider commitment and exchange of ideas. It may be that we are in the process of reproducing the monolithic routinised structures which 'Sticking With It' was concerned to dissolve.

4. Thin 'red lines'

The rationale for concentrating functions in the regional branches to avoid duplication of efforts/costs in the local branches is now well known. Local branches now operate largely a sales/marketing role, with reduced staff levels.

However, there are concerns about this policy in the reports. In particular, managers in the local branches and the regional centres emphasise that with staff spread so thinly in the former, they are vulnerable to staffing vacancies, from sickness, holidays, and so forth. In some local branches the situation is sufficiently 'tight' that the absence of a single individual markedly hampers process of work.

Regional branches have responded to this issue in different ways. In one case, management trainees are used as a reserve pool to be dispatched as emergency cover to local branches whenever needed. This has the advantage of increasing the experience of the trainee in a practical, local branch setting. From the viewpoint of the local branch, however, this outcome is not always satisfactory. In the region in question, the dispatched trainees have occasionally been inexperienced, so that the local branch have viewed their placement as worsening rather than lightening, their problem. 'Sometimes it's better to have no one in rather than someone who you've got to train up and supervise closely, even if it's only for a couple of days. It can be like having two left feet, if you know what I mean' (Branch Manager, Herts). This is an issue of some concern, since virtually all the local branch managers contacted could recount instances where sometimes serious errors were committed by inexperienced replacement staff covering for absent employees.

5. Pressures and preparation

The 'thin' staffing in the local branches is also reflected in some dilemmas of training. As part of the DCG report, and as detailed in the 'Sticking With It' project, local branch staff were to receive 'on the job' training, in new products, the new tasks, and so on. The training programmes have been co-ordinated by the training units in the regional branch centres. In order to implement this policy, individuals within local branches have been selected as branch trainers, and in conjunction with regional training personnel, have sought to implement training in their respective branches.

Many of the reports suggest that this policy has had distinctly patchy effects. Local branch trainers report difficulties in persuading branch managers to release staff even for short periods, to undertake training. The branch trainers themselves experience difficulties in getting release in order to train others or to liaise with regional training personnel, since training is an additional function added on to their existing tasks.

From their perspective, branch managers report that the work targets set by regional branches and their limited staff resources mean that it is difficult to release staff from immediate tasks in order to meet medium-term training objectives. This whole position is clearly exacerbated where staff are absent or being replaced. Apart from the subjective reports of participants, there may be some objective measures of this dilemma. Virtually all the branch trainers contacted in the reports note difficulties in persuading their managers to encourage training. Collected figures across the regions suggest a 32 per cent turnover in branch trainers. More significantly, a survey of regional reports suggests that during the summer months, when local branch staffing is stretched by holidays and so forth, training in the local branches virtually ceases.

Despite the emphasis upon continued change and development which is inherent in 'Sticking With It', it appears that staff training in the lower reaches of Tudor Rose is non-existent for four months in the year.

These points captured the more immediate issues noted by Cecil. In addition, he had constructed a series of notes concerning more long-term themes confronting the company. These notes are reproduced below.

Long-term (strategic) issues

(Confidential. Not to be released to other members of the board.)

The reports presented by Ed Young, and specialised management teams set up under my authority, have provided a picture of some emerging issues. To some extent these have confirmed my own observations from discussions in the regions, and the reports from my deputy, William Walsingham.

We should be clear that there are no clear issues here, only general trends which appear to be gradually emerging from 'Sticking With It'. Together they raise some deep issues concerning effective organisation and leadership in the company.

1 Integrating the regional teams

As a feature of the DCG report, the company is now concentrating its operational functions within regional branch centres, with local branches in support and HQ providing strategic overview.

Different regional centres are now at different stages in this logistical process of concentration. There appear to be three main stages involved:

1 formation of the new regional branch team, sometimes in 'greenfield' circumstances, sometimes with mainly extant facilities, materials and personnel;

2 transfer of functions from the local branches into the regional centre, and communication of new responsibilities into the local branches. This was/is a complex process demanding movement of functions while simultaneously retaining services to clients;

3 regular operation of the new structure once it is in place.

The intricacies of undertaking this three-stage process appear to have had different effects across different regions. In some – especially those beginning from 'greenfield' situations (largely new staff, new premises, and so on) –

the experience of struggling with these difficult issues, in circumstances of high workload, has generated a sense of shared identity among participants, in which association with their own efforts and the new regional grouping is strong. These pronounced group boundaries are also evident but less explicit where the regional teams are composed of previously established staff and/or utilise established premises and resources.

So in summary, the sheer efforts involved in implementing 'Sticking With It' over the last 18 months – the difficulties in managing the diverse operational details – have begun to foster a strong sense of team identity and common values among local and regional branch personnel. This has had advantages, more or less pronounced, in terms of high commitment, collective effort, adaptability, increased productivity, and so forth.

However, precisely as individual and group loyalties have focused in these new operational units, this process has begun to heighten cleavages *between* these units across the whole company. Consequently there is an emerging trend that integration between the regions may be weakening. At present these processes are not strong. There are no clear signs of interregional competition. Yet there is an 'unofficial' recognition by senior regional managers that they may occasionally benefit from 'putting one over' on other regions. Some of the more evident signs of this process are:

1 *Staff poaching*   There is some reference to regions seeking managerial talent from one another in the reports. Certain regions with a high record in management development and training are regularly 'approached' for applicants to managerial posts. The locus of these negotiations varies; sometimes these are informal contacts between senior regional managers who are asked to recommend talented people. At other times the individuals are approached themselves.

2 *Client poaching*   In theory, boundaries of regional operations are sharply defined, such that regions should not compete with one another for business. In practice, especially in the case of large corporate clients with multiple sites seeking to place business, local regional management may seek to negotiate with clients from beyond their own boundaries.

These are two instances of a more abstract problem. Ironically the exigencies of managing the difficult conditions of the last few months may have fostered strong localised allegiances which now need integration to ensure corporate collectivity.

2 Centre and periphery

This is a touchy subject. Sifting over the reports, plus the comments from various managers, it is clear that there are gathering tensions around the degree of decentralisation which would actually evolve out of 'Sticking With It'.

The intentions to devolve large decision-making powers down to regional management and even beyond have been strongly emphasised in the videos, the glossy reports, the management briefing and so on. The message has been that the old Tudor Rose style, with targets and operational directives formed in HQ and merely passed down as directives to the subordinate regions and branches, is over. Instead the 'Sticking With It' project has depicted regions as having high operational autonomy, with local management having wide powers within their localised domains, and HQ marshalling these within a broad strategic framework.

Furthermore the project has consistently echoed the need to create conditions for the release of local talent and ideas within regions and branches as well. Instead of ideas and orders coming from the top, senior management at HQ have emphasised the need to involve all staff members in decision making and to try to get their ideas coming up the organisational structure. An elaborate network of team briefings and management–employee meetings has been established – with greater or less effect – across the whole company. Openness and contribution to debate has been the statement of the day – the only way, management has argued, to avoid the rule-bound hierarchies which choked off growth previously.

This has been the rhetoric of 'Sticking With It'. Unfortunately there is some evidence to suggest that this decentralisation of powers is not occurring smoothly. That interests at the HQ levels may resist it and seek to retain controls which attribute them power. Again, evidence for this is so far sketchy, but some recurring themes are in evidence.

1 Despite the declared aim to give regional branch units strong underwriting autonomy, HQ has recently begun to impose sanction levels on some proposals. Regional units are finding that before they can underwrite proposals they must gain HQ clearance. Although the sanction ceilings are quite high at present, there is concern in some regions, and especially among underwriting specialists, that they will gradually be lowered, especially if the national economy becomes 'tight';

2 Regional management staffing policies are gradually coming under HQ influence and sanction. In one of Ed Young's reports for instance, he describes how senior regional managers from north-west England were formulating a manpower and training policy for the next 18 months. Two members of the board were present in this discussion, but they did not contribute. Ed Young reports his surprise when one of the board members later privately revealed details of a 'strategic human resources management plan' formulated at HQ which would set out these policies for the north-west management. This 'plan' went into considerable operational detail, and laid down personnel replacement targets and carefully listed training objectives for the period. Apparently these will be announced to north-west regional managers at a future meeting.

We should not make too much of these incidents. The elements of 'Sticking With It' are still moving through the system, and some regions will be quicker to respond to the new management style than others. Nevertheless it would be naive to imagine that after decades of centralised management control, various interests within the central HQ would be willing to relinquish their authority at the drop of a video. Indeed, there may be strong operational justifications for the maintenance of operational control.

What we may be seeing here, then, are various possibilities:

1 efforts by the HQ interests to gradually reimpose control systems similar to those existing before the DCG report. The point that it is underwriting sanctioning levels which have been imposed is significant in this respect;

2 this whole issue may highlight a carefully planned leadership strategy formulated at board level. The DCG report and the 'Sticking With It' project emerging from it may have been part of a constructed mission statement and a supporting set of images and rhetoric, designed to justify large-scale change, but with little real intention of achieving its aims of decentralisation.

From this perspective, senior executive management can be viewed as mobilising support and commitment to their policies by reference to different values, while yet seeking to retain, even to heighten, their power within the organisation. The decentralisation of functions to the regional branches, then, merely masks a greater concentration of control by the strategic elites. Of course, this raises interesting questions about the precise role of Thomas Cromwell too.

3 Twilight leadership

These points all suggest a particular assumption about present leadership and Tudor Rose. This is that a leadership elite exists, which by articulation of various norms, values, and so on, can control events; can generate legitimacy and mobilisation at will.

There is also evidence in the reports which is in almost direct contrast to this. There are various instances where HQ management, far from being the all-seeing, all-commanding leadership just previously described, are actually quite isolated from realities in the outlying parts of the network. Some illustrations of this might be as follows.

The 'over the hill' video

In recent weeks, the board has issued another video to all parts of the company, in which directors are interviewed by a team from *The Money Programme*. The theme of the video is that the main organisational changes are now largely accomplished: that Tudor Rose is now 'over the hill' of the necessary changes which it faced.

Intended as a morale booster and 'gung-ho' statement, the video was badly received virtually everywhere. Most of the regional officers were not 'over the hill' regarding the changes, but were, and are, still in the thick of the dislocations of the 'Sticking With It' project.

Comments that expenditure on this type of communication could be better utilised were rife. Even senior regional managers have indicated that this incident illustrates how the distance and poor communication between HQ and everyone else has merely continued under the new management policy.

The DCG report

Although this report had provided the basis for senior management planning, and the foundation for the whole 'Sticking With It' project, there is some concern in the regions that the study itself is superficial and based upon inadequate research.

In conducting the study, the DCG had not actually spent very much time in the regions and the operational units. There had been the occasional day's visit and 'study teams' of Tudor Rose managers had been established to identify important issues. Yet there is a view among some managers that the 'study teams' were really only designed to rubber stamp the DCG proposals and that the DCG had not itself undertaken deep study and did not understand the variations across different parts of the company.

The outcome – as several respondents see it – is that senior management at HQ are dealing with superficial information and do not even 'see' the issues confronting the structure of the organisation. The attempt to apply a blanket policy of regionalisation across the regional office is noted as one illustration of this. Increasingly, in this argument, the central leadership is 'out of touch with the trenches', so that the old style of company management is merely re-emerging again.

Changing societies

Although the DCG report has sharpened the awareness of Tudor Rose that it must continually review its commercial environment, the respondents in the reports suggest that there is uncertainty as to the degree that this has occurred. The example most frequently cited is the company's attitude to the building societies. While Tudor Rose is developing a segmented 'channel focus' approach, HQ responses to changes occurring within the building societies movement – the expansion of societies into home and personal insurance for instance – are ambivalent. The message from HQ appears to be 'wait and see'.

In the regional branches, however, management has various relationships with local building society outlets which they seek to develop. Uncertainty at the centre and perceived development opportunities at the regional level sometimes clash. One of the Midlands regions illustrates the dilemma. Here regional management had been aware of the entrepreneurial approach of one of the smaller local building societies, the Dudley Society. Responding to this, they have established various relationships with the society's management, mainly geared around sales of personal and household policies. In an effort to strengthen these further, Tudor Rose management had arranged for Dudley staff to take part in various broker and product training sessions. This news had not been welcomed at HQ. The Midlands region had been ordered to concentrate their training only on internal Tudor Rose staff and broker interests.

These are only small, isolated incidents, but they reflect a common theme. Among some regional staff there is a perception that HQ is somewhat distant from events beyond Hampton Court. Several recent events seem to reflect this. As a result there are gathering doubts about the effectiveness of HQ policy and credibility of senior managerial policies.

Some cracks

Finally, there is the issue of continued maximum effort. Over the last 18 months Tudor Rose has experienced considerable change. Virtually all staff have been required to work at full stretch, sometimes in circumstances of staff shortages (where personnel could not be quickly drafted into the new regional branches, for instance) and sometimes in conditions of uncertainty about their jobs. Staff have responded very well and performance is generally high.

There must be questions, however, as to whether the maximum required effort can be continued indefinitely. All of the regional management units report gathering strains in their own teams. Implications of the thin staffing levels in the local branches have already been noted. Moving around the regions there is the sense that everyone is exceptionally busy, that everyone is engaged in the intricacies of implementing the 'Sticking With It' project. Workloads are very high, with three of the new 'greenfield' regional units showing increasing staff turnover and absenteeism levels.

Ultimately there must be some drift in performance under these conditions. Similarly, with people so finely stretched, it is possible that developments occurring at local levels cannot be quickly identified and responded to. The outcome of that will be a company structure where strategic plans and decisions derive only from the top – no different, in fact, from the very process which 'Sticking With It' was intended to eliminate.

Postscript

Cecil's notes on this section end here. As he now reads them over, Cecil is aware that they contain some deep issues concerning change and leadership in Tudor Rose. They would require careful handling. Glancing through a recent copy of the (new) company newspaper, Cecil let his eyes rest upon the photograph of an urbane Thomas Cromwell on the front page . . .

Questions

1 Is the change programme an attempt to alter (a) the structure of Tudor Rose and (b) the culture of Tudor Rose? If so, what changes do senior executives want to implement?

2 How successful do you think the change programme has been so far?

3 How confident are you that the change programme will ultimately realise its objectives? Explain your answer.

4 Is 'Sticking With It' a new approach – or is it simply a repetition of the old pattern of centralised HQ control? What are the implications of your response to this question for future management policy in this company?

5 Is there a power struggle between Tudor Rose HQ and the decentralised regional branch management teams? Does your answer help to explain (a) the apparent incidence of centralisation (i.e. the sanctioning of new levels) and (b) the apparent incidence of insulation (i.e. the 'over the hill' video)?

6 What learning points are there in this case for those responsible for managing change in other organisations?

Acknowledgement

This case study was composed by Dr Ed Young, Health Services Management Unit, University Precinct, Oxford Road, Manchester M13.

THE MANAGEMENT OF CHANGE IN THE NHS: A STUDY OF THE RESOURCE MANAGEMENT INITIATIVE

We believe that a National Health Service that is run better, will be a National Health Service that can care better. Taken together, the proposals represent the most far-reaching reform of the National Health Service in its forty year history. They offer new opportunities, and pose new challenges, for everyone concerned with the running of the Service. I am confident that all who work in it will grasp these opportunities to provide even better health care for the millions of people who rely on the National Health Service.

(Margaret Thatcher, 1989)

Introduction to the NHS

Set up in July 1948 to manage and co-ordinate 2800 hospitals, by 1990/1 the National Health Service accounted for the second largest amount of Government expenditure (£23.3 billion), and with 1.25 million people on its payroll was the third largest organisation in the world. It was founded on six fundamental principles which effectively have not been altered over the past 43 years: (1) a separation of primary and secondary care medicine in which general practitioners provide frontline treatment and diagnosis while hospitals and local health authorities between them provide a comprehensive range of medical facilities; (2) health care is free at the point of consumption; (3) health care is paid for out of general taxation; (4) it provides a full and complete service from accident through surgery to provision for geriatric and mental care; (5) it is available to all; and (6) the Government is the owner and employer of staff.

The NHS is the responsibility of the Secretary of State for Health who has overall charge of it via the Department of Health which he or she heads. Under the Thatcher and Major Conservative Governments, the structure of the NHS was radically altered: purchasers in the form of GP fundholders and District Health Authorities (DHAs) were empowered to purchase medical care from provider institutions (hospital trusts) in a quasi-market arrangement. The Resource Management Initiative (RMI) was envisaged as facilitating this new organisational structure by improving the information and general management of hospitals. It is worth noticing that this newly rearranged NHS is now being subjected to a further series of restructurings by the Labour Government led by Tony Blair. These new alterations are primarily designed to limit the competitive practices that the market arrangements have introduced and are not, as such, an attack on the principles of good managment supposedly incorporated into the RMI.

Prelude to RMI

Since its inception the NHS has undergone a variety of structural changes, notably in 1974 and again in 1981 when the Government attempted to make it more accountable by means of annual discussions between Ministers and regional administrators. Continuing doubts at senior ministerial level concerning the NHS's efficient use of funds and effective provision of health care led to the commissioning of the *Griffiths Report* in 1983. Two of its most significant recommendations were that at each level (unit, district and region) a General Manager should be appointed to take overall responsibility, and that clinicians, who were then largely marginal to the management process, should be involved more closely in it. This latter objective was to be accomplished by a process of management budgeting in which clinicians would be provided 'with strictly relevant management information' which would facilitate 'some measurement of output in terms of patient care'.[15] A subsequent investigation of the impact of management budgeting in the four pilot sites where it had been implemented, by a team of consultants from Arthur Young, concluded that while some short-term advantages had been reaped, radical long-term change was extremely difficult to accomplish: 'Significant changes also require managerial revolution. They presuppose a willingness on the part of general managers to hire and fire, on the part of clinicians to change habits of a lifetime (e.g. treatment patterns, methods of training, medical teams, etc.).'[16] In other words, although considerable energy had been expended putting the technical systems in place, insufficient attention had been given to gaining the support of those individuals and groups on whom the success of the programme had depended.[17] After a further period of experimentation management budgeting was suspended.

The RMI

The Resource Management Initiative (RMI) was first announced in 1986 and subsequently piloted in six hospital and six community health service sites. The initiative was an integral part of a wide-ranging reform of the NHS, which allowed its hospitals to opt out of district control and become self-governing trusts, and imposed budgets on general practitioners, who would thenceforth advise District Health Authorities where to purchase hospital treatment in a deregulated internal market. With all the change programmes fully implemented, the budget-holding GPs would be free to refer their patients wherever they thought they would receive the best-quality treatment, giving them considerable power to make or break hospital units.

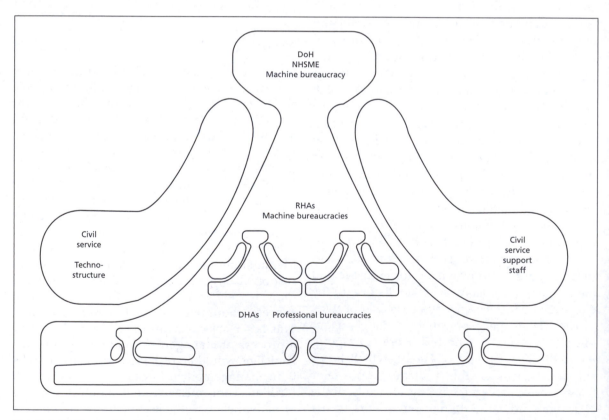

Fig. 7.1 NHS organisation structure
Source: reproduced with permission from Dearden, B. (1990)

According to various Government publications functions of the initiative were twofold:

1 to provide clinicians and other hospital managers with the information they required to use the resources they controlled to maximum effect, generally by introducing new information technology;

2 to encourage clinicians to take a greater interest and involvement in the management of the hospital and community units in which they worked, by making them responsible for the operational and strategic decisions taken in their place of work.

In other words, the Resource Management Initiative was going to help 'clinicians and other hospital managers to make better-informed judgements about how the resources they control can be used to maximum effect'.[18] The RMI was thus not only going to persuade clinicians to own the management process but to provide them with the accurate, up-to-date and relevant information they would require to cost medical activities and improve patient care. A multitude of Government publications suggested that the RMI would help clinicians identify areas of waste and inefficiency and those that could benefit from greater resource allocation, expose the health care consequences of given financial policies, and provide information that would inform the debate over future health care options. The response to this need to improve hospital information services was to develop and implement a sophisticated and extensive package of information technology called the 'Case-mix' system. Some important lessons had apparently been learned since the time of Griffiths and management budgeting, and documents explaining the role of the RMI emphasised that it would be a 'bottom-up' initiative involving the service providers at all stages in the design, planning and implementation process. It was also recognised that the fundamental organisational changes required by RMI and the other change programmes could not be imposed blanket-fashion on an organisation as large, diverse and heterogeneous as the NHS. Instead, each hospital unit was instructed to plan for the implementation of RMI on a local basis and in a way which best suited its unique structural features and cultural traits.

An overview

What follows is a series of impressionistic glimpses at some of the issues which those people most closely involved with RMI, either as implementors or as affectees, considered most significant.

The RMI project teams

The RMI project managers and their teams were mostly in very difficult political situations. On the one hand they were responsible for implementing complex structural and cultural change, had the backing of the Government and the overt support of senior NHS officials, and access to not inconsiderable funds. On the other hand, they were perceived by hospital employees as outsiders who had been 'bolted on' to their unit, they had few formal powers, and no means of enforcing change except through persuasion. The low esteem in which many project managers were held by virtue of the job they performed was often compounded by their lack of managerial and/or hospital experience. Two extremes are worthy of mention: in one hospital unit the project manager was extremely well connected with the decision-making hierarchy and RMI seemed to be making reasonable progress, while in another the project manager had only recently taken over the position and, what is more, had been appointed on a part-time basis. Interestingly, while many of the respondents interviewed for this case study implicitly touched on issues of 'leadership' and 'product championing', few recognised them as crucial to the success of RMI.

Clinician culture

The NHS in general and clinicians in particular had an identifiable, strong culture that many individuals regarded as being under threat from RMI. The points of conflict between RMI and employees' beliefs and values were several. First, the existing culture was primarily concerned with the quality of patient care, the maintenance of which was the concern of all. RMI, however, was generally viewed as a means of rationing limited resources that would have little positive impact on the quality of patient care offered. On the contrary, the view was expressed that the RMI was diverting valuable time and financial resources away from where they were most needed. As RMI was not perceived to be directly concerned with patient care, so this meant that clinicians felt they could legitimately ask the question 'What's in it for me?', and set about the task of negotiating terms and conditions, further complicating the process of policy implementation. Second, the clinician culture emphasised individual autonomy and flexibility of working practices, disregard for the formal hierarchy of management and respect for peers based on ability. Resource management was considered to be an attack on clinician integrity, as it dictated the need for strategic planning and budgetary controls that would systematise, rationalise and proceduralise the work of clinicians. This would effectively restrict their freedom to make individual decisions, and force them into collaboration not only with their peers but with administrators. Third, the clinician culture was one of high self-esteem and professional competence based on medical expertise not possessed by any other group. The RMI, which stressed the need for clinicians to learn new managerial skills, undermined their position as undisputed arbiters of what was good for patients, if not in the case of the individual, then at least for patients in general. In short, the RMI represented an attack on some of the central values of the NHS, and especially the clinician culture, that many had recognised in theory, but few had acted on to diffuse tensions and smooth the passage of change.

Structural reorganisation

The hospital units were undergoing considerable internal structural change. The Government model suggested that each hospital should be governed by a hospital management board to which would be answerable a number of clinical directorates, the directors of which would also have a place on the main hospital board. Each clinical directorate would probably be headed by a clinician, who would have the support of a business administrator and a nurse. These clinical directorates were destined to hold budgets of £2–£5 million, and would thus be responsible for resource allocation within a particular clinical specialism. The transition to clinical directorates was progressing slowly in the face of much resistance, limited funds and uncertainty. One primary concern for those appointed directors of the clinical directorates was that they were being given additional responsibilities without the authority they needed to control their peers. Structural reorganisation was, therefore, a political minefield which threatened to undermine a variety of entrenched interest groups, and in some hospitals employees were refusing to be co-opted into them.

IT systems

RMI requires the implementation of an integrated set of IT systems covering all aspects of hospital life, from planning patient care, recording treatments and tests, and ordering consumables, to stock and budget control, patient discharge and the co-ordination of primary health care (see Fig. 7.2 and 7.3). The introduction of these systems was still at an early stage, with no hospital possessing a fully developed and coherent set of IT systems. The most advanced hospitals had a variety of Patient Administration Systems, though these were usually able only to provide information at the ward level rather than that of the individual patient or doctor. In other instances the computer facilities that had been purchased were still in their original boxes. Some IT decisions, notably concerning the purchase of the main computer feeder systems, were taken at Regional Health Authority level. As the case was being written, firms capable of supplying the required systems were being selected and their equipment piloted. However, many IT decisions were also taken at the local unit level, and there was great divergence in approach to handling IT issues between hospitals: some had set up IT committees to co-ordinate purchasing agreements, while in others hardware and software were being purchased on an *ad hoc* basis with no concern for compatibility of specification. Even where IT systems had been set up these seemed to be prone to long downtimes due to insufficient maintenance support, itself a consequence of the low salaries paid in the NHS which impeded the recruitment of skilled IT staff. Furthermore some technical difficulties did not seem to have been thought through: for instance, while most clinical specialisms require a database that can store quantitative data, psychiatrists needed to be able to store large amounts of text. Add to these difficulties the poor communication, lack of training, technophobia, unwillingness to change work patterns, the changing balance of political power between young and old clinicians that IT seemed to invite, the general perception that the information the systems would produce would be of more use to accountants than to doctors, misgivings about patient confidentiality, and a host of other anxieties concerning change in the NHS, and the full scale of the difficulties involved with implementing RMI become apparent.

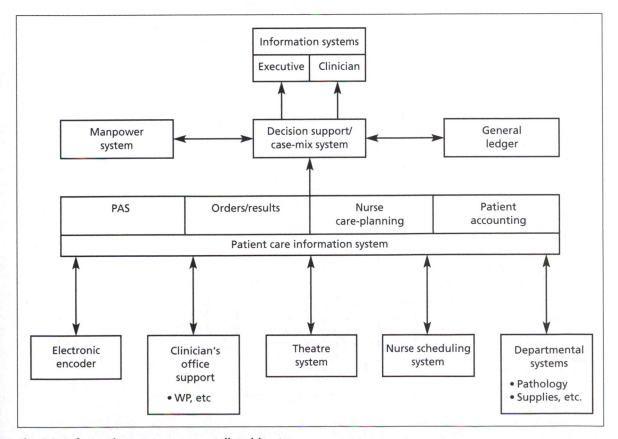

Fig. 7.2 Information systems – overall architecture

Source: reproduced with permission from original documentation by Victor Peel, HMSU, University of Manchester

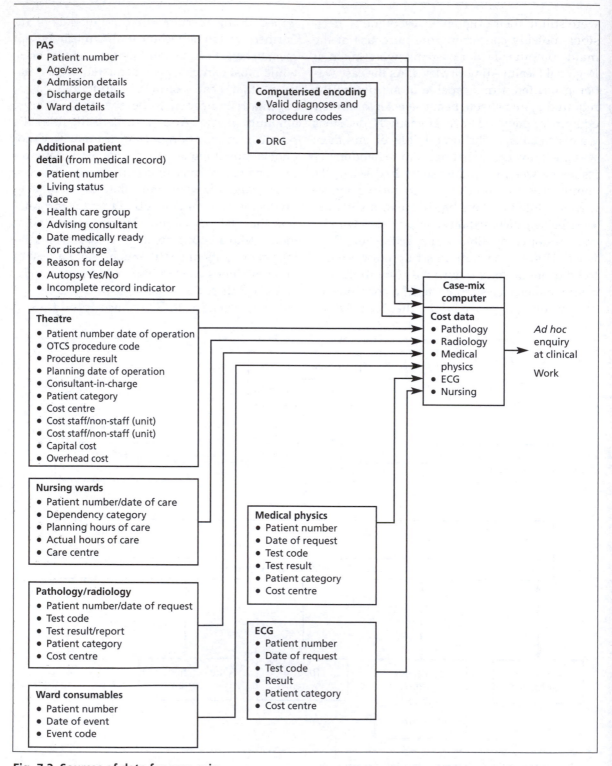

Fig. 7.3 Sources of data for case-mix

Source: reproduced with permission from original documentation by Victor Peel, HMSU, University of Manchester

Communication

One of the most striking findings of the study was the extent to which communications problems dominated individuals' accounts of the RMI implementation process. Even in those units where RMI was apparently well received by staff members, a variety of difficulties and inadequacies in information transmission were evident. While a few hospitals were characterised by too much formal written communication, mostly in the form of long and unprioritised circulars which had a tendency to get lost in the internal mail system and in-trays, and numerous time-consuming meetings, most were discovered to suffer from a dearth of worthwhile formal communication channels of any kind. Senior administrators and heads of departments were generally better informed than their subordinates, but even members of this cadre complained that the meetings they attended were often unhelpful and uninformative. Conversely, more junior members of staff had to rely on the standard video, sometimes supplemented by a few poor-quality seminars and leaflets, which did little other than raise their awareness of the fact that there was something called a 'Resource Management Initiative'. Most individuals' information concerning the RMI came by rumour and hearsay, and some RMI project teams, who had constituted almost no formal communication channels, seemed to rely entirely on informal networking to get their messages across. As a result, in some hospitals the various departments and the RMI project team were working on aspects of RMI in virtual isolation from each other.

The causes of these communications problems were many and varied. First, there were some problems that seemed to be 'intrinsic' to the NHS: job functions and patterns of work meant that everyone from nurses to clinicians were extremely busy people with little time to read circulars or attend meetings; the resources available to facilitate RMI were arguably less than adequate; and the nature, size and scale of

the communication task was vast. Second, there were problems associated with the hospital staff: substantial minorities of clinicians and nurses were openly opposed to the RMI, and were refusing to play an active role in making the initiative a success. And finally, there were problems associated with the RMI project team: some teams seemed unable to communicate adequately among themselves let alone to outsiders; few had developed comprehensive plans for disseminating information to those who needed or wanted it; and many teams appeared unable or reluctant to adopt the high-visibility leadership role that successful implementation of RMI was thought to require.

Morale

The level of enthusiasm for RMI varied considerably between hospital units and across internal hospital departments. Overall there was much support for the aims of RMI – for measuring outcomes, co-opting clinicians into the decision-making processes, instituting clear lines of responsibility, and generally 'making progress'. Levels of motivation were particularly high among senior administrators, staff in finance and IT departments, and others who perceived that they would personally benefit from the redistribution of power and resources that RMI entailed. This said, it should also be recognised that some clinicians and sections of the nursing staff held principled objections to the concept of RMI, which was seen as an 'external' Government programme and the first step towards a privatised NHS. The chief sources of discontent were, however, related to the mechanisms and styles by which RMI was being implemented in the hospital units. Many individuals, especially nursing staff, felt devalued and marginalised, while many clinicians were extremely ill-informed, apathetic, and possessed of numerous misconceptions. Perhaps the single greatest difficulty in maintaining high levels of staff morale in the face of the large-scale changes RMI entailed was the almost total lack of positive motivators (incentive schemes, bonuses for achieving targets, and so on) for most individuals. Thus, despite many individuals' receptiveness to change, poor leadership, planning and co-ordination by some of the RMI project teams meant that RMI was beginning to be recognised as yet another under-resourced, ill-conceived and poorly implemented programme of change that would ultimately come to have little impact on the effective working of the NHS.

Power, politics and conflict

While few, if any, hospitals have ever been apolitical, in those units where the implementation of RMI was being attempted, it was almost always accompanied by an increase in the level of political tensions. The traditional conflicts between clinicians and hospital administrators and clinicians and nursing staff were being accentuated by anxieties over budgets (which for many people were under threat), job functions (some of which were likely to disappear) and workloads (which were increasing). In addition, the appearance of RMI project teams had engendered a new set of political dynamics. The high salaries members of the RMI teams were rumoured to enjoy, the amount of secretarial support they employed and the seemingly limitless funds to which they had access won them few friends in the hospitals. Their privileged financial status, combined with their often uncoordinated attempts to implement a difficult series of structural and cultural changes which upset the status quo, placed many RMI project teams in impossible political positions. That these teams were answerable to the Unit General Manager of the hospital in which they operated, the Local Health Authority and the Regional Health Authority further complicated their positions. To some large extent, however, the RMI project teams were thought to be the architects of their own political problems: poor formal communication, little formal apparatus to facilitate conflict reduction, few attempts to involve junior members of staff or unions, and ill-conceived strategies for change all underpinned the conflict.

Understanding of RMI

The level of understanding of what RMI was, its implications for hospitals, and how it was being implemented was generally low. This said, individuals' understanding varied according to their position in the hospital hierarchy, the extent of their involvement with the RMI project team, and the department in which they worked, with those more senior people closely involved with the implementation of RMI, and the staff of finance, IT and medical records departments being best informed and most aware. The overwhelming majority of hospital staff considered RMI to be concerned with cutting costs, imposing budgetary controls, increasing efficiency, costing procedures, providing information and facilitating better decision making. In contrast, only a small minority of individuals, generally those occupying senior positions of authority with respect to RMI, identified the initiative as an attempt to change the organisation's culture and as a mechanism for improving patient care. In short, few individuals appreciated the full implications of RMI, and the fact that if it was to succeed a basic reorientation of beliefs, values and working practices was required. Furthermore, because most people conceived RMI as essentially a structural and procedural change programme that would do little to further key objectives, especially the improvement of patient care, confidence in and enthusiasm for it were more muted than might otherwise have been the case.

Resistance

There was considerable resistance to RMI from clinicians, nursing staff and hospital support staff. While the grounds for resistance were varied, the following generalisations can be made. Clinician resistance was motivated by fears that the real objective of RMI was to increase efficiency, possibly as a first step towards privatisation, and that the quality of patient care would be adversely affected. The resistance of the nursing staff was underpinned by fears that they were losing both status and control over budgets, while being required to work harder, especially with regard to the new technology, for which inadequate training had been given. Other hospital support staff were resistant to change for a variety of reasons, including ignorance, the absence of a feeling of 'ownership', fears that those departments not easily evaluated (such as Rehabilitation Services) would suffer undue budget cuts, and that unfair comparisons between the efficiency of functions would be used to allocate future funds. One special case of resistance was that concerning IT, which was widely regarded as diverting funds away from patient care, was causing much extra work for those whose job it was to key in data, and which was in many cases unreliable and prone to breakdown. Indeed, in one particular hospital the medical records staff had taken industrial action over the introduction of new technology, and many instances of 'technofear' were uncovered by the research.

Training

The overall picture was of a lack of good quality support training designed to facilitate the effective implementation of RMI. It was a very rare hospital unit that had a planned and co-ordinated training programme that met the needs of clinicians, nursing staff and others involved in making RMI a success. Even in those instances where some form of training was available nurses were often unable to attend relevant courses due to low staffing levels on the wards. Clinicians did not fare much better, with few being given the opportunity of attending more than two half-day sessions with a team of management consultants. One RMI project manager justified the lack of training provision for clinicians by arguing that they were a highly educated professional group that did not require further instruction. Such a view assumes that the medical skills possessed by clinicians are appropriate to the job of administration and strategic management, and many NHS employees considered this questionable, to say the least.

There were particular problems with the Information Technology training courses. Given that the success of RMI was contingent on individuals being able to use the IT being introduced under its auspices, the amount and quality of relevant training being provided was surprisingly low. There was at least one case reported where a shortage of qualified staff meant that someone who had recently taught herself to use some equipment was now teaching others. There were other instances where frustrated individuals keen to receive training funded their own attendance on courses in their own time. More generally, there was a lack of appropriate computing facilities in many hospitals, which effectively limited the amount of training that could be conducted in the short term. The consequences of these problems were as predictable as they were unwelcome: technophobia was widespread among certain groups, resistance to change was strengthening, and commitment to RMI and trust in the project teams were being undermined.

Style of change

The RMI project teams, and the Government literature on RMI, all stressed that the process of change was consultative, participative and re-educative. However, there was little evidence that much consultation had taken place within the hospital units themselves, other than with the most senior administrators and clinicians. One of the greatest barriers to more consultation was the lack of formal communication channels linking the RMI implementing teams with other members of their hospitals, the absence of which effectively precluded a two-way flow of information. The extent of employee participation in the process of RMI implementation was also limited. Most people, including many clinicians, described RMI as being imposed upon them in a top-down, almost coercive fashion. The espoused goal of pursuing a re-educative implementation strategy was also questionable in practice, given the inadequacy of much of the training available to hospital staff. In fact, the overwhelming majority of NHS employees interviewed considered RMI to be an alien initiative for which they were not responsible, over which they had little control, and in which they had minimal confidence.

The future

While Government plans indicated that by the end of 1991 260 hospital units should have fully implemented RMI, predictably none of the hospitals in the region studied realised all the structural, cultural and strategic objectives of the RMI by this date. It had long been recognised that the RMI was being rushed through in the minimum amount of time, and that the programme was considerably under-resourced. At each site where RMI was being implemented £910 000 at 1989/90 prices was made available from the Department of Health over a period of three years to cover the costs of a project team, training, and the purchase of a case-mix and nursing computer system. The large-scale nature of the changes envisaged, the complexity of the hospital environment, and the spoiling tactics of various entrenched interest groups, combined with the speed of implementation and a lack of funds, were not a recipe for unequivocal smooth success.

The final paragraph of the Government's discussion paper on change in the NHS, *Working for Patients*, boldly asserted that:

> Throughout this programme, the Government will hold to its central aims: to extend patient choice, to delegate responsibility to those who are best placed to respond to patients' needs and wishes, and to secure the best value for money. The result will be a better deal for the public, both as patients and as taxpayers. The Government will build further on the strengths of the NHS, while tackling its weaknesses. This will ensure that the NHS becomes an even stronger, more modern Service, more committed than ever to working for patients.[19]

By late 1997, however, these words had something of a hollow ring. The Conservative Government of John Major had been replaced by a Labour Government with a somewhat different vision for the NHS, and the RMI programme had already began to dip into the realms of history.

Questions

1 On the basis of information contained in this case and your own general knowledge provide a brief account of the culture of the NHS.

2 What are the essential differences (cultural and in other ways) between the NHS and large commercial organisations? What special problems and opportunities do these differences entail for the NHS?

3 What are the objectives of the Government, the clinicians and the RMI project managers concerning the NHS/RMI as revealed by the case? Are these objectives based on irreconcilable conflicts of interest?

4 You are a newly appointed RMI project manager. How will you seek to maximise your effectiveness within your hospital? What do you think your principal difficulties will be? Can you devise a three-year plan for managing the changes required to ensure the successful implementation of RMI?

5 Does the successful implementation of the RMI presuppose a change in NHS culture, and if so will this damage the organisation?

6 According to what criteria should the success of change programmes such as RMI be measured?

STANHOF SYSTEMS - A MERGER MADE IN HEAVEN

Introduction

Alliances across national boundaries are likely to become an increasingly common feature of life for UK companies, both as a natural consequence of membership of the EU and also as a result of the 'globalisation' of markets which require the deployment of very large resources. While synergy in technology and marketing strategy will, of course, be important to the success of such arrangements, the ability of the participants to accommodate each other's culture and style, both corporate and national, will be equally important. Organisations with strongly embedded cultures and inflexible styles may find it a severe challenge to work effectively with others of a different persuasion.

This case offers a glimpse of two companies with different corporate cultures, based in different countries, which were brought together through a merger.

The new company's parents

The new company, Stanhof Systems Ltd, was formed in the early 1990s by merging the UK marketing subsidiaries of two large corporations, one British (Standard Holdings plc), the other German (Hofberg AG).

Standard Holdings plc

With a turnover of almost £10bn, Standard Holdings plc was a powerful British group with a commanding position in several domestic markets. Standard had diverse engineering and consumer products interests. It had grown essentially by acquisition, absorbing smaller companies and using the technology and expertise so acquired to take the corporation into new markets. Standard was essentially a collection of separate businesses, each of which was required to stand on its own two feet. Standard's management saw their first duty as being to

shareholders and did not hesitate to take strong action with units that did not produce satisfactory returns. The corporation was very decentralised and corporate control consisted chiefly of a close and regular review of financial performance. Corporate headquarters was extremely small and had neither the time nor the inclination to hand down corporate policies on non-financial issues. Accordingly, outside its unremitting demand for financial health from its constituent businesses, Standard Holdings gave its business general managers a great deal of freedom in how they achieved their results. Standard devoted relatively little resource to 'blue-sky' R&D, believing that it was the role of an industrial corporation to apply technology rather than to invent it.

Hofberg AG

Hofberg AG was even larger than Standard, having annual sales of DM 80bn and substantial capabilities in a variety of markets in Germany and in other countries around the world. Hofberg's growth had been mainly organic; it had moved in a measured and deliberate way into new markets as its substantial investment in R&D yielded technological advancements which could be exploited. While it was now large and diversified, its expansion had always followed a logical path, developing new business out of established expertise. The corporation prided itself on its ethical and rational approach to business, to which it ascribed its sustained growth and profitability over many years.

The corporation had a strong sense of history, revering its founders and celebrating the contribution of long-serving staff and managers. The Hofberg museum, open to the public, was a fascinating assembly of the corporation's vast product diversity and a monument to the corporation's innovative excellence over more than a century.

The corporation enjoyed a high degree of loyalty from its managers, and for an established manager lifetime employment within the corporation was the norm. The corporation invested substantially in training and a residential management college served the needs of managers at each stage in their career; an invitation to attend a programme there was taken as a strong indication that a manager was moving up in his or her career. The corporation's serious concern for staff health and welfare was widely demonstrated, not least by the fact that the corporation also had its own health farm, to which senior staff recuperating from illness or those in need of physical revitalisation could be recommended.

A substantial central staff was available to advise line managers in all operating businesses. Published policies guided key activities to achieve a consistency of action across all divisions. Hofberg was of a size to enable almost every manager to realise his or her ambitions within the corporation. Managers with potential were moved regularly from business to business throughout Germany to develop their skills. Such transfers were almost always successful. However, it has to be admitted that postings to fledgling operations overseas were a different matter and not every manager found an overseas posting an easy experience.

In common with other very large and growing corporations, Hofberg had reviewed its organisation structure in the late 1980s. Recognising the need to achieve greater focus but not wishing to lose the economies of scale, it had divided the previous very large industrial groupings into a number of smaller, product/market focused divisions. It was felt that these divisions would be better able to focus on business opportunities in their sector worldwide. Nevertheless the new divisions were still very large, employing up to 30 000 people.

The subsidiaries forming the new company

The two marketing subsidiaries from which the new company was to be formed had been direct competitors prior to the merger, a merger agreed between Standard Holdings and Hofberg as part of a wider pattern of co-operation in product development and marketing within a particular, specialised field of engineering. Both subsidiaries operated exclusively in the UK but their histories were very different.

Standard Systems Ltd

Standard Systems Ltd, with 1600 employees, was firmly established in its UK market where it had been well known for many years. Although marketing some products made outside the Group, Standard Systems was effectively the tied marketing channel of one of Standard Holdings' main manufacturing divisions. Standard Systems' management had long felt that the unit would function more successfully if it were allowed to operate at arm's length from the manufacturing division, in a true supplier–customer relationship. However, attempts to achieve this goal had been thwarted by the superior muscle of the manufacturing division's management. This had led to constant friction between the business and the division. Much against its will, Standard Systems had been forced to transfer its HO activities to the main plant of the manufacturing division in the 1970s. This move, intended to bring about an improvement in relations between the marketing unit and the manufacturing division, had, if anything, brought disagreements into sharper focus. In particular, the management of the marketing unit became more convinced than ever that they were being prevented from pursuing the optimum marketing strategy. Moreover the siting of a sales-orientated unit within a factory complex only served to highlight the contrast in priorities between the two units; for instance, Standard Systems' management was regularly required to placate customers given a cool reception by the manufacturing plant's security staff, who saw their prime duty as protecting the industrial premises from unauthorised entry.

Hofberg Systems Ltd

Hofberg Systems Ltd was smaller than Standard Systems, having just 400 employees. It had entered the Hofberg family by an unusual (for Hofberg AG) route, having been acquired as a going concern in the mid-1980s. Hofberg AG had acquired ownership as a result of the threatened failure of its UK distributor, an independent UK marketing company (Sutton Systems) which had relied mainly on German-manufactured Hofberg products for its portfolio. Hofberg had moved in to take over Sutton when cash flow problems threatened to overwhelm it. The German-led management team which Hofberg AG installed at what was renamed Hofberg Systems Ltd enjoyed considerable freedom of action. There were two reasons for this: first, expertise in guiding overseas operations was not one of Hofberg's greatest strengths and those Hofberg executives with overseas experience were given wide powers; second, Hofberg's divisional senior management in Germany were heavily committed to other initiatives, both in Germany and in developing a new and challenging business alliance in the important US market. While not a sideshow, the UK operation was not seen as being an issue of the order of magnitude of some other initiatives. Moreover it was felt to be in the safe hands of seasoned expatriates and as such not requiring constant supervision. Hofberg was nevertheless committed to Hofberg Systems and demonstrated it by providing the funds to acquire a brand new office block on a prestigious site to house the company's HO operation.

At the time of the merger, the management styles and cultures of Standard Systems and Hofberg Systems differed considerably.

In general, the style in Standard Systems could be described as consultative and participative, with staff enjoying easy and friendly relations with their senior managers. Communication on first-name terms was the norm even between secretaries and the most senior management. There were few written policies and the general style of spoken and written communication was informal and friendly and implied an underlying trust. Most people did not feel the need for a rule book to tell them what the company expected in terms of conduct. Conflict between individual members of management was rare and disagreements were usually focused on issues rather than personalities. A more negative side to these close and easy internal relationships was that management tended to be tolerant of undistinguished performance by individuals. In fact, management's commitment to the concept of teamwork led them to overlook significant disparities in the performance levels of individuals. As promotion was commonly on the basis of seniority, there was a tendency for high fliers to leave the company to seek more rapid career advancement elsewhere.

Because of the larger size, more established roots and wider customer base of their business, the senior managers of Standard Systems assumed that they would automatically become the primary influence in the merged company and further expected that they would occupy most of the key roles in the company. Accordingly, they welcomed the merger both as a career opportunity for themselves and also as a heaven-sent chance to get 'out from under' the manufacturing division which had limited their freedom for so long.

The management style in Hofberg Systems was more formal and disciplined than that in Standard Systems. The three most senior managers in Hofberg Systems were German nationals sent by Hofberg AG to turn the company around. These managers already had experience of overseas troubleshooting on at least one previous occasion, although not in the UK. At the time of the takeover of Sutton, these incoming managers had inherited an operation in serious need of business control and discipline; as the first UK company with which they had come into close contact, Sutton had made a very poor impression.

A substantial number of the Sutton managers had been quickly removed and in their place had been recruited people who possessed not only professional skill but also a no-nonsense approach to control and discipline. Staff remaining were treated well in a material sense but greater demands were placed on them to achieve results and to conform to organisationally specified norms of behaviour; a new level of accountability and professionalism was required. Controls over people and processes were introduced on a broad front. In a relatively short period of time, the lax management regime of the former management had been eliminated and a new atmosphere of consistency, predictability and accountability had been substituted. Staff were left in no doubt that each individual's performance was under continuous scrutiny. The word 'requirements' was much in evidence in letters from management to staff and in the company's Personnel Policy handbook. Probably as a consequence of all these initiatives, there was a more pronounced sense of hierarchy and a greater psychological distance between the senior management and staff in Hofberg Systems than was the case in Standard Systems.

Preparations for the merger

Although the idea of a merger had a clear logic – the two companies were direct competitors and wasting energies fighting each other – the parents were not willing to agree to a merger without a proper plan and management arrangements which would assure a route to market for their respective product ranges. It was decided that the key issues of people, products and trading procedure needed to be addressed before a final decision was made on whether to proceed with a merger. Joint teams would work on these issues as a matter of urgency. Meetings would be held at parent company premises, alternating between Germany and Britain. Speed was clearly important as rumours were already spreading among staff

and customers and there was a need to make a positive statement one way or the other.

Standard fielded a very small team of managers, all but one being from the Standard Systems business unit itself. These managers continued to carry out their normal operational duties as well as addressing the strategic requirements of the proposed merger. The Standard managers were given minimal guidance by corporate staff on how to proceed in the planning meetings: corporate management took it as read that the team running Standard Systems would be perfectly capable of planning the birth of the new company, which would after all be only 25 per cent larger than the one they already ran. Moreover Standard executives at corporate and divisional level felt that Standard held the high ground in the negotiations, being the UK-based partner and the UK market leader to boot.

Hofberg AG fielded a larger team. None of them worked in Hofberg Systems, all of them being corporate or divisional staff rather than business unit staff. Almost all were Germans, based in Germany, and most were specialists in marketing and business planning. They were armed with well-researched market information and up-to-date performance data on both companies and on the UK market. They had clear objectives but also had room to manoeuvre. Their team included a member whose sole purpose was to create an agreed work agenda and to clarify and record agreed actions.

All the planning meetings were conducted in English, regardless of where they were held and regardless of the fact that the number of German speakers participating always outnumbered those whose first language was English. The Hofberg team undertook to produce minutes of meetings and were assiduous in faxing them to the members of both teams within 24 hours of the end of each meeting.

The members of the two teams found that they interacted well and meetings were both productive and amicable. To a large extent, this spirit was created by the warmth of the welcome extended by the German hosts at the first meeting, which was held in Germany. The parties found that they complemented each other well, the managers from Standard bringing first-hand experience of the UK market and contributing imaginatively to the formulation of an organisational and customer strategy for the merger, the Hofberg managers excelling in numerical analysis and co-ordination and in formulating a product strategy. The Standard managers were delighted to discover that Hofberg AG was primarily concerned with realising a long-term vision rather than seeking short-term profitability. The members of both teams felt that they saw eye to eye on most important strategic issues and found it relatively straightforward to reach consensus on most matters. Social contacts outside the meetings were enjoyed by all and some cross-company friendships were formed.

The team from Standard felt particularly pleased by this initial contact with Hofberg and were much encouraged by the attitudes displayed by Hofberg executives, especially their enlightened approach to marketing and willingness to take the long view in developing the new business unit. They felt that their original optimism had been entirely justified and that a bright future was assured for the merged company and for themselves in it.

Appointing the management team

Once the plans had reached a satisfactory state of completion and the parents assented to the merger, a senior management team had to be formed for the new company, which was to be known as Stanhof Systems Ltd. The parent organisations agreed that as the new company was to be owned 50 : 50 by the parents, the team should comprise managers drawn in equal numbers from Standard Systems and Hofberg Systems. The appointee to the position of chairman was made by Standard Holdings. The chairman already had wide responsibilities in Standard Holdings plc and these he retained,

giving such time as he could afford to the new company. The position of managing director was thus to be filled by Hofberg AG, who selected a German national of some seniority who had previously functioned as an overseas troubleshooter for one of Hofberg's largest divisions. The remaining senior management positions (the functional directors) were filled by senior managers from Standard Systems and Hofberg Systems with half the positions going to managers from each. Although this was achieved without much difficulty, the new MD insisted that the position of commercial director (CD) – seen in German corporations as occupying a role approaching partnership with the MD – should go to the incumbent commercial director of Hofberg Systems. This manager would be the sole remaining German national from the original Hofberg Systems senior management team, as Hofberg AG were assigning the others to new duties in Germany, a move which would relieve the surplus of senior managers that the merger inevitably produced.

Running the new company

The new MD insisted that the prestigious offices which had formerly been the Hofberg Systems HO should be the HO of the merged company. As a result of the erstwhile occupancy by Hofberg Systems, large offices for the MD and commercial director were already *in situ*, adjacent to each other on the top floor, commanding an impressive view of the surrounding country. Smaller offices for all the other senior managers were *in situ* on the lower floors, collocated with the senior managers' HO staff. The joint MD/CD office was run in a polite, correct and very formal way, in the German style. The MD's and CD's executive secretaries observed a respectful formality towards the MD and CD, yet were informal in their dealings with the other senior managers, whom they addressed by their first names when invited to do so and with whom they shared informal and friendly relations when work issues brought them into contact.

None of the former Standard Systems managers spoke German, whereas the MD and CD were both exceptionally fluent in English, having worked in English-speaking territories on previous assignments for Hofberg. They lapsed into German only occasionally when speaking to each other in front of colleagues, for instance when one of them, answering a telephone call from the Hofberg HO in Germany, needed to consult the other on a point under discussion. At all other times they conversed in English when in the company of colleagues.

In line with the established practice in Germany, the MD not only relied on advice from his CD on all commercial and financial matters but also consulted him routinely on many other strategic and operational matters. This meant that the MD and CD spent much time together. Whenever the MD was absent the CD was always left in charge of day-to-day affairs. Observing this *modus operandi*, the managers from Standard Systems felt that there was effectively a two-tier senior management structure, with the MD and commercial director occupying the first tier. To mitigate this impression, the MD refrained from producing the internally circulated management organisation chart in the German fashion, that is with the names of the MD and CD shown together in the top organisational box. Nevertheless the charts produced for the German parent company had to be produced according to the German convention.

The newly appointed MD quickly established the *modus operandi* for the new company. He had risen in Hofberg AG by reason of ability and hard work and had volunteered for difficult overseas assignments before. Both he and the CD had survived some tough challenges far from home and they quickly fell into a way of working together which they found effective. The MD had no doubt that he could make a success of this assignment and that this success would be beneficial to his career with Hofberg, whose employee he, of course, remained. His style was brisk and highly professional. Thorough preparation and an intimate knowl-edge of the subject in hand were prerequisites for any meeting in which he was involved, whether formal or 'informal'. Formal management meetings were held regularly, but were always conducted to a timed agenda; they consisted essentially of formal presentations on the agenda items, with only a little time allowed for subsequent discussion. 'Drop in' discussions and unstructured exchanges of views, which had been a feature of life in Standard Systems, did not seem to be encouraged by the MD.

The other senior managers appointed from Hofberg Systems, who, since the return to Germany of the original Hofberg senior management 'task-force', were all British, accepted this management style without difficulty. However, the senior managers appointed from Standard Systems found the lack of intimacy, formality of working relationships and 'distance' between themselves and the MD unexpected and disconcerting. Even though they much admired his vision and business judgement, they felt distinctly uncomfortable with his style of management. It seemed to them that, far from decreasing the distance between him and them, time served to increase it.

In respect of a wide range of business documents and procedures, the new MD insisted on a strict adherence to a formally prescribed way of working. Agendas, minutes and organisation charts all had to conform exactly to a prescribed format and the required typeface and layout of letters and memos was specified in detail. The ex-Hofberg Systems managers accepted this move as a necessary step towards regulation and control, whereas the ex-Standard Systems managers saw it as an obsession with order which brought little commercial advantage. Many of these procedures were derived from procedures that had been established in Hofberg Systems when it had become a Hofberg company. The former Standard Systems managers concluded that the MD believed there was one 'right' way to run a company, down to the smallest detail. The ex-Hofberg Systems managers showed little sympathy with the ex-

Standard Systems managers' desire for more participation in decisions on systems and procedures. The ex-Standard Systems managers did not understand the attitude of the Hofberg managers, who seemed to put such a high value on compliance and conformity.

Whereas the ex-Standard Systems managers appeared to their new colleagues to be too *laissez-faire*, even naive, in their approach to managing staff, the ex-Hofberg managers appeared to their new colleagues to be obsessed with control systems, apparently believing staff could not be relied upon to act or function conscientiously without such mechanisms.

One by one, the ex-Standard Systems managers became disenchanted with the environment of the new company. Within two years, no senior manager of Standard Systems provenance remained in the new company.

Moreover relations between the new company and the associated Standard manufacturing division persisted, apparently unresolved, in the merged company.

Questions

1 Provide brief overviews of the cultures of (a) Standard Systems and (b) Hofberg Systems.

2 Why did the proposed merger appear to be well starred at the outset?

3 Why were there no problems evident at the planning stage?

4 From where did the differences of attitude and perception in the merged company spring?

5 Could the conflicts of culture have been avoided and if so how?

6 Whom would you blame most for the conflicts?

NOTES

1 I spent several days in November 1993 conducting interviews and visiting the site at Renault Véhicules Industriels in Vénissieux. I would like to thank all those who agreed to participate in the project. In particular, I am grateful to François Blanc, Director of Training and Conditions of Service, for granting me access, answering my questions, and providing detailed comments and assistance in the writing of this case study, and to Christine DuDragne for arranging the interviews.

2 Georges Leprince (1991), *Les Travailleurs Berliet-RVI Vénissieux 1915–1991*, Messidor, 150.

3 RVI (1993), *Chiffres 92, Renault VI*, Lyon: Renault VI.

4 RVI (1993), *Chiffres 92, Renault VI*, Lyon: Renault VI.

5 Broad employment categories at RVI are 'ouvrier', 'technicien' and 'cadre'. These categories indicate status rather than occupation. A technicien may be employed as a supervisor on the shopfloor, as an administrator or even as a manager.

6 'Cadre' is a peculiarly French concept. It is not adequately translated by 'manager' as a cadre is not necessarily a manager and a manager is not necessarily a cadre. As with technicien, that it is a category refers to status rather than occupation, so a cadre may be a manager, an engineer or an administrator.

7 RVI (1992), *Bilan Social d'Entreprise*, Lyon: Renault VI.

8 RVI (1992), *Bilan Social d'Entreprise*, Lyon: Renault VI.

9 RVI (1992), *Bilan Social d'Entreprise*, Lyon: Renault VI.

10 Renault was a volume producer strongest in southern Europe, and Volvo was a maker of large executive cars focused on northern Europe and with a presence in North America.

11 It should be observed that while all of Renault was included in the proposed merger, only Volvo's automotive operations were at stake, with the Volvo parent company intending to retain separate control over its marine, aero engine and food processing businesses, and its pharmaceutical interests.

12 Message to the press from a Volvo spokesman.

13 The idea was that the French Government would retain the right to limit any investor to 20% of the merged company's capital in the event of a breakdown of the shareholders agreement. The Government stated that the golden share would only be used to protect the group from a hostile takeover. However, in theory it meant that Volvo's share could be cut down to 20% at any time after the merger.

14 The Ecole Nationale d'Administration is the training ground for the elite of the French Government service.

15 National Health Service Management Enquiry: 1983. *The Griffiths Report*. London: Department of Health and Social Security.

16 Arthur Young: 1986. *Practical Management Budgeting for the NHS: a new initiative for successful implementation*. Glasgow.

17 Pollitt, C. *et al.* (1988) The reluctant managers: clinicians and budgets in the NHS. *Financial Accountability and Management*, 4 (3) pp. 213–233.

18 Health Notice (1986), 34.

19 *Working for Patients*. 1989. London: HMSO.

CHAPTER 8

Conclusion

OBJECTIVES

To enable students to:

- reflect on the information contained in the previous seven chapters;
- understand that the material presented in this book provides an overview of just some of the knowledge, models and frameworks that have been   produced, and that further reading is essential in order to fully appreciate this field of study;
- draw their own conclusions concerning the use and value of the cultural perspective on organisations.

INTRODUCTION

This final brief chapter has three main sections. First, it attempts to summarise some of the most interesting points made in the first seven chapters. Second, some additional intricacies and complexities regarding organisational culture as an academic field of interest are considered. Third, some general conclusions about the organisational culture perspective are drawn. This and the preceding seven chapters together provide a useful basis on which students may build in their consideration of cultural issues through further reading and research.

REVIEWING ORGANISATIONAL CULTURE

In Chapter 1 it was suggested that the current interest in organisational culture stemmed from research into national cultures and organisational climate. The current focus on organisational culture also reflects a perception that people are the most important element in organisations and the realisation that social factors need to be taken into account by frameworks for understanding organisational performance. Intellectually, organisational culture has principally been fed by anthropology and organisational sociology, and has many similarities with those perspectives that emphasise the importance of power and politics in organisations. There is an important distinction to be drawn between organisational culture as a metaphor for understanding organisational life and as an objective property of organisations or people. In this book organisational culture was defined as: *the pattern of beliefs, values and learned ways of coping with experience that have developed during the course of an organisation's history, and which tend to be manifested in its material arrangements and in the behaviours of its members.*

Schein's three-level model (artefacts, beliefs and basic assumptions) represents a convenient means of classifying the many different elements of an organisation's culture. It should, however, be recalled that organisational cultures are complex and dynamic entities. In order to avoid confusion a distinction therefore needs to be drawn between an organisation's espoused culture and its culture-in-practice. Organisational culture is important because it is through the medium of culture that employees make sense of their workplaces and work activities and attribute meaning to organisational experiences.

In Chapter 2 it was shown that there are a large number of sources of organisational culture, four of the most significant of which are national culture, the organisation's leaders, the nature of its business activities and its environment. The perpetuation of organisational culture over time is achieved through effective recruitment, selection and socialisation of compatible individuals and the rejection of those who do not fit in. It was suggested that organisational cultures differ in terms of their transparency/opaqueness and simplicity/complexity, and that these factors determine how easy it is for new recruits to learn how to survive in the organisation they have joined.

One continuing problem for those interested in organisation studies is how best to research issues of culture. On the one hand, quantitative approaches seem able to yield precise and convincing results regarding dominant beliefs and values without offering penetrating insights into the culture as it is *lived* by employees. On the other hand, qualitative approaches offer interesting and empathetic interpretations of cultures which are hard to quantify or to use as the basis for interventions aimed at solving problems. Similarly, the various typologies and means for assessing culture strength that have been formulated are only partially satisfactory, providing starting points for description rather than incisive analysis.

In Chapter 3 the difficulties associated with attempts to conceive of organisations as homogeneous entities were exposed. Most organisations, especially those that are large and have a lengthy history, are likely to have numerous embedded subcultures.

The nature of these subcultures, how they have formed, and whether they are enhancing, orthogonal or conflicting are important considerations for scholars and practitioners alike. Another vexed question concerns the functions that have been attributed to organisational cultures. These include: conflict reduction, co-ordination and control, the reduction of uncertainty, motivation and sustaining competitive advantage. It should always be recalled that culture is not an inherently positive force in organisations. Indeed, there are organisations that possess dysfunctional cultures, which increase conflict, reduce co-ordination and control, increase uncertainty, diminish motivation and undermine competitive advantage. It is also true that most individuals devote only a fraction of their time and energy to their work organisations, and that while some employees unequivocally adhere to their organisation's culture, others will exhibit strained adherence, secret non-adherence or open non-adherence. As organisations make increasing use of part-time employees and continue to contract out non-core activities so organisational cultures are likely to become more complicated and confused.

As the culture field has expanded there have been increasing attempts to link the issues that a focus on culture raises to other aspects of organisational inquiry, such as gender, learning, groupthink, ethics and postmodernism. There is considerable evidence to suggest that the nature of an organisation's culture has profound implications for how women are regarded and treated, and the propensity of the organisation to learn. Perhaps most intriguingly, postmodern accounts of culture suggest that it is a transient episode in the field of organisation studies, and that the term culture is more notable as a legitimating device for particular research agendas than as anything very new.

In Chapter 4 five models for understanding the process of culture change were considered. None of these models was especially convincing, a fact which reflects the complexity of culture change processes, the newness of this field of interest and the paucity of good-quality research so far conducted. The models had four principal common themes: all of them suggested that the notions of perceived crisis, leadership, perceived success and relearning were crucial for understanding culture change. In future, more plausible models of culture change may be developed which take account of the nature of the culture undergoing change. Three aspects of a culture which require attention from a more sophisticated model are: how available alternative cultures are, the participants' level of commitment to the current culture, and the fluidity of the current culture.

In Chapter 5 methods of managing culture change were reviewed. There is broad scope for disagreement concerning whether culture can be managed, depending on how the term 'culture' is understood. Rather than become embroiled in these academic debates the most fruitful way forward is to attempt to assess the possibilities for culture management given various constraints: for example, the influence of environmental variables, and the scarcity of resources like competent leaders, finance and mechanisms for co-ordination, communication and control. A general framework for managing culture suggests that the actual culture of an organisation should be identified, the ideal culture sketched in theory, and then practical steps taken to align them. One interesting approach to bringing about this alignment involves adopting a consistent cues approach with respect to human resource policies, programmes, systems and procedures: recruitment and selection, induction, socialisation and training, performance appraisal and reward, transfers and secondments, and opportunities for participation, communication and counselling can all play a role in a strategy for managing culture.

A second significant approach to managing culture centres on the role of organisational leaders, especially the individual at the apex of the organisation. Leaders have considerable scope for exercising power over the development of a culture through symbolic means. How leaders use their time, their use of language, their performance in meetings and skill at manipulating agendas and interpreting minutes, and their sensitivity to different settings can send vital messages to their subordinates and encourage employees to think and act in particular ways. Similarly, leaders' use of rites of passage, enhancement, degradation, conflict reduction, integration and renewal can have a central impact on the cultural evolution of an organisation. It may, however, be true that established leaders are more likely to attempt to preserve the status quo than induce change, and can thus be an obstacle to be overcome where culture change is required. As Bate has demonstrated, there are many different strategies available to leaders to promote culture change. Where a large-scale programme of culture change is planned Silverzweig and Allen's normative systems model may be employed as a guide for developing an effective change management strategy.

In Chapter 6 the relationships between organisational culture, strategy and performance were considered. While some commentators have suggested that culture and strategy refer to the same sets of phenomena, it is probably more useful to define them as separate entities. The strategy of an organisation is its long-term plans for achieving its ultimate objectives while its culture (cognitions, behaviours and artefacts) influences both strategy formulation and implementation in a variety of ways. The performance of an organisation may be evaluated according to a multiplicity of different criteria (various economic indicators, the number of people employed, the sophistication of its internal systems and procedures, control over the environment, stability and survival), depending on the interests of the stakeholder group concerned.

Culture influences strategy formulation through its influence on scanning procedures, selective perception, interpretation, ethical and moral considerations, the effects of assumptions, and the power of various subcultures. Culture influences strategy implementation through its influence over employee behaviour. It should be noted that culture is not the only influence on organisational strategy and that it is often the case that an organisation's strategy is at variance with its culture. As a general rule, the more an organisation's strategy is at variance with its culture the greater the likelihood is that it will not be effectively implemented. Another general heuristic is that the richer (in terms of the number of stories) and more consistent an organisation's culture is, the more reliable will be the implementation of that organisation's strategy. It is important to realise that culture and strategy are mutually interdependent and that the formation and implementation of a strategy (a cultural artefact) is likely to have an ongoing influence on the evolution of an organisation's culture (in terms of its dominant beliefs, values and assumptions). The considerable influence that culture exerts over how organisations function means that it is imperative that cultural issues are taken into account when planning mergers and acquisitions.

The culture of an organisation has an important impact on its performance. It is possible that strong (in the sense of consistent) cultures which are strategically appropriate (fit both the organisation's strategy and the environment), adaptable (and so able to cope with change), which value both key stakeholders and leadership at all levels, and which have a strong sense of mission may be associated with high performance over sustained periods of time. This conclusion has yet to be verified. What is certain is that the nature of the relationships between culture, strategy and performance are complex, and that all conclusions concerning their patterns of interaction should be made cautiously. These, then, were some of the most notable findings of the first seven chapters.

ORGANISATIONAL CULTURE: AN ACADEMIC FIELD OF INTEREST

This book has focused on organisational culture as a subject of interest to students on taught courses. Thus while it has drawn on the wealth of material generated by scholars interested in organisational culture it has not specifically dealt with the many complex research issues which dominate the field. Indeed, in the interests of conciseness and clarity these issues have deliberately been bypassed and suppressed. For any student wishing to consider organisational culture as a field of research the bibliography provided at the back of this book provides a number of leads.

This said, in Chapter 1 we surveyed some of the many definitions of organisational culture that scholars and practitioners in this field have produced. The diversity of views evident here provides us with some insight into what Martin (1992) has termed the 'state of conceptual chaos' that currently afflicts the academic study of cultural phenomena in organisations. And while this book has not concerned itself with these scholarly debates it is, however, worth briefly considering the three competing perspectives on organisational culture employed by researchers. These three perspectives Martin describes as *integration, differentiation, and fragmentation*.

1 *Integration* Researchers working within this perspective tend to suggest that cultural manifestations (artefacts, beliefs, values and so forth) are consistent with one another, and thus are mutually reinforcing. It is generally held that all members of an organisation share in a common culture, and that there is an organisation-wide consensus in terms of beliefs held and behaviours expected. Exponents of this perspective also usually subscribe to the view that the culture of organisations is relatively clear, straightforward and unambiguous.

2 *Differentiation* Researchers who have adopted this perspective are inclined to submit that cultural manifestations can sometimes be inconsistent. For example, they point out that managers can often be found saying one thing and doing another. This perspective also readily admits the existence of subcultures and suggests that consensus is only likely to be found within these groupings. While some element of ambiguity and uncertainty in the study of culture is allowed, it is largely ignored.

3 *Fragmentation* This is the most difficult of the three perspectives to characterise adequately in a few sentences. Researchers working within this perspective can detect little if any consensus in the cultures they study. Rather than identify specific subcultures these researchers claim that what consensus there is concerns specific issues, and will be in a more-or-less constant state of flux. Ambiguity is central to their endeavours to understand cultures, which are said to lack clear consistencies and inconsistencies, being a jungle of different, often competing, and always uncertain meanings.

Martin's classification of approaches to the study of organisational culture has been outlined only to provide a feel for some of the intellectual complexities which underpin much of the material presented in this book. To some extent this complexity reflects the fact that scholars from a variety of different disciplines (including sociology, psychology, anthropology, linguistics and folklore studies) are contributing to culture research (Alvesson and Berg, 1992). It should, though, be noticeable that this book has been written from within a combination of the integration and differentiation perspectives. The reader interested in pursuing more scholarly debates in organisational culture is here referred to the wealth of academic texts and journal articles that have been (and continue to be) produced.

CONCLUSIONS

Organisational culture is one of the most exciting perspectives on organisations currently available, and opens up a whole new way of understanding how organisations behave. It suggests that people rather than systems and structures should be the key focus of attention, and that understanding employees' interpretations of processes and events is more important than attempting to formulate general social scientific laws. The current interest in organisational culture reflects increasing consensus that what matters in organisations is often 'informal', 'political', 'ambiguous' and subject to multiple interpretations. While academics have tended to think of culture as a means of gaining more detailed diagnoses of how organisations work, managers have sought to capitalise on insights generated by the cultural perspective to wield greater control over their organisations. What is clear is that the identification of organisational cultures has wide ramifications, for it means shedding a humanistic light upon organisations, and encourages us to treat their members not as roles but as full human beings.

REFERENCES

Adam-Smith, D. & Peacock, A. (eds) (1994), *Cases in Organisational Behaviour*, London: Pitman Publishing.

Albert, M. & Silverman, M. (1984a), 'Making Management Philosophy a Cultural Reality, Part 1: Getting Started', *Personnel*, **61** (1), 12–21.

Albert, M. & Silverman, M. (1984b), 'Making Management Philosophy a Cultural Reality, Part 2: Design Human Resources Programs Accordingly', *Personnel*, **61** (2), 28–35.

Allen, R. F. & Kraft, C. (1987), *The Organizational Unconscious*, Morristown, NJ: Human Resources Institute.

Alvesson, M. (1993), *Cultural Perspectives on Organizations*, Cambridge: Cambridge University Press.

Alvesson, M. & Berg, P. O. (1992), *Corporate Culture and Organizational Symbolism*, Berlin: Walter de Gruyter.

Anthony, P. (1994), *Managing Culture*, Buckingham: Open University Press.

Argyris, C. (1976), 'Theories of Action that Inhibit Individual Learning', *American Psychologist*, **39**, 638–54.

Argyris, C. (1982), *Reasoning, Learning, and Action*. San Francisco, Calif: Jossey Bass.

Argyris, C. & Schon, D.A. (1978), *Theory in Practice*, San Francisco: Jossey Bass.

Ash, M. K. (1981), *Mary Kay*, New York: Harper & Row.

Barnatt, C. (1990), 'Managing 'Hit and Run' Workers within Organizational Cultures and Subsystems', unpublished paper.

Barney, J. (1986), 'Organizational Culture: Can it be a Source of Sustained Competitive Advantage?', *Academy of Management Review*, II (3), 656–65.

Bate, P. (1994), *Strategies for Cultural Change*, Oxford: Butterworth Heinemann.

Beach, L. R. (1993), *Making the Right Decision: Organizational Culture, Vision, and Planning*, Englewood Cliffs, NJ: Prentice Hall.

Berg, P. O. (1985), 'Organization change as a Symbolic Transformation Process', in: P. J. Frost, L. F. Moore, M. R. Louis, C. C. Lundberg, & J. Martin (eds), *Organizational Culture*, Beverly Hills, Calif.: Sage, 281–99.

Berg, P. O. & Kreiner, K. (1990), 'Corporate Architecture: Turning Physical Settings into Symbolic Resources', in P. Gagliardi (ed.) *Symbols and Artifacts: Views of the Corporate Landscape*, New York: Aldine de Gruyter, 41–67.

Beyer, J. M. & Trice, H. M. (1988), 'The Communication of Power Relations in Organizations through Cultural Rites', in: M. D. Jones, M. D. Moore & R. C. Sayder (eds), *Inside Organizations: Understanding the Human Dimension*, Newbury Park, Calif.: Sage, 141–57.

Beyer, J. M. & Trice, H. M. (1993) *The Cultures of Work Organizations*, Englewood Cliffs, NJ: Prentice Hall.

Blauner, R. (1967), *Alienation and Freedom*. Chicago, Ill.: The University of Chicago Press.

Boje, D. M., Fedor, D. B. & Rowland, K. M. (1982), 'Myth Making: A Qualitative Step in OD Interventions', *The Journal of Applied Behavioral Science*, **18** (1), 17–28.

Bowles, M. L. (1989), 'Myth, Meaning and Work Organization', *Organization Studies*, **10** (3), 405–21.

Boyett, I. & Finlay, D. (1993), 'The UK's East Midlands Company of the Year 1992 – A State Funded Secondary School?' School of Management & Finance, University of Nottingham.

Brewis, J. (1994), 'The Role of Intimacy at Work: Interactions and Relationships in the Modern Organization', in D. A. Smith & A. Peacock (eds), *Cases in Organisational Behaviour*, London: Pitman Publishing.

Brown, A.D. & Starkey, K. (1994), 'The effect of organizational culture on communication and information'. *Journal of Management Studies*, **31** (6), 807–28.

Burack, E. H. (1991), 'Changing the Company Culture – the Role of Human Resource Development', *Long Range Planning*, **24** (1), 88–95.

Business Week (1984), 'Who's Excellent Now?', 5 November, 76–78.

Cadbury, A. (1987), 'Ethical Managers Make their Own Rules', *Harvard Business Review*, Sept.–Oct., 69–73.

Carby, K. & Stempt, P. (1985), 'How Hambro Changed its Name and Much More Besides', *Personnel Management*, October, 58–60.

Dalmau, T. & Dick, R. (1991), 'Managing Ambiguity and Paradox: The Place of Small Groups in Cultural Change', paper presented to the 8th International SCOS Conference on Organizational Symbolism and Corporate Culture, Copenhagen, Denmark, 26–28 June.

Dandridge, T. C., Mitroff, I. & Joyce, W. F. (1980), 'Organizational Symbolism: A Topic to Expand Organizational Analysis', *Academy of Management Review*, **5** (1), 77–82.

Davis, S. M. (1984), *Managing Corporate Culture*, Cambridge, Mass.: Ballinger.

Davis, S. M. (1985), 'Culture is not just an internal affair', in: R. H. Kilmann, M. J. Saxton, R. Serpa & associates (eds), *Gaining Control of the Corporate Culture*, San Francisco, Calif.: Jossey Bass, 137–47.

Davis, T. R. V. (1985), 'Managing Culture at the Bottom', in: R. H. Kilmann, M. J. Saxton, R. Serpa & associates (eds), *Gaining Control of the Corporate Culture*, San Francisco, Calif.: Jossey Bass, 163–83.

Deal, T.E. & Kennedy, A.A. (1982), *Corporate Cultures: the Rites and Rituals of Corporate Life*, Reading, Mass.: Addison-Wesley.

Dearden, B. (1990), *Resource Management and the Shape of the Organisation*. NHS Training Authority: Bristol.

Denison, D. (1990), *Corporate Culture and Organizational Effectiveness*, New York: John Wiley.

Dobson, P. & Starkey, K. (1993), *The Strategic Management Blueprint*, Oxford: Blackwell.

Drennan, D. (1992), *Transforming Company Culture*, London: McGraw-Hill.

Dyer, W. G. (1984), 'The Cycle of Cultural Evolution in Organizations', unpublished paper, Sloan School of Management, Massachusetts Institute of Technology.

Dyer, W. G. (1985), 'The Cycle of Cultural Evolution in Organizations', in: R. H. Kilmann, M. J. Saxton, R. Serpa & associates (eds), *Gaining Control of the Corporate Culture*, San Francisco, Calif.: Jossey Bass, 200–29.

Dyer, W. G. (1986), *Cultural Change in Family Firms: Anticipating and Managing Business and Family Transitions*, San Francisco, Calif.: Jossey Bass.

Eldridge, J. E. T. & Crombie, A. D. (1974), *A Sociology of Organizations*, London: Allen & Unwin.

Feldman, S. P. (1988), 'How Organizational Culture can Affect Innovation', *Organizational Dynamics*, 17 (1), 57–68.

Fitzgerald, T. H. (1988), 'Can Change in Organizational Culture Really be Managed?', *Organizational Dynamics*, 17 (2), 5–15.

Fortune, (1983), October, 17.

Gagliardi, P. (1986), 'The Creation and Change of Organizational Cultures: A Conceptual Framework', *Organization Studies*, 7 (2), 117–34.

Gagliardi, P. (1990), *Symbols and Artifacts: Views of the Corporate Landscape*, New York: Aldine de Gruyter.

Geertz, C. (1973), *The Interpretation of Cultures*, New York: Basic Books.

Gherardi, S. (1995), *Gender, Symbolism and Organizational Cultures*, London: Sage.

Gold, K. A. (1982), 'Managing for Success: A Comparison of the Private and Public Sectors', *Public Administration Review*, Nov.–Dec., 568–75.

Golden, K. A. (1992), 'The Individual and Organizational Culture: Strategies for Action in Highly-Ordered Contexts', *Journal of Management Studies*, 29 (1), 1–21.

Goldsmith, W. & Clutterbuck, D. (1985), *The Winning Streak*, Harmondsworth: Penguin.

Goodstein, L. D. & Burke, W. W. (1991), 'Creating Successful Organization Change', *Organizational Dynamics*, spring, 5–17.

Gordon, G. G. (1985), 'The Relationship of Corporate Culture to Industry Sector and Corporate Performance', in: R. H. Kilmann, M. J. Saxton, R. Serpa & associates (eds), *Gaining Control of the Corporate Culture*, San Francisco, Calif.: Jossey Bass, 103–25.

Green, S. (1988), 'Understanding Corporate Culture and its Relation to Strategy', *International Studies of Management and Organization*, 18 (2), 6–28.

Gregory, K. (1983), 'Native-View Paradigms: Multiple Culture and Culture Conflicts in Organizations', *Administrative Science Quarterly*, 28, 359–76.

Guest, D. E. (1990), 'Human Resource Management and the American Dream', *Journal of Management Studies*, 27 (4), 377–97.

Guest, D. E. (1992), 'Right Enough to be Dangerously Wrong: An Analysis of the "In Search of Excellence" Phenomenon', in: G. Salaman (ed.), *Human Resources Strategies*, London: Sage.

Hampden-Turner, C. (1990), *Corporate Culture: From Vicious to Virtuous Circles*, London: Economist Books.

Handy, C. B. (1978), *The Gods of Management*, Harmondsworth: Penguin.

Handy, C. B. (1985), *Understanding Organizations*, Harmondsworth: Penguin.

Harrison, R. (1972), 'Understanding Your Organization's Character', *Harvard Business Review*, 50, May–June, 119–28.

Hassard, J. & Parker, M. (1993), *Postmodernism and Organisations*, London: Sage.

Hassard, J. & Sharifi, S. (1989), 'Corporate Culture and Strategic Change', *Journal of General Management*, 15 (2), 4–19.

Hennestad, B. W. (1991), 'Reframing Organizations: Towards a Model', Unpublished manuscript, Norwegian School of Management, Sandvika.

Heskett, J. (1989), *Philips, a Study of the Corporate Management of Design*, London: Trefoil Publications.

Hirsch, P. M. & Andrews, J. A. Y. (1983), 'Ambushes, Shootouts, and Knights of the Round Table: The Language of Corporate Takeovers', in: L. R. Pondy, P. J. Frost, G. Morgan & T. C. Dandridge (eds), *Organizational Symbolism*, Greenwich, Conn.: JAI, 145–55.

Hofstede, G. (1980), *Culture's Consequences: International Differences in Work-related Values*, Beverly Hills, Calif.: Sage.

299

Hofstede, G. (1991), *Cultures and Organizations, Software of the Mind*, Maidenhead: McGraw-Hill.

Hofstede, G., Neuijen, B., Ohayv, D. & Sanders, G. (1990), 'Measuring Organizational Cultures: A Qualitative Study Across Twenty Cases', *Administrative Science Quarterly*, **35**, 286–316.

Isabella, L. A. (1990), 'Evolving Interpretations as a Change Unfolds: How Managers Construe Key Organizational Events', *Academy of Management Journal*, **33** (1), 7–41.

Ishizuna, Y. (1990), 'The Transformation of Nissan – Reform of Corporate Culture', *Long Range Planning*, **23** (3), 9–15.

Jackall, J. (1988), *Moral Mazes: The World of Corporate Managers*, Oxford: Oxford University Press.

Janis, I. L. (1972), *Victims of Groupthink*, Boston, Mass.: Houghlin Mifflin.

Jaques, E. (1952), *The Changing Culture of a Factory*, New York: Dryden Press.

Jeffcutt, P. (1994), 'From interpretation to representation in organizational analysis: postmodernism, ethnography and organizational symbolism', *Organization Studies*, **15** (2), 241–74.

Johnson, G. (1990), 'Managing Strategic Change: The Role of Symbolic Action', *British Journal of Management*, **1** (1), 183–200.

Johnson, G. & Scholes, K. (1993), *Exploring Corporate Strategy*, 3rd edn, Hemel Hempstead: Prentice Hall.

Jones, R. & Gal, P. (1994) 'Reality catches up with Aussie Co', in: D.A. Smith and A. Peacock (eds), *Cases in Organisational Behaviour*, London: Pitman.

Jones, J. E. & Pfeiffer J. W. (eds) (1975), *The 1975 Annual Handbook for Group Facilitators*, San Diego, Calif.: Pfeiffer & Co.

Kan, S. (1989), *Symbolic Immortality*, Washington, DC: Smithsonian Institution Press.

Kanter, R. M. (1983), *The Change Masters*, New York: Simon & Schuster.

Katz, D. & Kahn, R. L. (1966), *The Social Psychology of Organizations*, New York: John Wiley.

Keenoy, T. & Anthony, P. D. (1992), 'HRM: Metaphor, Meaning and Morality', in: P. Blyton & P. Turnbull (eds), *Reassessing Human Resource Management*, London: Sage.

Kennedy, C. (1993), 'Changing the Company Culture at Ciba-Geigy', *Long Range Planning*, **26** (1), 18–27.

Kerr, J. & Slocum, J. W. (1987), 'Managing Corporate Culture through Reward Systems', *Academy of Management Executive*, **1** (2), 99–108.

Kilmann, R. H. (1984), *Beyond the Quick Fix: Managing Five Tracks to Organizational Success*, San Francisco, Calif.: Jossey Bass.

Kleinfield, S. (1981), *The Biggest Company on Earth: A Profile of AT&T*, New York: Holt, Rinehart & Winston.

Koch, S. & Deetz, S. (1981), 'Metaphor Analysis of Social Reality in Organizations', *Journal of Applied Communication Research*, **9**, 1–15.

Kotter, J. P. & Heskett, J. L. (1992), *Corporate Culture and Performance*, New York: The Free Press.

Krefting, L. A & Frost, O. J. (1985), 'Untangling webs, surfing waves, and wildcatting, a multiple-metaphor perspective on managing organizational culture', in: P. J. Frost *et al.*, *Organization Culture*, Beverly Hills, Calif.: Sage, 155–68.

Lakoff, G. & Johnson, M. (1980), *Metaphors We Live By*, Chicago, Ill.: University of Chicago Press.

Lewin, K. (1952), *Field Theory in Social Science*, London: Tavistock.

Lewicki, R. (1981), 'Organization seduction: building commitment to organizations', *Organizational Dynamics*, **10** (2), 5–21.

Lorsch, J. W. (1986), 'Managing Culture: The Invisible Barrier to Strategic Change', *California Management Review*, **28** (2), 95–109.

Louis, M. R. (1980), 'Organizations as culture-bearing milieux', in: L. R. Pondy *et al.* (eds), *Organizational Symbolism*, Greenwich, Conn.: JAI; quoted in M. R. Louis (1985), 'An Investigator's Guide to Workplace Culture', in: P. J. Frost, L. F. Moore, M. R. Louis, C. C. Lundberg & J. Martin (eds), *Organizational Culture*, Newbury Park, Calif.: Sage, 73–93.

Lundberg, C. C. (1985), 'On the Feasibility of Cultural Intervention', in: P. J. Frost, L. F. Moore, M. R. Louis, C. C. Lundberg & J. Martin (eds), *Organizational Culture*, Newbury Park, Calif.: Sage, 169–85.

McDonald, P. (1991), 'The Los Angeles Olympic Organizing Committee: Developing Organizational Culture in the Short Run', in: P. J. Frost, L. F. Moore, M. R. Louis, C. C. Lundberg & J. Martin (eds), *Reframing Organizational Culture*, London: Sage, 26–38.

McDonald, P. & Gandz, J. (1992), 'Getting Value from Shared Values', *Organizational Dynamics*, winter, 64–77.

McGregor, D. (1960), *The Human Side of Enterprise*, New York: McGraw-Hill.

MacIntyre, A. (1981), *After Virtue: A Study in Moral Theory*, London: Duckworth.

Mangham, I. L. (1990), 'Managing as a Performing Art', *British Journal of Management*, **1**, 105–15.

Mangham, I. L. & Overington, M. A. (1983), 'Dramatism and the Theatrical Metaphor: Really Playing at Critical Distances', in: G. Morgan (ed.), *Beyond Method: Social Research Strategies*, Beverly Hills, Calif.: Sage.

Marcuse, H. (1955), *Eros and Civilization*, Boston, Mass.: Beacon Press.

Marks, M. & Mirvis, P. H. (1986), 'The Merger Syndrome: When Corporate Cultures Clash', *Psychology Today*, October, 36–42.

Martin, J. (1985), 'Can Organizational Culture be Managed?', in: P. J. Frost, L. F. Moore, M. R. Louis, C. C. Lundberg & J. Martin (eds), *Organizational Culture*, Beverly Hills, Calif.: Sage, 95–8.

Martin, J. (1992), *Cultures in Organizations: Three Perspectives*, New York: Oxford University Press.

Martin, J., Feldman, M. S., Hatch, M. J. & Sitkin, S. B. (1983), 'The Uniqueness Paradox in Organizational Stories', *Administrative Science Quarterly*, **28**, 438–53.

Martin, J. & Siehl, C. (1983), 'Organizational Culture and Counterculture: An Uneasy Symbiosis', *Organizational Dynamics*, autumn, 52–64.

Martin, J., Sitkin, S. B. & Boehm, M. (1985), 'Founders and the Elusiveness of a Cultural Legacy', in: P. J. Frost, L. F. Moore, M. R. Louis, C. C. Lundberg & J. Martin (eds), *Organizational Culture*, London: Sage, 99–124.

Maruyama, M. (1984), 'Alternative Concepts of Management: Insights from Asia and Africa', *Asia Pacific Journal of Management*, January, 100–11.

Maslow, A. H. (1943), 'A Theory of Human Motivation', *Psychological Review*, **50**, 370–96.

Meek, V. L. (1988), 'Organizational Culture: Origins and Weaknesses', *Organization Studies*, **9** (4), 453–73.

Merton, R. K. (1957), *Social Theory and Social Structure*, Glencoe, Ill.: The Free Press.

Miles, R. E. & Snow, C. C. (1978), *Organizational Strategy, Structure and Process*, New York: McGraw-Hill.

Miller, D. & Mintzberg, H. (1983), 'The case for configuration', in: G. Morgan (ed.), *Beyond Method: Strategies for Social Research*, Beverly Hills, Calif.: Sage.

Mills, A. J. (1988), 'Organization, gender and culture', *Organization Studies*, **9** (3), 351–69.

Mintzberg, H. (1973), *The Nature of Managerial Work*, New York: Harper & Row.

Mintzberg, H. (1987), 'Crafting strategy', *Harvard Business Review*, July–August, 66–75.

Mirvis, P. H. & Marks, M. (1985a), 'Merger Syndrome: Stress and Uncertainty, Part 1'. *Mergers and Acquisitions*, **20** (3), 50–5.

Mirvis, P. H. & Marks, M. (1985b), 'Merger Syndrome: Management by Crisis. Part 2'. *Mergers and Acquisitions*, **20** (3), 70–6.

Morgan, G. (1986), *Images of Organization*, Beverly Hills, Calif.: Sage.

Morgan, G. (1997), *Images of Organization*, Thousand Oaks, CA: Sage.

Nord, W. R. (1985), 'Can Organizational Culture Be Managed, A Synthesis', in: P. J. Frost, L. F. Moore, M. R. Louis, C. C. Lundberg & J. Martin, (eds), *Organizational Culture*, Beverly Hills, Calif.: Sage, 187–96.

Ogbonna, E. (1992), 'Organization Culture and Human Resource Management: Dilemmas and Contradictions', in: P. Blyton & P. Turnbull (eds), *Reassessing Human Resource Management*, London: Sage.

Ogbonna, E. (1992/3), 'Managing Organizational Culture: Fantasy or Reality?', *Human Resource Management Journal*, **3** (2), 42–54.

Olins, W. (1978), *The Corporate Personality: An Inquiry into the Nature of Corporate Identity*, London: Design Council.

Orwell, G. (1949), *1984*, New York: New American Library.

O'Toole, J. J. (1979), 'Corporate and Managerial Cultures', in: C. L. Cooper (ed.), *Behavioral Problems in Organizations*, Englewood Cliffs, NJ: Prentice Hall.

Ott, J. S. (1989), *The Organizational Culture Perspective*, Pacific Grove, Calif.: Brooks/Cole.

Ouchi, W. (1981), *Theory Z: How American Business can Meet the Japanese Challenge*, Reading, Mass.: Addison-Wesley.

Ouchi, W. & Wilkins, A. L. (1985), 'Organizational Culture', *Annual Review of Sociology*, **11**, 457–83.

Pacanowsky, M. E. & O'Donnell-Trujillo, N. (1982), 'Communication and Organizational Culture', *The Western Journal of Speech Communication*, **46** (spring), 115–30.

Pascale, R. T. (1984), 'Perspectives on Strategy: The Real Story behind Honda's Success', *California Management Review*, **26** (3), 47–72.

Pascale, R. & Athos, A. (1981), *The Art of Japanese Management*, New York: Simon & Schuster.

Payne, R. L. (1990), 'The Concepts of Culture and Climate', Working Paper 202, Manchester Business School.

Perrow, C. (1979), *Complex Organizations: A Critical Essay*, 2nd edn, Glenview, Ill.: Rand McNally.

Peters, T. J. (1978), 'Symbols, Patterns, and Settings: An Optimistic Case for Getting Things Done', *Organizational Dynamics*, autumn, 3–23.

Peters, T. & Waterman, R. (1982), *In Search of Excellence*, New York: Harper & Row.

Pfeffer, J. (1981a), 'Management as Symbolic Action: The Creation and Maintenance of Organizational Paradigms', in: L. L. Cummings & B. M. Staw (eds), *Research in Organizational Behavior*, **3** (1), 1–52. Greenwich, Conn.: JAI.

Philips, F. (1978), *45 Years with Philips: an Industrialist's Life*, Poole: Blandford Press.

Podmore, D. & Spender A. (1986), 'Gender in the labour process – the case of men and women lawyers', in; *Gender and the Labour Process*. Aldershot: Gower.

Porter, M. E. (1990), *Competitive Strategy: Techniques for Analysing Industries and Competitors*, New York: The Free Press.

Purcell, J. (1989), 'The Impact of Corporate Strategy on Human Resource Management', in: J. Storey (ed.), *New Perspectives on Human Resource Management*, London: Routledge.

Quinn, J. B. (1978), 'Strategic Change, Logical Incrementalism', *Sloan Management Review*, **20**, 7–21.

Quinn, R. E. & McGrath, M. R. (1985), 'The Transformation of Organizational Cultures: A Competing Values Perspective', in: P. J. Frost, L. F. Moore, M. R. Louis, C. C. Lundberg & J. Martin (eds), *Organizational Culture*, Newbury Park, Calif.: Sage, 315–34.

Reed, M. (1990), 'From paradigms to images: the paradigm warrior turns post-modern guru', *Personnel Review*, **19** (3); 35–40.

Reed, M. & Hughes, M. (1992), *Rethinking Organization*, London: Sage.

Roberts, H. & Brown, A. D. (1992), 'Cognitive and Social Dimensions of IT Implementation', paper presented at the British Academy of Management Sixth Annual Conference, Bradford 14–16 September.

Rokeach, M. (1973), *The Nature of Human Values*, New York: The Free Press.

Rosenfeld, R., Whipp, R. & Pettigrew, A. (1987), 'Processes of Internationalization: Regeneration and Competitiveness', paper presented to the ESRC/EIASM Seminar on Competitiveness and Internalization, European Institute for Advanced Studies in Management, Brussels, 11 June.

Rowlinson, M. & Hassard, J. (1993), 'The Invention of Corporate Culture: A History of the Histories of Cadbury', *Human Relations*, **46** (3), 299–326.

Saffold, G. S. (1988), 'Culture Traits, Strength, and Organizational Performance: Moving Beyond "Strong" Culture', *Academy of Management Review*, **13** (4), 546–58.

Sathe, V. (1985a), *Culture and Related Corporate Realities*, Homewood, Ill.: Irwin.

Sathe, V. (1985b), 'How to Decipher and Change Corporate Culture', in: R. H. Kilmann, M. J. Saxton, R. Serpa & associates (eds), *Gaining Control of the Corporate Culture*, San Francisco, Calif.: Jossey Bass, 230–61.

Schein, E. H. (1964), 'The Mechanism of Change', in Bennis, Schein, Steels and Berlew (eds), *Interpersonal Dynamics*, Homewood, Ill.: Dorsey Press, 199–213.

Schein, E. H. (1981), 'Does Japanese Management Style have a Message for American Managers?', *Sloan Management Review*, **23**, 55–68.

Schein, E. H. (1985a), 'How Culture Forms, Develops and Changes', in R. H. Kilmann, M. J. Saxton, R. Serpa & associates (eds), *Gaining Control of the Corporate Culture*, San Francisco, Calif.: Jossey Bass, 17–43.

Schein, E. H. (1985b), *Organizational Culture and Leadership*, San Francisco, Calif.: Jossey Bass.

Schneider, S. C. (1989), 'Strategy Formulation: The Impact of National Culture', *Organization Studies*, **10** (2), 149–68.

Scholz, C. (1987), 'Corporate Culture and Strategy – the Problem of Strategic Fit', *Long Range Planning*, **20** (4), 78–87.

Schuler, R. S. & Huber, V. L. (1993), *Personnel and Human Resource Management*, 5th edn, St Paul, Minn.: West Publishing, 258.

Schwartz, H. & Davis, S. M. (1981), 'Matching Corporate Culture and Business Strategy', *Organizational Dynamics*, **10**, 30–48.

Selznick, P. (1957), *Leadership and Administration*, Evanston, Ill.: Row, Peterson.

Siehl, C. (1985), 'After the Founder, an Opportunity to Manage Culture', in: P. J. Frost, L. F. Moore, M. R. Louis, C. C. Lundberg & J. Martin (eds), *Organizational Culture*, Beverly Hills, Calif.: Sage, 125–40.

Siehl, C. & Martin, J. (1990), 'Organizational Culture: A Key to Financial Performance?', in: B. Schneider (ed.), *Organizational Culture and Climate*, San Francisco, Calif.: Jossey Bass.

Silverzweig, S. & Allen, R. F. (1976), 'Changing the Corporate Culture', *Sloan Management Review*, **17** (3), 33–49.

Smircich, L. (1983), 'Concepts of Culture and Organizational Analysis', *Administrative Science Quarterly*, **28**, 339–58.

Sutton, C. D. & Nelson, D. L. (1990), 'Elements of the Cultural Network: The Communicators of Corporate Values', *Leadership and Organization Development Journal*, **11** (5), 3–10.

Tagiuri, R. (1968), 'The Concept of Organizational Climate', in: R. Tagiuri & G. Lituin (eds), *Organizational Climate: Explorations of a Concept*, Boston, Mass.: Harvard University Graduate Business School.

Tobias, A. (1976), *Fire and Ice*, New York: William Morrow.

Trice, H. M. & Beyer, J. M. (1984), 'Studying Organizational Cultures through Rites and Ceremonials', *Academy of Management Review*, **9**, 653–69.

Trice, H. M. & Beyer, J. M. (1990), 'Using Six Organizational Rites to Change Culture', in: R. H. Kilmann, M. J. Saxton, R. Serpa & associates (eds), *Gaining Control of the Corporate Culture*, San Francisco, Calif.: Jossey Bass, 370–99.

Trice, H. M. & Beyer, J. M. (1993) *The Cultures of Work Organisations*, Englewood Cliffs, N.J.: Prentice Hall.

Trilling, L. (1974), *Sincerity and Authenticity*, London: Oxford University Press.

Tunstall, W. B. (1983), 'Cultural Transition at AT&T', *Sloan Management Review*, 25 (1), 15–26.

Tylor, E. B. (1971), *Primitive Culture: Researches into the Development of Mythology, Philosophy, Religion, Language, Art and Custom*, first pub. 1903, 2 vols, London: Murray (1871).

Ulrich, W. L. (1984), 'HRM and Culture: History, Ritual and Myth', *Human Resource Management*, 23 (2), 117–28.

Uttal, B. (1983), 'The Corporate Culture Vultures', *Fortune*, 17 October, 66–72.

Van Maanen, J. (1991), 'The Smile Factory: Work at Disneyland', in: P. J. Frost, L. F. Moore, M. R. Louis, C. C. Lundberg & J. Martin (eds), *Reframing Organizational Culture*, Newbury Park, Calif.: Sage, 58–76.

Walsh, J. P. & Ungson, G. R. (1991), 'Organizational memory', *Academy of Management Review*, 16 (1): 57–91.

Weick, K. E. (1985), 'The Significance of Corporate Culture', in: P. J. Frost, L. F. Moore, M. R. Louis, C. C. Lundberg & J. Martin (eds), *Organizational Culture*, Beverly Hills, Calif.: Sage, 381–9.

Weick, K. E. (1987), 'Organizational Culture as a Source of High Reliability', *California Management Review*, 29 (2), 112–27.

Whipp, R. (1987), 'Technology Management, Strategic Change and Competitiveness', in: M. Dorgham, (ed.), *Proceedings of the Fourth International Vehicle Design Congress*, Geneva: Inderscience.

Whipp, R., Rosenfeld, R & Pettigrew, A. (1989), 'Understanding Strategic Change Processes: Some Preliminary British Findings', in: A. Pettigrew (ed.), *The Management of Strategic Change*, Oxford: Blackwell.

Whipp, R., Rosenfeld, R. & Pettigrew, A. (1989b), 'Culture and Competitiveness: Evidence from Two Mature UK Industries', *Journal of Management Studies*, 26 (6), 561–85.

Whitley, R. (1990), 'The Comparative Analysis of Business Recipes', Working Paper 191, Manchester Business School.

Whitley, R. (1992), *Business Systems in East Asia: Firms, Markets and Societies*, Beverly Hills, Calif. Sage.

Wiener, Y. (1988), 'Forms of Value Systems: A Focus on Organizational Effectiveness and Cultural Change and Maintenance', *Academy of Management Review*, 13 (4), 534–45.

Wilkins, A. L. (1983), 'Organizational Stories as Symbols which Control the Organization', in: L. R. Pondy, P. J. Frost, G. Morgan & T. C. Dandridge (eds) *Organizational Symbolism*, Greenwich, Conn.: JAI, 81–92.

Wilkins, A. L. & Patterson, K. J. (1985), 'You Can't Get There From Here: What will Make Culture-Change Projects Fail', in: R. H. Kilmann, M. J. Saxton, R. Serpa & associates (eds), *Gaining Control of the Corporate Culture*, San Francisco, Calif.: Jossey Bass, 262–91.

Wilkins, A. L. & Dyer, W. G. (1988), 'Toward Culturally Sensitive Theories of Culture Change', *Academy of Management Review*, 13 (4), 522–33.

Wilkins, A. L., Perry, L. T. & Checketts, A. G. (1990), ' "Please don't Make me a Hero": A Re-examination of Corporate Heroes', *Human Resource Management*, 29 (3), 327–41.

Williams, A., Dobson, P. & Walters, M. (1993), *Changing Culture, New Organizational Approaches*, 2nd edn, London: Institute of Personnel Management.

Wuthnow, R. J., Davison, H., Bergesen, A. & Kurzweil, E. (1984), *Cultural Analysis*, London, Routledge & Kegan Paul.

NAME INDEX

INDEX